# Diabetic Complications: Early Diagnosis and Treatment

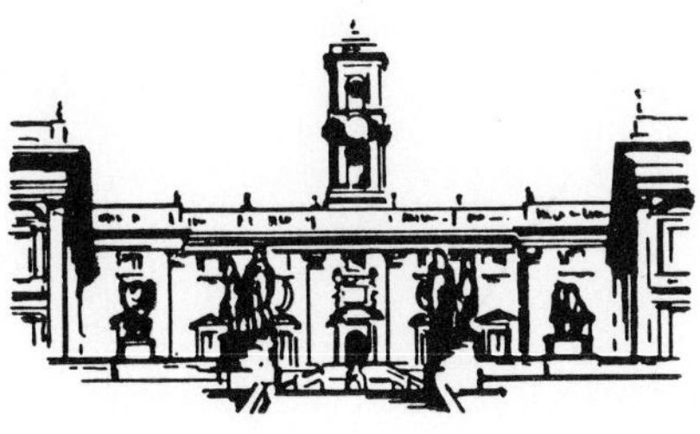

The publication of this book was made possible by the generous sponsorship of FIDIA RESEARCH LABORATORIES and NOVO INDUSTRI A/S

# *Contents*

# *Scientific Committee Members and Guest Contributors*

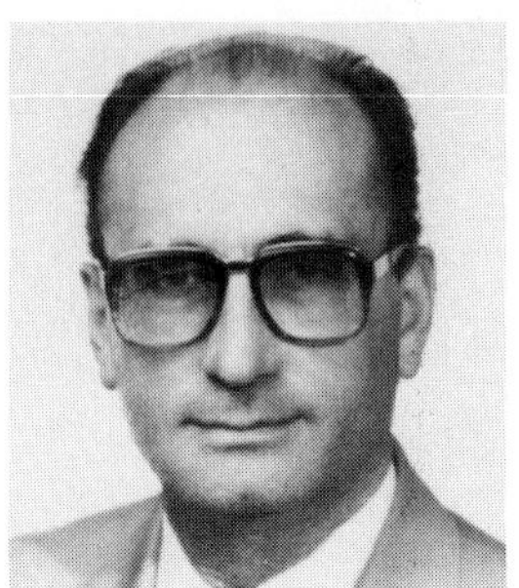

D. Andreani (*Rome, Italy*)

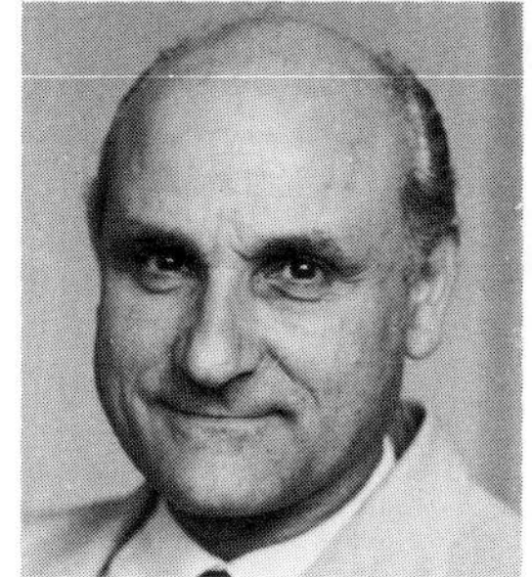

R. Brancato (*Milan, Italy*)

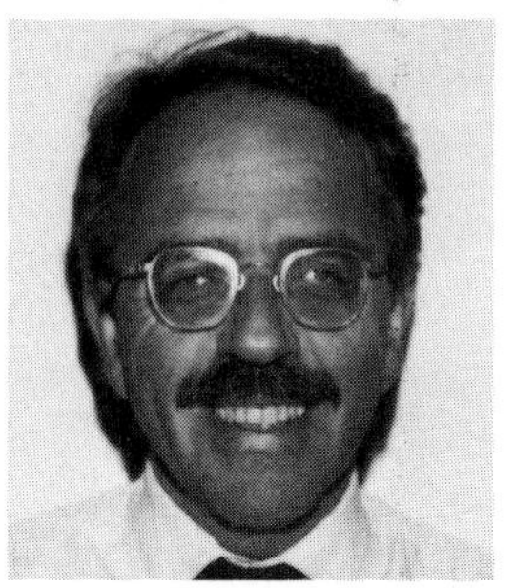

G. H. Bresnick (*Madison, USA*)

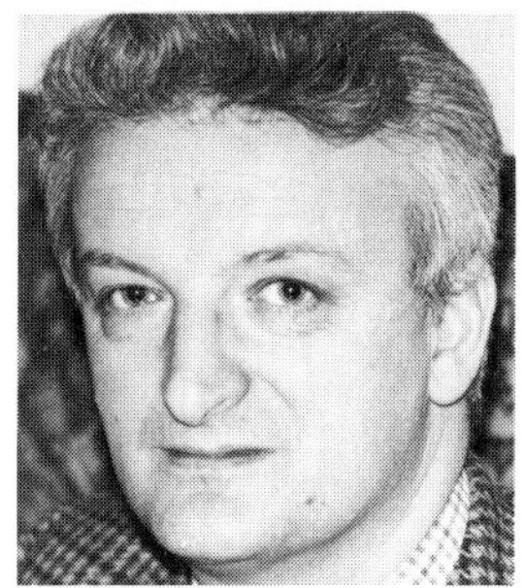

N. Canal (*Milan, Italy*)

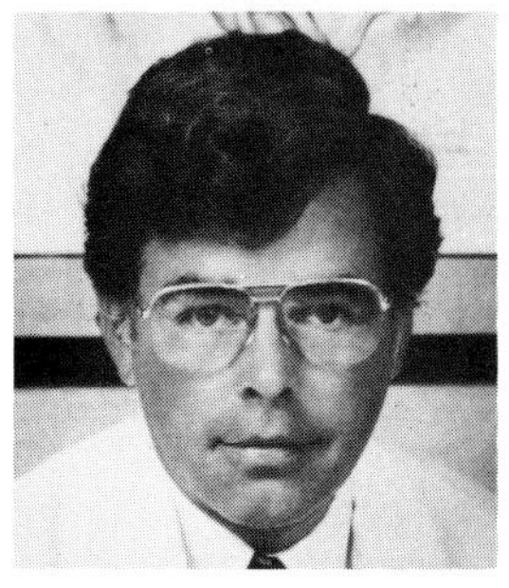

R. S. Clements, Jr (*Alabama, USA*)

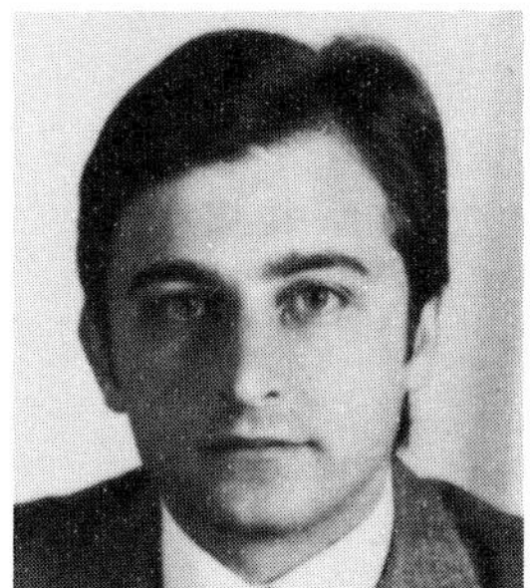

G. Comi (*Milan, Italy*)

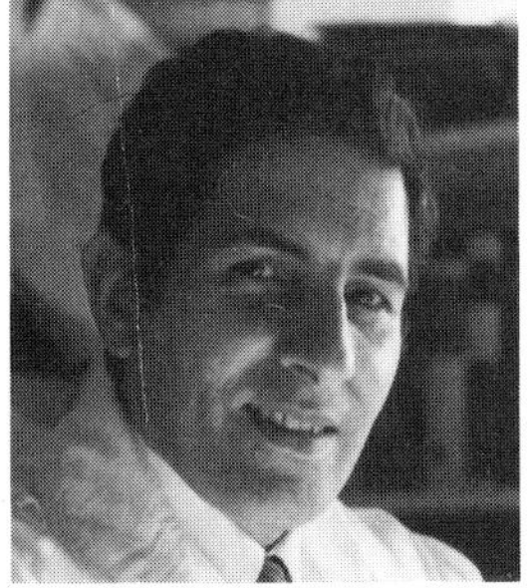

G. Crepaldi (*Padua, Italy*)

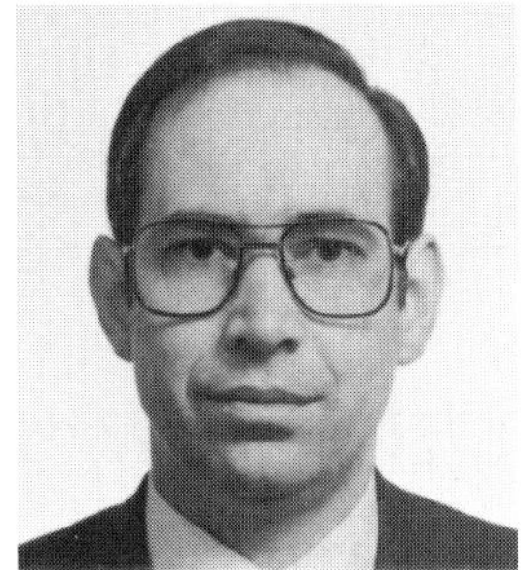

J. G. Cunha-Vaz (*Coimbra, Portugal*)

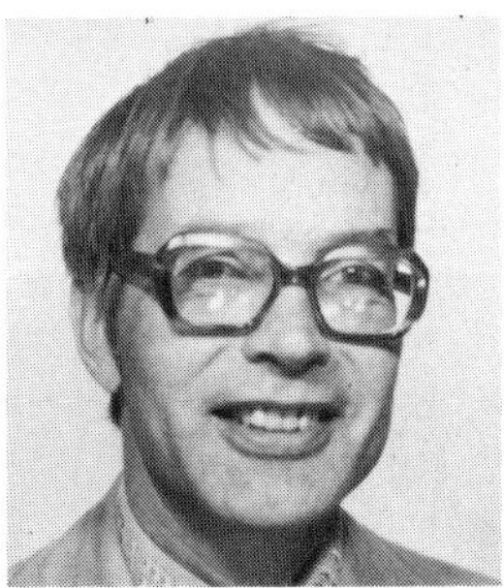

T. Deckert (*Gentofte, Denmark*)

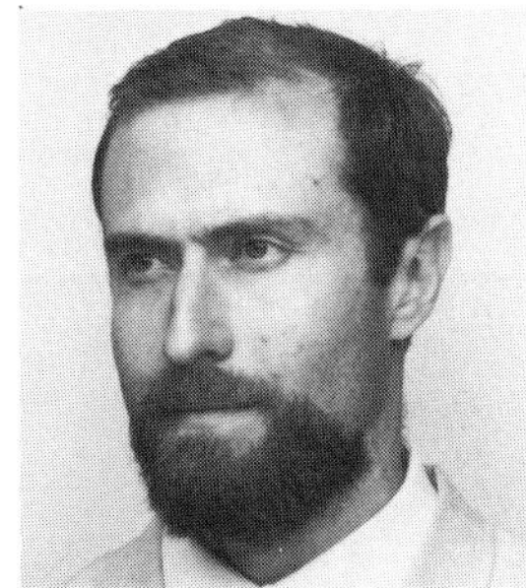

U. Di Mario (*Rome, Italy*)

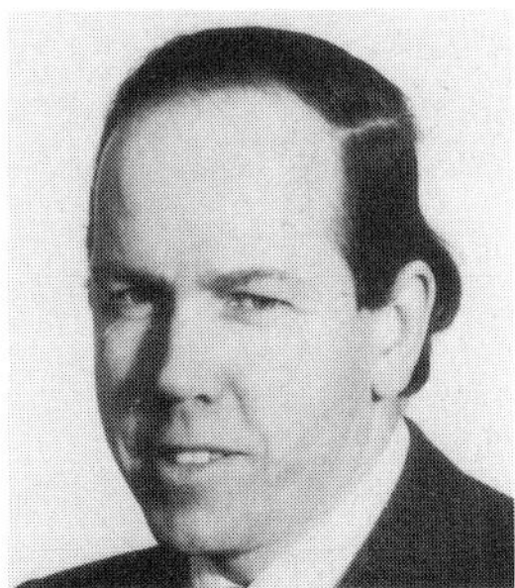

D. J. Ewing (*Edinburgh, UK*)

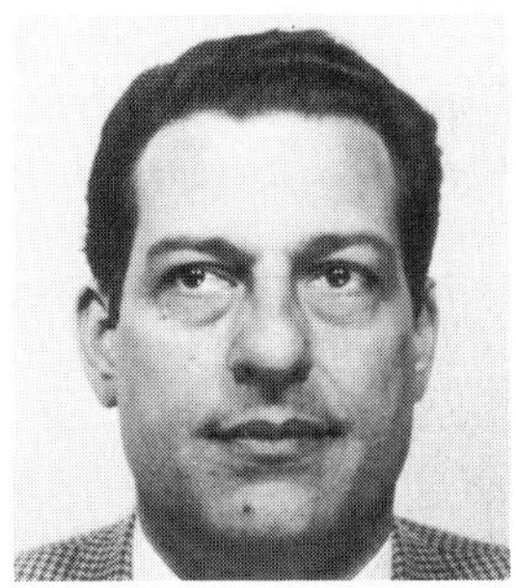

D. Fedele (*Palermo, Italy*)

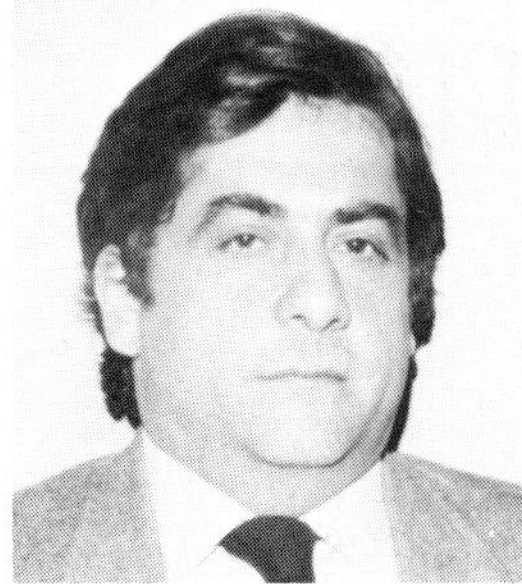

S. Gambardella (*Rome, Italy*)

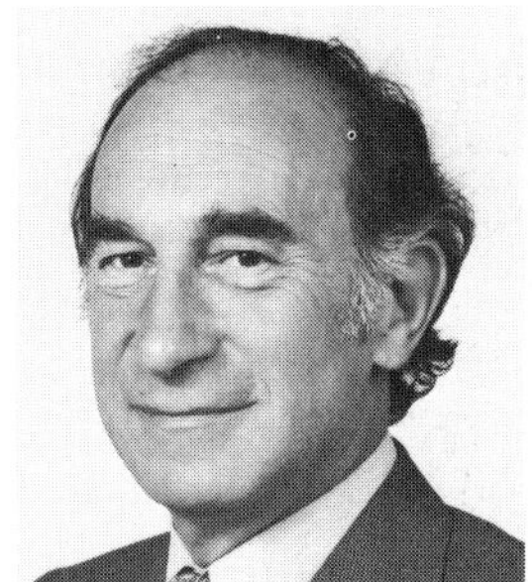

H. Keen (*London, UK*)

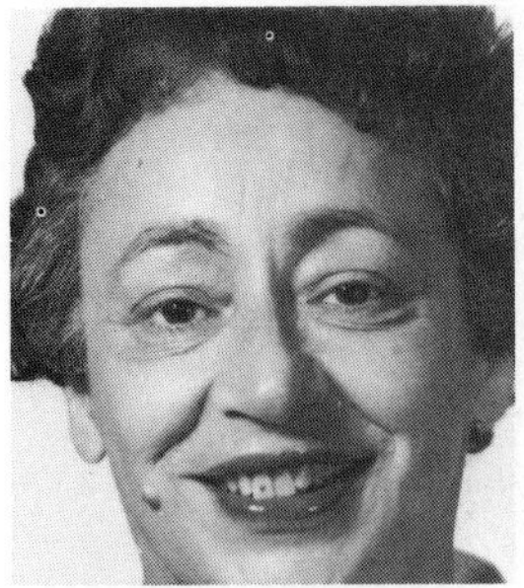

E. M. Kohner (*London, UK*)

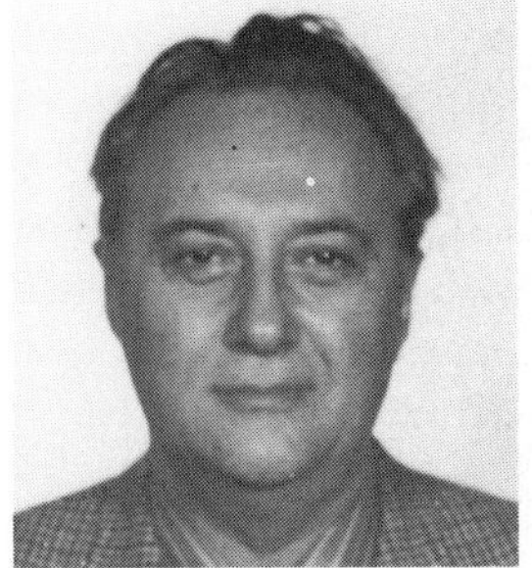

G. Menzinger (*Rome, Italy*)

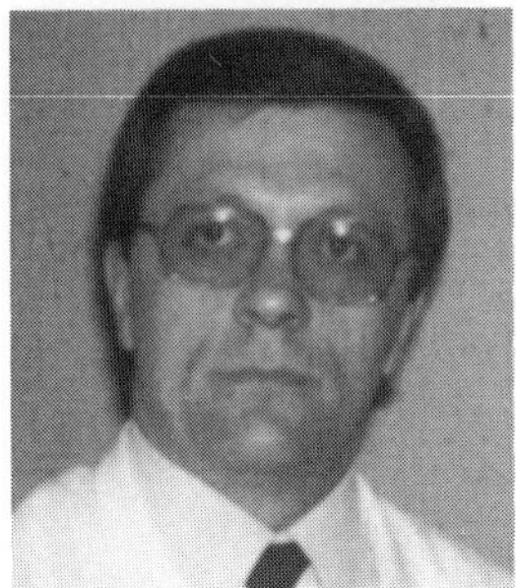

P. Micossi (*Milan, Italy*)

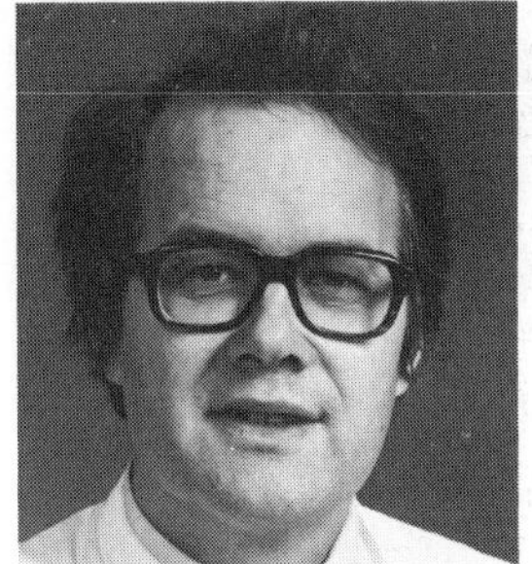

C. E. Mogensen (*Aarhus, Denmark*)

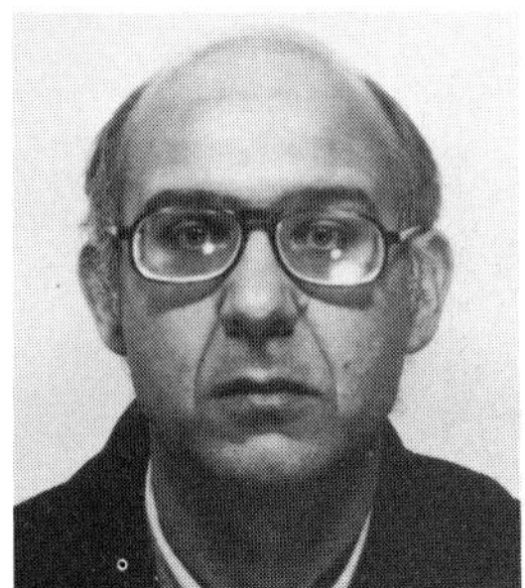

R. Nosadini (*Padua, Italy*)

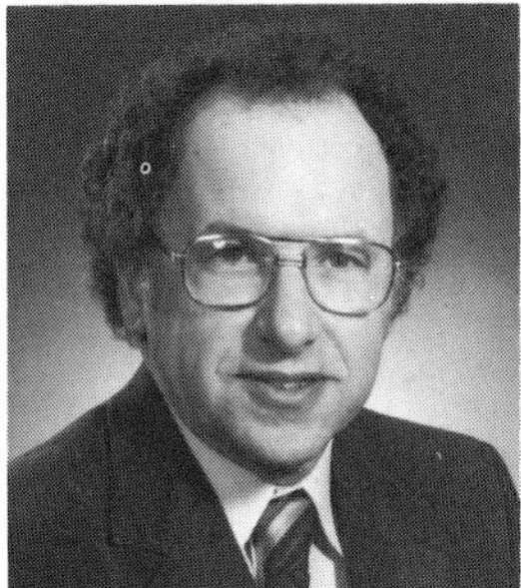

D. Porte, Jr (*Seattle, USA*)

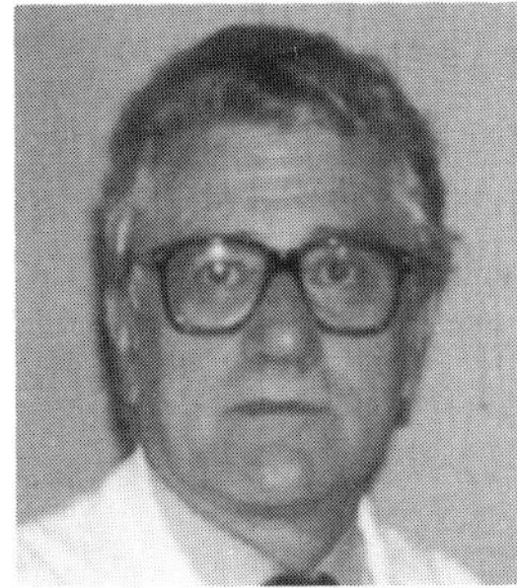

G. Pozza (*Milan, Italy*)

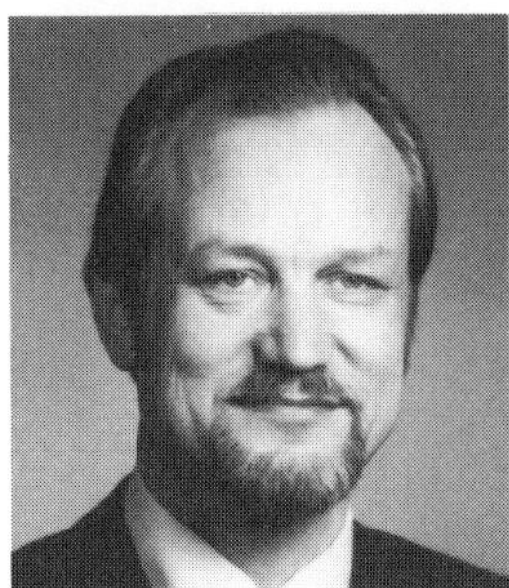

K. Pyörälä (*Kuopio, Finland*)

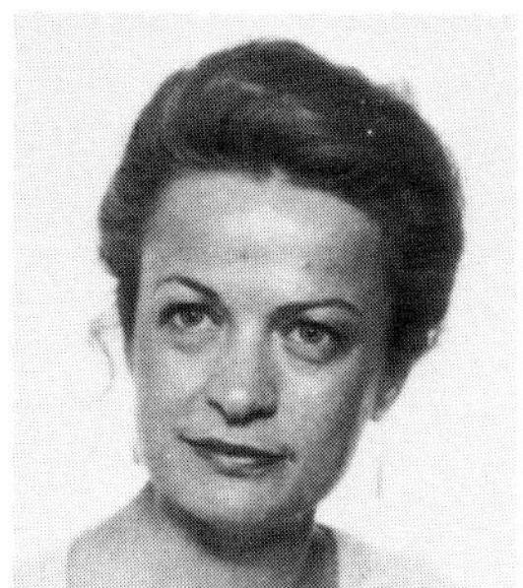

T. Segato (*Padua, Italy*)

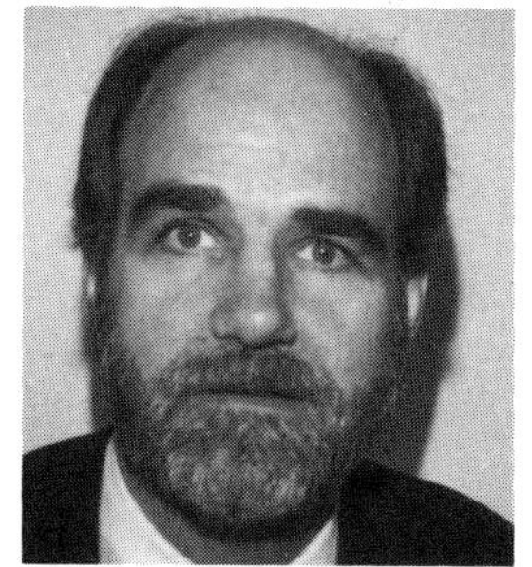

M. W. Steffes (*Minneapolis, USA*)

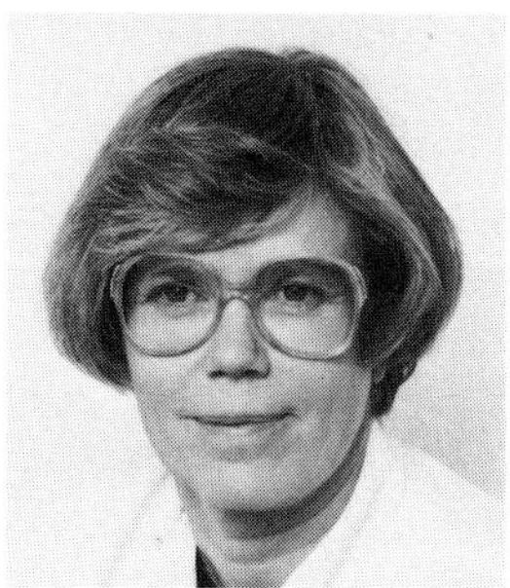

M.-R. Taskinen (*Helsinki, Finland*)

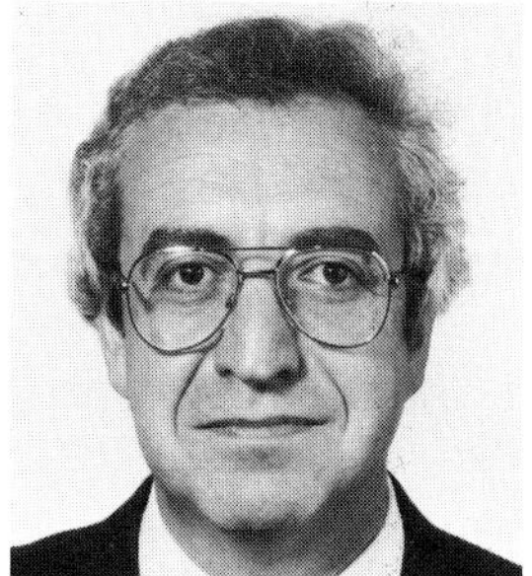

G. Viberti (*London, UK*)

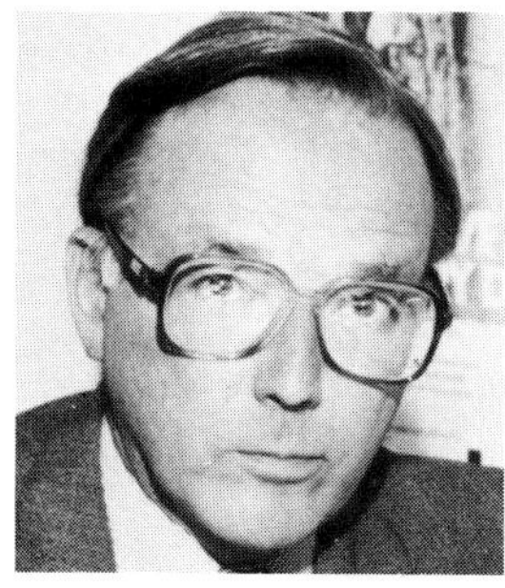

J. D. Ward (*Sheffield, UK*)

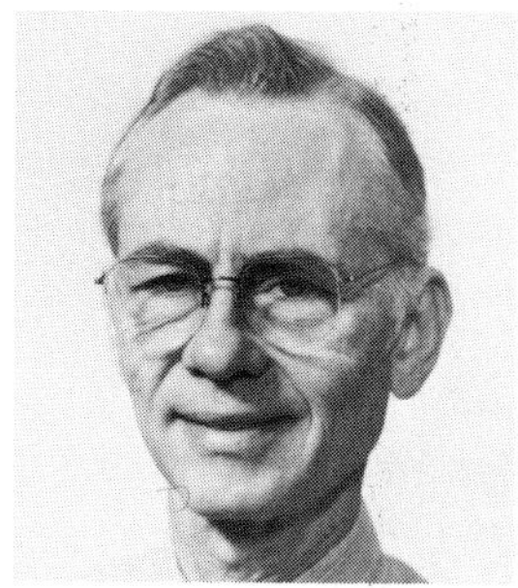

J. R. Williamson (*St Louis, USA*)

# *Addresses of First-named Contributors*

D. Andreani, *Cattedra Endocrinologia, Clinica Medica 2, Policlinico Umberto I, 00161 Rome, Italy*

R. Brancato, *Clinica Oculistica, Ospedale S. Raffaele, Via Olgettina 60, 20132 Milan, Italy*

G. H. Bresnick, *Department of Ophthalmology F4/338, Clinical Science Center, University of Wisconsin, 600 Highland Avenue, Madison, WI 53792, USA*

N. Canal, *III Piano A Neurologia, Ospedale S. Raffaele, Via Olgettina 60, 20132 Milan, Italy*

R. S. Clements, Jr, *Diabetes Hospital, Suite 414–415, University of Alabama at Birmingham, 1808 Seventh Avenue South, Birmingham, AL 35294, USA*

G. Comi, *Clinica Neurologica, Ospedale S. Raffaele, Via Olgettina 60, 20132 Milan, Italy*

G. Crepaldi, *Istituto di Medicina Interna, Università di Padova, Via Giustiniani 2, 35128 Padova, Italy*

J. G. Cunha-Vaz, *Clinica Ofthalmologica, Hospitais da Universitade, 3049 Coimbra, Portugal*

T. Deckert, *Steno Memorial Hospital, Niels Steensensvej 2, 2820 Gentofte, Denmark*

U. Di Mario, *Clinica Medica 2, Policlinico Umberto I, Viale del Policlinico, 00161 Rome, Italy*

D. J. Ewing, *Department of Medicine, The Royal Infirmary, Edinburgh EH3 9YW, UK*

D. Fedele, *Istituto di Medicina Interna, Università di Padova, Via Giustiniani 2, 35128 Padova, Italy*

S. GAMBARDELLA, *Clinica Medica 2, Policlinico Umberto I, Viale del Policlinico, 00161 Rome, Italy*

H. KEEN, *United Medical and Dental Schools of Guy's and St Thomas's Hospitals, University of London, London SE1 9RT, UK*

E. M. KOHNER, *Diabetic Retinopathy, Hammersmith Hospital, Du Cane Road, London W12 0HS, UK*

G. MENZINGER, *Cattedra di Malattie del Ricambio, II Università 'Tor Vergata', 00133 Rome, Italy*

P. MICOSSI, *Direzione Scientifica, Ospedale S. Raffaele, Via Olgettina 60, 20132 Milan, Italy*

C. E. MOGENSEN, *Second University Clinic of Internal Medicine, Kommune-hospitalet, DK-8000 Aarhus, Denmark*

R. NOSADINI, *Istituto di Medicina Interna, Università di Padova, Via Giustiniani 2, 35128 Padova, Italy*

D. PORTE, JR, *Division of Endocrinology and Metabolism, VA Medical Center, 1660 South Columbian Way, Seattle WA 98108, USA*

G. POZZA, *Clinica Medica, Ospedale S. Raffaele, Via Olgettina 60, 20132 Milano, Italy*

K. PYÖRÄLÄ, *Department of Medicine, University of Kuopio, 70210 Kuopio 21, Finland*

T. SEGATO, *Istituto di Clinica Oculistica, Università degli Studi di Padova, Via Giustiniani 2, 35128 Padova, Italy*

M. W. STEFFES, *Department of Laboratory Medicine and Pathology, Box 198 Mayo Memorial Building, 420 Delaware Street SE, Minneapolis MN 55455, USA*

M.-R. TASKINEN, *Second Department of Medicine, University of Helsinki, Haart-maninkatu 4, 00290 Helsinki 29, Finland*

G. C. VIBERTI, *United Medical and Dental Schools of Guy's and St Thomas's Hospitals, University of London, London SE1 9RT, UK*

J. D. WARD, *Royal Hallamshire Hospital, Glossop Road, Sheffield S10 2JF, UK*

J. R. WILLIAMSON, *Department of Pathology, Washington University School of Medicine, 660 South Euclid Avenue, St Louis MO 63110, USA*

# *Editors' Preface*

Abundant literature on diabetic complications has continued to be published since the scientific community became aware that the real problem facing modern diabetology is the prevention and proper treatment of the complications of diabetes which blight the lives of the majority of long-standing diabetic patients. There is thus a need periodically to reconsider the achievements of research in this field, which is spread along so many different lines, and to re-evaluate where our efforts should be directed in the next few years.

The present volume represents an attempt to bring together on paper researchers and clinicians who are actively challenging diabetes and its complications. The expected result is to highlight the state of the art, the pace and the scope of the exciting progress in this area and to provide a good account of diabetic complications for readers who wish to obtain an up-to-date view of the most important issues at stake. Moreover, this volume must be considered a contribution of a special kind in so far as it is purposely related to an international symposium (Rome 1987) at which the contributors to this book and a good number of distinguished diabetologists, who have been working on diabetic complications for years, have gathered together.

The volume is intended to deal especially with the early phases of diabetic complications: microvascular (retina and kidney), macrovascular and neurological. In this respect each complication is presented in such a way as to give concise and essential information on the early stages of the disorder and a brief overview of the natural history of the disease with the aim of achieving satisfactory prevention, whenever possible, and treatment. Most reports contain some original data from the authors as well.

We most heartily hope that the book may provide active diabetologists with a statement of where our understanding in this field lies, and in what directions further advances are expected, and that it may be of some help to, and above all stimulate interest in, all those young researchers and clinicians who want to come on-stage.

D. Andreani
G. Crepaldi
U. Di Mario
G. Pozza

# Macroangiopathy

Diabetic Complications: Early Diagnosis and Treatment
Edited by D. Andreani, G. Crepaldi, U. Di Mario and G. Pozza


CHAPTER 1

# *Macrovascular Disease in Diabetes Mellitus*

H. Keen
*United Medical and Dental Schools of Guy's and St Thomas's Hospitals, London, UK*

It has become a clinical axiom that macrovascular disease represents a major threat to the health and life of people with diabetes mellitus (1). However, like many other clinical truisms, the broad generalization requires to be looked at with some care. This is necessary because, by understanding the elements which go to make up the enhanced impact of cardiovascular disease upon the diabetic, its mechanisms may become clearer and methods for its detection, prevention and therapy may also become more evident. Further, the special case of diabetes may have general applicability in promoting understanding in the population at large.

## Definitions

The term macrovascular disease has come to be identified in the diabetic (as has atherosclerosis in the non-diabetic) with a set of structural changes in the vessel wall, with a series of clinical syndromes and with a collection of functional investigative findings (e.g. ECG abnormality, doppler ultrasound flow patterns). These different indices of arterial disease, while generally correlated, should not be used interchangeably, particularly in the description of vascular disease in the diabetic. Dissociation between structural changes in the arterial wall and the frequency of the clinical manifestations of coronary heart disease have long been appreciated in non-diabetic subjects. Some of the abnormalities, clinical and investigational (e.g. congestive heart failure, changes in the repolarization (ST/T) segment of the electrocardiogram) which are usually lumped into the macrovascular disease category, are themselves non-specific. Though frequently a consequence of coronary artery disease, they are by no means necessarily so. A specific diabetic cardiopathy may be responsible for impaired cardiac performance and metabolic changes may affect the ST segment of the ECG. Abnormalities of flow in peripheral arteries, demonstrated by doppler ultrasound studies, are clearly significantly associated with an increased risk of later clinical manifestations of peripheral vascular disease (e.g. claudication and gangrene) but that risk in the individual falls considerably short of 100%. The collective term 'macrovascular disease' like 'atherosclerosis' should be used with circumspection and the precise phenomenon under discussion should be specified.

In considering macrovascular disease in diabetes it is important to distinguish between the two major clinical types of diabetes: the insulin-dependent and the non-insulin-dependent. Apart from age differences between the two types, they also differ in respect of clinical cardiovascular manifestation and associated risk factors such as patterns of circulating lipoproteins, raised arterial pressure and the presence of diabetic kidney disease.

## CLINICAL SYNDROMES AND THEIR PREVALENCE

### Ischaemic Heart Disease

Increased risk of the clinical syndromes of myocardial infarction and angina pectoris has been associated with the diabetic state for many decades (2). Evaluating the strength and the nature of the association is complicated. Events of myocardial infarction may well be underestimated in the diabetic population because of the liability to painless events, often associated with autonomic neuropathy but sometimes occurring without it (3). They may be overestimated because of biased interpretation of non-specific symptoms in diabetic patients 'known' to be associated with atherosclerosis. However, when both standardized clinical and objective electrocardiographic data are included, coronary heart disease is considerably increased in insulin-dependent patients and significantly so in non-insulin-dependent patients compared with age- and sex-matched non-diabetic populations, an excess which is particularly evident in the diabetic female who in some, but not all, such comparisons lose the relative sparing of the female seen in non-diabetic populations.

### Prospective Study

In the insulin-dependent diabetic, recent studies in a Danish cohort of insulin-treated patients diagnosed before the age of 31 years have demonstrated a striking increase in total and cardiovascular mortality compared with like-aged and -sexed individuals in the general population. It has also been shown that most of this increased risk is experienced by the subgroup of the cohort who, during the course of their diabetes, become proteinuric, indicating the development of clinical diabetic nephropathy (4). The mortality ratio in proteinuric IDDM (insulin-dependent diabetes mellitus) patients is ten or more times higher than in non-proteinuric patients of similar age and duration of diabetes. A recent case-control study of surviving patients in this IDDM cohort (5) demonstrated that the risk of a clinical event or the development of silent electrocardiographic evidence of myocardial ischaemia was eight times higher in clinically proteinuric than in age-, sex- and duration-matched non-proteinuric IDDM patients when cumulative incidence over 6 years was compared by life-table methods. The annual risk of such an event in proteinurics was of the order of 7% per annum compared with less than 1% per annum in non-proteinurics. The reasons for this heightened susceptibility in proteinuric diabetics are not yet clear. In part, it may be secondary to the raised arterial pressure and altered lipoprotein patterns associated with chronic renal disease, but this is unlikely to account for most of the excess. Proteinuria may be the renal marker of a more general vascular vulnerability in diabetes which may affect vessels of arterial size and structure as well as small vessels such as the renal glomerular vasculature.

### Microalbuminuria and Coronary Heart Disease in Non-Insulin-Dependent Diabetes Mellitus

Further support for the 'predictive' importance of proteinuria and some suggestive extension of its relationship with arterial disease comes from studies in non-insulin-dependent diabetics. In two retrospective studies (6, 7) it was possible to demonstrate that even the presence of microalbuminuria (i.e. the subclinical increase of urinary albumin excretion rate above the normal 2–15 μg/min but below the 200–250 μg/min at which clinical tests become positive) was a strong predictor of total and cardiovascular mortality and morbidity (8). Although some of this association could be explained by an effect of raised blood pressure on both arterial disease and albumin excretion rates, multivariate analyses showed that at least part of the urinary albumin hyperexcretion prediction with cardiovascular disease and death was independent of associated elevation of blood pressure.

Preliminary analyses of a recent cross-sectional study of urinary albumin excretion rates and indices of coronary heart disease (CHD) in 136 unselected non-insulin-dependent diabetic patients aged 35–64 years (9) indicate statistically significant associations between urinary albumin excretion rates on the one hand and clinical evidence (WHO questionnaire and Minnesota-coded electrocardiography (10)) of cardiovascular disease on the other (Table 1). Albumin excretion rates are positively and significantly correlated with blood pressure values and with 'hypertension' (WHO definition), and with atherogenic patterns of plasma lipids and lipoproteins, but multivariate analysis in the group as a whole demonstrated that the association between albumin excretion rates and CHD was independent of these and the other risk factors (smoking, adiposity, age) measured in the study.

Table 1. Overnight urinary albumin excretion rate (AER) in non-insulin-dependent diabetics with and without clinical/ECG evidence of coronary heart disease (Mattock et al., 1987)

| | Overnight AER* (μg/min) | | |
|---|---|---|---|
| | CHD Negative | CHD Positive | *P* |
| Men (54) | 12.4 (8.8–17.5) | 38.2 (20.8–70.4) | <0.01 |
| Women (56) | 5.9 (4.4– 7.8) | 12.1 ( 9.2–16.0) | <0.05 |

* Geometric means (95% confidence intervals).

## Mechanisms of Proteinuria–CHD Association

We are no further than at the beginning of our understanding of this newly recognized association, and explanation is presently speculative at best. The operation of third factors responsible for both proteinuria and vascular disease, such as raised blood pressure, has already been referred to. Such 'confounding' associations certainly do not explain the whole of the relationship. The association of raised plasma lipids with proteinuric renal disease, notably the hypercholesterolaemia of the nephrotic syndrome, is well recognized but poorly understood. Interestingly, and at present inexplicably, the relationship with plasma lipid abnormalities appears to extend down to the low levels of increased albumin excretion.

## Microalbuminuric

It has been suggested that penetration of the glomerular barrier by negatively charged albumin particles may be an indication of a much more generalized increase in permeability of the vascular wall; indeed there is evidence of increased passage of labelled albumin from the circulation into the tissues generally in association with raised urinary excretion rates (11). The diabetic state may unmask some inadequacy, perhaps genetically determined, of the production of agents (e.g. charged proteoglycans, such as heparan sulphate) or the operation of mechanisms (e.g. $Na^+H^+$ cell membrane counter-transport) which ordinarily maintain the integrity of the vascular endothelial barrrier. Thus, microalbuminuria may be a marker of a host susceptibility state which is manifested both by raised glomerular permeability to plasma albumin and also by increased vulnerability of the arterial wall to penetration by atherogenic lipoproteins or macrophage foam cells from the circulation. This concept of enhanced vascular susceptibility to what might otherwise be innocuous stimuli could explain the overall increase and liability to arterial disease exhibited by the diabetic. However, it requires much further exploration and research.

## Diabetic Cardiopathy

Several clinical and experimental studies have supported the notion that non-coronary factors may contribute to heart disease in the diabetic patient (12, 13). In the Framingham Study (14), the excess of heart disease in long-term diabetic subjects appeared to be due in large part to congestive heart failure occurring in long-term insulin-dependent diabetic women without clear evidence of prior coronary disease. Angiocardiographic investigation of a number of insulin-dependent patients with anginal pain failed to show evidence of coronary artery obstruction sufficient to account for the symptoms (15), and functional studies of left ventricular performance (16, 17) have lent weight to the suggestion that there may be a specific defect of cardiac muscle function associated with the diabetic state. This may be a consequence of disturbed myocardial metabolism secondary to the diabetic state since it improves as the diabetes comes under control (18). There is also histological evidence of obstructive disease of vessels of arteriolar size (19) and also of capillary microaneurysms (20) associated with diffuse myocardial fibrosis, presumably secondary to generalized ischaemia. Autonomic neuropathy may also contribute to total cardiovascular mortality with increased risk of sudden cardiorespiratory arrest in severely neuropathic diabetic patients, particularly after the administration of respiratory depressant drugs or anaesthesia (21). For a given degree of myocardial ischaemia following upon coronary obstruction, the clinical outcome is decidely more adverse in the diabetic than in the non-diabetic, with approximately twice the mortality rate in the former compared with the latter (22). Outcome after infarction appears to be related to the severity of diabetic metabolic upset which accompanies it (23) though efforts to normalize metabolism in this situation may not strikingly improve the outcome (24).

### Peripheral Vascular Disease

Peripheral vascular disease has been much less well documented in diabetic populations and compared with general population experience than has coronary heart disease. In the Framingham population the incidence of intermittent claudication in diabetics (without distinction by type) was 12.6 and 8.4 per $10^3$ patient-years for men and women respectively, compared with 3.3 and 1.3 per $10^3$ patient-years in non-diabetics (25). Nilsson *et al.* (26) found 9.9% of the diabetic population with absent foot pulses, compared with 2.6% of the non-diabetic population, allowing for age and sex differences.

Ischaemic gangrene affecting the lower extremity is difficult to quantitate. Mortality is high in patients with gangrene so prevalence is relatively low. Incidence is a better indicator but data are scarce. In Rochester, Minnesota, USA, the rate of new episodes of gangrene in diabetic subjects, originally without evidence of peripheral vascular disease, was 4.5 per $10^3$ person-years (27).This may be compared with overall estimates of rates in the general US population of about 0.2 per $10^3$ population per year as estimated from hospital discharges for gangrene (28). Major lower-limb amputations in diabetics (below or above knee) are very likely to be the consequence of obstructive arterial disease. Hospital discharge data from six States in the USA (29) indicated that 45% of all lower extremity amputations were in diabetics.

Many factors may contribute to the greater impact of obstructive arterial disease upon the diabetic foot and leg. With a given degree of arterial obstruction, the associated presence of sensory and autonomic neuropathy will increase the vulnerability of the tissues of the foot to low-grade physical or thermal trauma; failure of autonomic vascular control may interfere with the normal local blood-flow responses to such local insults. Add to this vascular and neurological disturbance the liability of the devitalized diabetic foot to chronic infection and the high relative risk for chronic ulceration and gangrenous tissue destruction, and lower limb amputation is largely explained.

## EPIDEMIOLOGICAL CONSIDERATIONS

The WHO Multinational Study of Vascular Disease in Diabetics (30) recruited from each of four national centres approximately 500 representative diabetic patients aged

35–54 years, stratified by age subgroups, sex and known duration of diabetes (Figure 1). They were submitted to systematic and standardized enquiry, examination and investigations. Subjective evidence of cardiovascular disease was recorded using the validated WHO questionnaire (but intercultural comparisons of such symptomatic enquiries are hazardous). The study also required a standard 12-lead electrocardiogram for each patient. The records were subjected to Minnesota ECG coding (31) by two experienced coders working independently. Disagreements were adjudicated by a third observer. A history of stroke and of amputation for ischaemic disease of toe, foot or leg was also systematically recorded.

Table 2 gives a general overview of arterial disease rates and associated risk factors in the 14 cohorts and indicates the considerable variation between centres. Figure 1 shows the rates (for the sexes separately) of ECG evidence of probable coronary disease (major Q-wave items or left bundle branch block) and of possible coronary disease (minor Q-wave items and ST/T wave items) for individual centres. Figure 2 shows the rates for claudication and amputation. The rates of both of these major indices of macrovascular morbidity varied considerably between centres with notably low rates for both Hong Kong and Tokyo and high rates for CHD in some European centres. The low rates of abnormality in Japanese diabetics and also in the Chinese diabetics of Hong Kong support other less standardized evidence from autopsy data of the relative infrequency of coronary artery disease as a cause of death among Japanese diabetics. This parallels the low frequency of CHD in the general Japanese population. The parallel though higher rates of atherosclerosis in diabetics in relation to the rates for arterial disease in their respective general population was also noted in the International Atherosclerosis Project (32) based upon quantitative estimations of the extent and severity of atherosclerotic disease in autopsy material from general populations varying widely in their natural prevalence of atherosclerosis.

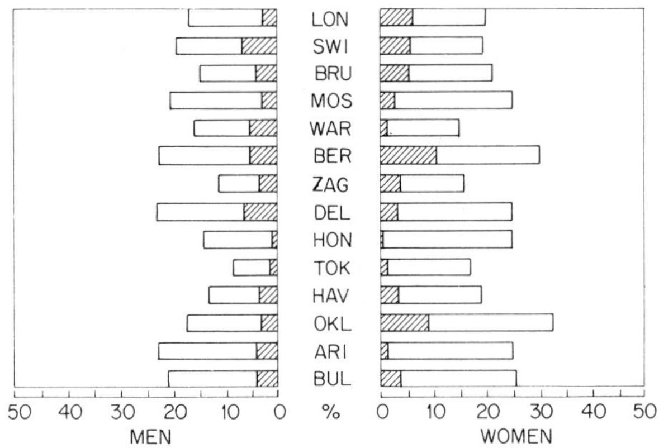


Figure 1. WHO Multinational Study of Vascular Disease in Diabetics. Prevalence rates for ECG categories 'ECG Coronary Possible' and 'ECG Coronary Probable' by centre and sex. ▨ ECG coronary possible; □ ECG coronary probable. See Table 2 for full names of the centres.

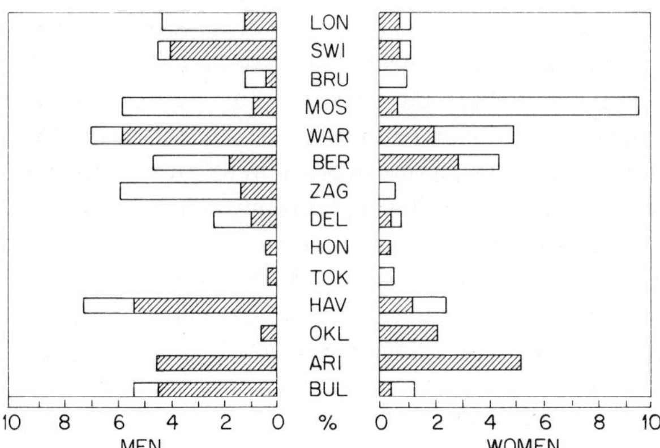


Figure 2. WHO Multinational Study of Vascular Disease in Diabetics. Prevalence rates for Leg Vascular Disease categories, amputation and intermittent claudication by centre and sex. ▨ amputation; □ intermittent claudication. See Table 2 for full names of the centres.

This relative sparing of the Japanese diabetic for CHD is unlikely to be a genetically mediated ethnic characteristic, for rates of CHD reported for diabetic Japanese migrants to Hawaii are much higher and indistinguishable from the rates of the Europid population (33). The factors responsible for this increase in risk in these migrants are not clearly understood, but an associated rise in mean blood cholesterol concentration and 'Westernization' of dietary practices may play an important role. Data on changes in other major risk factors (e.g. smoking habits, arterial pressure, adiposity, physical activity, alcohol intake) are not readily available. However, the inference is that high rates of arterial disease are not a necessary accompaniment of the diabetic state. Recognition in the Westernized setting of the responsible environmental agents and their successful reversal might well reduce arterial disease risk in the Europid diabetic to the levels obtaining in indigenous Japanese diabetics.

## CONCLUSION

There is now clear evidence of the enhanced susceptibility of both insulin-dependent and non-insulin-dependent diabetics to arterial disease though, in the latter, the relative importance of diabetes is increasingly overhauled by the effects of age per se. It remains uncertain whether the enhanced susceptibility of the diabetic is a direct consequence of the metabolic abnormality of diabetes itself or, as Jarrett has convincingly argued, perhaps a result of parallel factors acting independently of the metabolic abnormality (34). There is also strong reason to conclude that, in the diabetic as in the non-diabetic, the major risk factors for arterial disease—hypertension, hyperlipidemia and cigarette smoking—are operative and determinant of risk, their effects being amplified approximately two-fold overall (Table 2). The intervention of arteriopathic influences peculiar to the diabetic state, such as alterations in clotting factors, platelet behaviour or tissue metabolic disturbances, may well contribute to the enhancement of risk in the diabetic, but a new and interesting direction has been given to research in this field by the demonstration of the strong association of quite small increases in urinary albumin excretion rate with increased arterial disease risk. This will be the subject of much investigation in the next few years. However, from the point of view of practical clinical decision making, it is clear that energetic attempts to control the levels of the known risk factors, by the correction of hypertension and hyperlipidemia and the cessation of cigarette smoking, represent a most important approach, potentially able to reduce very considerably the impact of arterial disease in the susceptible diabetic population.

Table 2. WHO Multinational Study risk factors for arterial disease and prevalence of 'large vessel disease'

| | *n* | HT* % | SMOKE** % | HCHOL*** % | LVD**** % |
|---|---|---|---|---|---|
| London | 497 | 25.8 | 37.6 | 20.2 | 29.0 |
| Switzerland | 534 | 36.3 | 33.1 | 36.2 | 28.4 |
| Brussels | 422 | 34.8 | 37.8 | 16.2 | 22.7 |
| Moscow | 499 | 43.1 | 21.8 | 31.1 | 39.0 |
| Warsaw | 486 | 32.2 | 36.2 | 12.3 | 38.5 |
| Berlin | 560 | 37.3 | 35.6 | 32.3 | 42.8 |
| Zagreb | 402 | 42.5 | 28.4 | 34.3 | 29.1 |
| New Delhi | 555 | 29.8 | 16.7 | 33.8 | 39.6 |
| Hong Kong | 422 | 29.3 | 35.7 | 13.1 | 23.9 |
| Tokyo | 436 | 28.1 | 41.3 | 10.6 | 18.2 |
| Havana | 515 | 36.0 | 52.3 | 33.8 | 45.6 |
| Oklahoma | 653 | 35.3 | 43.3 | 11.1 | 39.0 |
| Arizona | 241 | 29.6 | 34.2 | 4.7 | 32.5 |
| Bulgaria | 473 | 33.5 | 20.9 | 9.8 | 34.4 |
| Total | 6695 | 33.9 | 33.1 | 22.3 | 33.5 |

* BP(syst) ⩾ 160 or BP(diast) ⩾ 95 mmHg or ON TREATMENT.
** Current smoking > 1 cigarette/day.
*** Hypercholesterolaemia ⩾ 6.7 mmol/l.
**** WHO questionnaire evidence of CHD/PVD or history of completed stroke or amputation/ischaemia, gangrene or Minnesota code, ECG coronary possible or probable (Whitehall criteria).
Figures in table are adjusted for age.

## REFERENCES

1. Jarrett RJ, Keen H, Chakrabarti R (1982) Diabetes, hyperglycaemia and arterial disease. In: Keen H, Jarrett J (eds) Complications of diabetes, second edition. Edward Arnold, London, pp 179–203
2. Levine SA (1982) Angina pectoris; some clinical consideration. J Am Med Assoc 79: 928–933

3. Hume L, Oakley GD, Boulton AJM, et al. (1986) Asymptomatic myocardial ischemia and its relation to diabetic neuropathy: an exercise electrocardiography study in middle-aged diabetic men. Diabetes Care 9: 384–388
4. Borch-Johnsen K, Kragh Andersen P, Deckert T (1985) The effect of proteinuria on relative mortality in Type 1 (insulin-dependent) diabetes mellitus. Diabetologia 28: 590–596
5. Jensen T, Borch-Johnsen A, Kofoed-Enevoldsen A, Deckert T (1987) Coronary heart disease in young Type 1 (insulin-dependent) diabetic patients with and without diabetic neuropathy: incidence and risk factors. Diabetologia 30: 144–148
6. Jarrett RJ, Viberti GC, Argyropoulos A, et al. (1984) Microalbuminuria predicts mortality in non-insulin-dependent diabetes. Diabetic Med 1: 17–19
7. Mogensen CE (1984) Microalbuminuria predicts clinical proteinuria and early mortality in maturity-onset diabetes. N Engl J Med 310: 356–360
8. Viberti GC, Keen H (1984) The patterns of proteinuria in diabetes mellitus. Diabetes 33: 686–692
9. Mattock M, Keen H, Viberti GC, et al. (1987) Microalbuminuria, coronary heart disease and its risk factors in non-insulin-dependent diabetes: a prevalence study (submitted for publication)
10. Rose GA, Blackburn H (1982) Cardiovascular survey methods. WHO Monogr Ser No 56
11. Feldt-Rasmussen B (1986) Increased transcapillary escape rate of albumin in Type 1 (insulin-dependent) diabetic patients with microalbuminuria. Diabetologia 29: 282–286
12. Rubler S, Dlugash J, Yuceoglu YZ, et al. (1982) New type of cardiomyopathy associated with diabetic glomerulosclerosis. Am J Cardiol 30: 595–602
13. Hamby RI, Zoneraich S, Sherman S (1974) Diabetic cardiomyopathy. J Am Med Assoc 229: 1749–1754
14. Kannel WB, Hjortland M, Castelli WP (1974) Role of diabetes in congestive heart failure: The Framingham Study. Am J Cardiol 34: 29–34
15. Regan TJ, Lyons MM, Ahmed SS, et al. (1977) Evidence for cardiomyopathy in familial diabetes mellitus. J Clin Invest 60: 885–899
16. Shapiro LM, Howat AP, Calter MM (1981) Left ventricular function in diabetes mellitus. I. Methodology and prevalence and spectrum of abnormalities. Br Heart J 45: 112–128
17. Shapiro LM, Leatherdale BA, Mackinnon J, et al. (1981) Left ventricular function in diabetes mellitus. II. Relation between clinical features and left ventricular function. Br Heart J 45: 129–132
18. Sykes CA, Wright AD, Malins JM, et al. (1977) Changes in systolic time intervals during treatment of diabetes mellitus. Br Heart J 39: 255–259
19. Blumenthal HT, Alex M, Goldenberg S (1960) A study of lesions of the intramural coronary by branches in diabetes mellitus. Arch Pathol 70: 27–42
20. Factor SM, Okun EM, Minase T (1980) Capillary microaneurysms in the human diabetic heart. N Engl J Med 302: 384–388
21. Ewing DJ, Campbell IE, Clarke BF (1980) The natural history of diabetic autonomic neuropathy. Quart J Med 49: 95–108
22. Gwilt DJ, Petri M, Lewis PW, et al. (1985) Myocardial infarct size and mortality in diabetic patients. Br Heart J 54: 466–472
23. Soler NG, Pentecost BL, Bennett MA, et al. (1974) Coronary care for myocardial infarction in diabetics. Lancet i: 475–478
24. Gwilt DJ, Petri M, Lamb P, et al. (1984) Effect of intravenous insulin infusion on mortality among diabetic patients after myocardial infarction. Br Heart J 51: 626–631

25. Kannel WB, McGee DL (1979) Diabetes and cardiovascular disease. The Framingham Study. J Am Med Assoc 241: 2035–2038
26. Nilsson SE, Nilsson N, Frostberg N, Emilson T (1967) The Krisstad Survey. II. Acta Med Scand Suppl 469: 1–42
27. Melton LJ, Macken KM, Palumbo PJ, Elveback LR (1980) Incidence and prevalence of clinical peripheral vascular disease in a population based cohort of diabetic patients. Diabetes Care 3: 650–654
28. US Department of Health and Human Services (1980) Detailed diagnosis and surgical procedures for patients discharged from short-stay hospitals: United States 1978. DHHS Publ No (PHS) 50-1274 Washington DC
29. Most RS, Sinnock P (1983) The epidemiology of lower extremity amputations in diabetic individuals. Diabetes Care 6: 87–91
30. Diabetes Drafting Group (1985) Prevalence of small vessel and large vessel disease in diabetic patients from 14 centres. The World Health Organization Multinational Study of Vascular Disease in Diabetics. Diabetologia 28: 615–640
31. Blackburn H, Keys A (1960) The electrocardiogram in population studies. A classification system. Circulation 21: 1160–1175
32. Robertson WB, Strong JP (1969) Atherosclerosis in persons with hypertension and diabetes mellitus. Lab Invest 18: 538–551
33. Kawate R, Yamakido M, Nishimoto Y, et al. (1979) Diabetes mellitus and its vascular complications in Japanese migrants on the island of Hawaii. Diabetes Care 2: 161–170
34. Jarrett R (1984) Type 2 (non-insulin-dependent) diabetes mellitus and coronary heart disease—chicken, egg or neither? Diabetologia 26: 99–102

Diabetic Complications: Early Diagnosis and Treatment
Edited by D. Andreani, G. Crepaldi, U. Di Mario and G. Pozza


# CHAPTER 2

# *Excess Mortality in Diabetes*

P. Micossi, G. Gallus* and G. Pozza
*Istituto Scientifico S. Raffaele, *Cattedra di Biometria e Statistica, Cattedra di Clinica Medica, University of Milan, Italy*

Various studies (1−8) show a persistent excess mortality in diabetes compared to the population in general, despite the benefits brought by the discovery of insulin (Table 1).

However, the specific problem of excess mortality in diabetes has not yet received the required attention. In spite of the abundant literature in some way related to mortality, it is still difficult to answer basic questions such as: Is the life expectancy of a Type 1 diabetic subject not developing renal disease comparable to that of a normal person (9, 10)? Is diabetes not relevant to life expectancy when age at diagnosis is above 70 years (11)? Is the dependency of excess mortality on age at diagnosis in maturity-onset diabetes an indication of heterogeneity, or is it a simple consequence of the fact that a late onset prevents the disease from manifesting its effects on mortality?

Most papers dealing with excess mortality in diabetes are concerned with the association with cardiovascular risk factors, because cardiovascular diseases are by far the most important cause of death among diabetic patients (11).

It is currently thought that Type 1 and Type 2 diabetes contribute to overall mortality as two distinct nosological entities with different etiopathological mechanisms and this has justified dealing with each of them separately.

The reliability of death certification data in estimating the impact of diabetes on population mortality will not be considered here. Statistics obtained from death certificates, which provide extremely important epidemiological data for many other diseases, are virtually useless for diabetes as they grossly underestimate the real impact of diabetes on mortality (12).

## TYPE 2 DIABETES MELLITUS

There is evidence that excess mortality in maturity-onset diabetes mellitus is related to many factors (age at diagnosis, sex, treatment, calendar time, etc.), but there are

Table 1. Excess mortality in diabetes from different sources

| Study | Period | Type of diabetes | Risk | Excess mortality | | |
|---|---|---|---|---|---|---|
| | | | | Males | Females | All |
| Pittsburgh (1) | 1950–81 | Insulin-dependent diabetes | O/E (c) | 5.4 | 11.5 | |
| Funen County (2) | 1973–81 | Insulin-treated diabetes | O/E (c) | — | — | 3.6 |
| Equitable Life Insurance Society (3) | 1951–70 | All diabetes | O/E (c) | — | — | 3.4 |
| Rancho Bernardo (4) (a) | 1972–80 | All diabetes | CSR (d) | 2.4 | 3.5 | — |
| Joslin Clinic (5) | 1930/1956–60 | All diabetes | SMR (e) | 1.7 | 2.2 | 2.0 |
| Framingham (6) (a) | 1948–68 | All diabetes | RR (f) | 1.7 | 3.3 | — |
| Oslo (7) (a) | 1956–61 | All diabetes | O/E (c) | 2.9 | 2.6 | — |
| Birmingham (8) (b) | — | All diabetes | O/E (c) | 1.6 | 1.8 | — |

(a) heart disease mortality
(b) disease of the circulatory system mortality
(c) observed/expected death rate ratio
(d) Cox standardized risk ratio
(e) Standardized mortality ratio
(f) Relative risk

only a few studies which attempt to perform a proper control of the major determinants of excess mortality. This is also due to the difficulty of following up unselected cohorts of incident cases. Therefore, relatively little is known about the real causes of excess mortality.

In economically developed Western societies, the principal cause of death in diabetic patients is ischemic heart disease which is responsible for more than half of all diabetic deaths (13, 14). This reflects the trend in the general population, and is also observed in Asia and Africa where a low incidence of cardiovascular mortality is found in both the diabetic and non-diabetic population.

What should be underlined, however, is that excess cardiovascular mortality still occurs more often in diabetic than in non-diabetic subjects.

The longitudinal Framingham Study has shown that excess mortality due to cardiovascular diseases in diabetic subjects is twice as high in men and three times as high in women (15). A higher excess mortality in women is confirmed in several other studies (4, 6, 7, 16–19).

Cardiovascular disease is the natural consequence of atherosclerosis, partly reflecting its increased frequency in the diabetic population (20, 21). Excess mortality, however, may be due not only to the susceptibility of diabetic patients to atherosclerosis, but also to the increased risk of their dying during the acute phase of myocardial infarction (22, 23). Atherosclerosis in the diabetic subject, although not qualitatively different from that in the non-diabetic subject, presents more serious characteristics because of a greater involvement of the coronary microcirculation (23). Efforts to estimate cardiovascular mortality have provoked studies which attempt to identify specific risk factors for coronary heart disease in diabetic patients or in subjects with impaired glucose tolerance. Excess mortality has been attributed to arterial hypertension, hyperlipidemia, obesity and hyperglycemia per se, but the actual independent role of each one of these factors remains an unresolved and elusive question, and the possibility of a potentially synergic action cannot be excluded.

## Age at Diagnosis

The different life expectancy observed in subgroups of diabetic patients, according to the age of onset, has been taken as an indication of heterogeneity (5, 7, 8).

Panzram and Zabel-Langhennig (11) have shown that excess mortality decreases along with the increase in age at diagnosis, it being double that of the general population in those who had diabetes diagnosed between the age of 40 and 49 years; mortality is almost normal when diabetes is diagnosed after the age of 75 years. The existence of a relationship between excess mortality and age at diagnosis was confirmed by Krolewski et al. (19) and by ourselves (Gallus et al. unpublished data). Our study shows that in individuals who have diabetes diagnosed after the age of 60 years, excess mortality almost disappears. Panzram reports that excess mortality is already evident in the first year of the disease, whereas our preliminary observation seems to indicate a latency period of about 10 years before the negative influence of diabetes becomes evident.

## Hyperglycemia

It is still difficult to establish how much excess mortality depends on the metabolic derangements associated with hyperglycemia. The evidence that individuals with impaired glucose tolerance (23) and recently diagnosed diabetes (17) have a higher risk of coronary heart disease may give weight to the hypothesis of a genetic association of multiple risk factors, or alternatively to the hypothesis of an independent role of glucose.

Various studies have attempted to substantiate the independent role of glucose by showing that the action of other risk factors only partly explained the observed excess mortality (24). However, according to Jarrett, 'It is more likely that diabetes develops in individuals who already possess characteristics which increase the risk of coronary heart disease in addition to the risk of developing diabetes' (25). In both cases it is possible that environmental factors cause genetically predetermined pathological conditions to become manifest. Furthermore, a recent survey in our epidemiological unit (26) has shown that risk factors for coronary heart disease are increased in the non-diabetic relatives of diabetic subjects.

## Hypertension

It is known that hypertension is more frequent in the diabetic than in the non-diabetic subject (23). The Tecumseh prospective study (27) has shown that the frequency of clinically evident diabetes increases progressively from the fifth of the population with the lowest values of arterial pressure, through the three-fifths of the population with intermediate values, to the remaining fifth with the highest values.

There is still much debate on the determining role of hypertension in causing atherosclerosis. Pell and D'Alonzo have concluded that the excess of coronary heart disease is mainly attributable to arterial hypertension and that this causes a mortality rate approximately twice as high in hypertensive diabetic patients compared to normotensive diabetic subjects (28).

In a previous study the same authors found that, as far as the different rate of mortality in diabetic and non-diabetic individuals was concerned, excess mortality only occurred among diabetic hypertensive subjects. Thus, the susceptibility of diabetic patients to cardiovascular disease may be entirely explained by the increased incidence of hypertension in the diabetic population (29).

The Schwabing Study (30), carried out on 600 non-selected caucasian diabetic subjects, showed that systolic pressure was significantly associated with cardiovascular morbidity in non-insulin-dependent diabetic men, while in women high levels of triglycerides also appeared to be a predictive factor.

Further evidence pointing to the independent role of hypertension is that arterial pressure shows no tendency to increase with the duration of the disease (31).

Certain studies favour the hypothesis of interaction between the two pathological entities in the genesis of atherosclerosis, rather than of independent roles. This would indicate that diabetic subjects are unable to tolerate pressure rises which would be of no harm to normoglycemic individuals (32).

Debate occurs in the literature concerning the primum movens: 'Is diabetes the cause of hypertension?', or 'Is there a predisposition to both types of disease pathology?', or 'Is hypertension a risk factor in determining diabetes?'

These last two questions could point to the existence of a common genetic etiology; hypertension itself, as well as diabetes mellitus, may be a polygenic disorder (33).

## Obesity

Obesity has been shown to be a risk factor for coronary heart disease in the general population (34); consequently, the presence of more overweight subjects in the diabetic population, as opposed to the general population, has led to investigations into the possible relationship between overweight, heart disease and mortality. There is very little evidence of an increasing risk of coronary heart disease with increasing obesity, while certain studies describe a more complex relationship between these two factors. In the Chicago People's Gas Company Study (35), it was found that those at greater risk were near their ideal weight or markedly obese, while the lowest mortality rate belonged to subjects who were in the intermediate condition.

The Whitehall Study (36), which, like the Chicago Study, dealt only with the male sex, found a positive relationship between death due to coronary heart disease and body mass index. It should be remembered that obesity is usually associated with hypertension, hyperlipidemia and diabetes, and when the role of these factors was investigated through a multiple analysis, obesity did not show any independent contribution (36). A report on the data in the Framingham Study (37) contradicts the above and concludes that obesity is a serious and independent risk factor, especially in women.

It is clear that present evidence concerning the role of obesity in coronary heart disease remains equivocal and further studies on its independent role should be undertaken.

## Dyslipidemia

Various studies have shown that atherogenic changes in lipids and lipoproteins are closely associated with diabetes mellitus (38, 39). There is evidence of a higher incidence of lipid disorders in diabetes, and that these disorders are more evident in diabetic females than males. This could explain why excess mortality is higher in diabetic women (39, 40).

However, total cholesterol levels do not seem to play a significant role in the genesis of cardiovascular diseases in diabetic subjects (41) and, furthermore, conflicting results have been reported concerning the levels of $HDL_2$ cholesterol and triglycerides (39, 42) although there is agreement on the reduction of lipoprotein lipase activity in Type 2 diabetic patients (38, 39, 43).

Recently attention has been focused on apoproteins, whose role is thought to be critical in lipoprotein clearance, and mathematical models of lipoprotein turnover have been developed to investigate this aspect (43).

The effect on mortality of the interaction between hyperglycemia and hyperlipidemia is not completely understood. The co-existence of genes on chromosomes 11 and 19 which control insulin and insulin-receptor synthesis and apoprotein and apoprotein-receptor synthesis would support the hypothesis of a genetic linkage.

## TYPE 1 (INSULIN-DEPENDENT) DIABETES MELLITUS

The introduction of insulin in clinical practice for treating juvenile-onset, insulin-dependent diabetes mellitus dramatically changed the natural history of this disorder. The overall mortality from diabetic ketoacidosis sharply decreased, and life expectancy was significantly improved for these patients. A recent report from Denmark indicates that the prognosis of Type 1 diabetes has improved considerably during the last 40 years and that duration is the most important determinant of excess mortality (44).

However, longer survival was associated with an increased risk of developing chronic complications of insulin-dependent diabetes, some of which are eventually fatal. Despite continued efforts to optimize the treatment over the past six decades, mortality is still higher among these patients compared to the general population, and their life expectancy is thus much shorter. It should be considered that most of the papers dealing with excess mortality in insulin-dependent diabetes refer to countries in the northern part of Europe and to the United States. There is a three- to seven-fold increase in mortality in insulin-dependent diabetes (2, 45). These results may not reflect the situation in other areas, like the Southern European countries.

### Age at Diagnosis

It has been shown that excess mortality is inversely related to age at diagnosis by comparing those diagnosed above and below the age of 30 years (2), or above and below the age of 20 years (46). These observations are limited in that insulin-treated diabetic subjects were included in the study without distinguishing between Type 1 and Type 2 individuals.

However, when follow-up studies are restricted to insulin-dependent diabetic subjects, attained age, rather than age at onset and/or duration of the disease, showed a stronger relationship to mortality (47). A twenty-fold excess mortality was found in insulin-dependent diabetic subjects aged 25–40 years (45).

## Causes of Death

Ketoacidosis, hypoglycemic coma, infections and primary disorders without any apparent relation to diabetes only account for 25% of the overall mortality in the insulin-dependent diabetic population (10, 47), the most prevalent cause of death being end-stage renal failure and cardiovascular diseases. Thus, chronic complications of insulin-dependent diabetes, i.e. diabetic nephropathy and macroangiopathy, are the main determinants of excess mortality in this type of diabetes.

## Proteinuria

Recent epidemiological observations suggest that not all of the patients may have the same mortality risk. The onset of persistent proteinuria shows a peak incidence of 3–5% per year in individuals with a duration of insulin-dependent diabetes between 10 and 25 years, thereafter decreasing to less than 1% per year in those with a duration of the disease of 30–35 years (10). Furthermore, the cumulative incidence of diabetic nephropathy is 30–40%, indicating that as many as 60% of insulin-dependent diabetic subjects are unlikely to develop this complication (48).

The relative mortality among patients with persistent proteinuria steeply increases in the age groups over 20 years, reaching a peak of 100 in the age group from 30 to 40 years.

The incidence of persistent proteinuria reaches a peak after 10–20 years of duration of disease, and this is directly related to excess mortality; a markedly smaller increase in mortality is observed in patients without persistent proteinuria (10). Persistent proteinuria is associated with elevated mortality caused by end-stage renal failure, but the relative mortality caused by cardiovascular disease was also found to be significantly higher among these patients compared to non-proteinuric subjects (10). Taken together these observations generated the hypothesis that only one subset of insulin-dependent diabetic subjects, by developing clinical proteinuria, has a high mortality risk.

A urinary albumin excretion in excess of 30 μg/min predicts clinical proteinuria in insulin-dependent diabetes (49) and is associated with increased mortality. Similar results were obtained in two independent studies (50, 51). Interestingly, microalbuminuria was also shown to predict mortality in non-insulin-dependent diabetic subjects, although in these patients death mainly occurs because of cardiovascular disease (52, 53), whereas death from uremia is uncommon. Indeed, persistent proteinuria occurs also in non-insulin-dependent diabetes mellitus, but the phenomenon has been less extensively investigated than in insulin-dependent diabetes.

The finding of a higher prevalence of cardiovascular disease in nephropathic insulin-dependent diabetic subjects and the predictive value of renal abnormality for cardiovascular death in non-insulin-dependent diabetic subjects render speculative the existence of a common factor in the pathogenesis of both complications of diabetes and, hence, of excessive mortality.

Arterial hypertension is a strong determinant of the risk of cardiovascular damage (54) and it was found to be related both to coronary heart disease and to persistent proteinuria in insulin-dependent diabetic subjects; the chronological relationship between the onset of proteinuria and hypertension suggested a renal origin for the latter (47). However, insulin-dependent diabetic patients with an albumin excretion rate greater than 30 $\mu$g/min, i.e. 'at risk' microalbuminuria, were found to have elevated (although non-hypertensive) blood pressure compared to a group of insulin-dependent diabetic patients matched for age, sex and duration of diabetes, but with a lower albumin excretion rate (55), raising the possibility that elevated blood pressure may precede clinical impairment of renal function.

## CONCLUSIONS

This brief review indicates that a wide range of uncertainties still exists as to the impact of diabetes on mortality.

Studies showing an independent role of glucose in increasing the rates of cardiovascular mortality in the diabetic population, or those of mortality due to end-stage renal disease, are counterbalanced by evidence that the genetic background is probably equally important for life expectancy.

One is dealing with diabetes probably not as a definite disease but rather as a complex syndrome with stratified genetic linkage with other disorders, implicating an increased tendency to develop degenerative diseases.

There is also no agreement on the individuals who should be considered to be at increased risk, so as to identify precise targets for public health service policies aimed at reducing excess mortality associated with diabetes.

It should be recalled that most of the studies have been undertaken on populations aged over 40 years, often without controlling for factors implicated with increased mortality.

It is therefore concluded that carefully designed studies are still needed to provide clear evidence on the true dimension of the issue of excess mortality in diabetes in the different areas, age groups, families, sexes, etc., and on the causative factors. This is the preliminary step which would then allow public health policies and even therapeutic strategies to be designed.

## REFERENCES

1. Dorman JS, Tajima N, LaPorte RE, Becker DJ, Cruickshanks KJ, Wagener DK, Orchard TJ, Drash AL (1985) The Pittsburgh insulin-dependent diabetes mellitus (IDDM) morbidity and mortality study: case-control analyses of risk factors for mortality. Diabetes Care 8 (Suppl 1): 54–60
2. Green A, Hougaard P (1984) Epidemiological studies of diabetes mellitus in Denmark:

5. Mortality and causes of death among insulin-treated diabetic patients. Diabetologia 26: 190–194
3. Goodkin G, Wolloch L, Gottcent RA, Reich F (1975) Diabetes: a twenty-year mortality study. Trans Assoc Life Ins Med Dir Am 58: 217–271
4. Barrett-Connor E, Wingard DL (1983) Sex differential in ischemic heart disease mortality in diabetics: a prospective population-based study. Am J Epidemiol 118: 489–496
5. Kessler II (1971) Mortality experience of diabetic patients. Am J Med 51: 715–724
6. Kannel WB, McGee DL (1979) Diabetes and glucose tolerance as risk factors for cardiovascular disease: the Framingham Study. Diabetes Care 2: 120–126
7. Westlund K (1969) Mortality of diabetics, report 13. Life Insurance Companies Institute for Medical Statistics at the Oslo City Hospitals. The Norwegian Research Council for Science and the Humanities, Oslo. PJ Schmidts Bogtrykkeri, Vojens
8. Hayward RE, Lucena BC (1965) An investigation into the mortality of diabetes. J Inst Act 91: 286–336
9. Green A, Borch-Johnsen K, Kragh P, Hougaard P, Keiding N, Kreiner S, Deckert T (1985) Relative mortality of Type 1 (insulin-dependent) diabetes in Denmark: 1933-1981. Diabetologia 28: 339–342
10. Borch Johnsen K, Kragh Andersen P, Deckert T (1985) The effect of proteinuria on relative mortality in Type 1 (insulin-dependent) diabetes mellitus. Diabetologia 28: 590–596
11. Panzram G, Zabel-Langhennig (1981) Prognosis of diabetes mellitus in a geographically defined population. Diabetologia 20: 587–591
12. Fuller JH, Elford J, Goldblatt P, Aldestein AM (1983) Diabetes mortality: new light on an underestimated public health problem. Diabetologia 24: 336–341
13. Marks HH, Krall LP (1971) Onset, course, prognosis and mortality in diabetes mellitus. In: Marble A, White P, et al. (eds) Joslin's diabetes mellitus. Lea & Febiger, Philadelphia, pp 209–254
14. Entmaker PS (1975) Long-term prognosis in diabetes mellitus. In: KE Sussman, RJS Metz (eds) Diabetes mellitus. Committee on Professional Education, American Diabetes Association, New York, pp 191–196
15. Gordon G, Castelli WP, Hjortland MC, et al. (1977) Predicting coronary heart disease in middle-aged and older persons. The Framingham Study. J Am Med Assoc 238: 497–499
16. Butler WJ, Ostrander LD Jr, Carman WJ, Lamphiear DE (1985) Mortality from coronary heart disease in the Tecumseh study: Long-term effect of diabetes mellitus, glucose tolerance and other risk factors. Am J Epidemiol 121: 541–547
17. Jarrett RJ, McCartney P, Keen H (1982) The Bedford Survey: ten year mortality rates in newly diagnosed diabetics, borderline diabetics and normoglycaemic control and risk indices for coronary heart disease in borderline diabetics. Diabetologia 22: 79–84
18. Mihara T, Oohashi H, Hirata Y (1986) Mortality in Japanese diabetics in a seven-year follow-up study. Diabetes Res Clin Pract 2: 139–144
19. Krolewski AS, Czyzyk A, Janeczko D, Kopczynski J (1977) Mortality from cardiovascular disease among diabetics. Diabetologia 13: 345–350
20. Ostrander LD Jr, Francis T Jr, Hayner NS, Kjelsberg MO, Epstein FH (1965) The relationship of cardiovascular disease to hyperglycaemia. Ann Intern Med 62: 1188-1199
21. Keen H, Rose GA, Pyke DA, Boyns DR, Chlouverakis, Mistry S (1965) Blood-sugar and arterial disease. Lancet ii: 505–508
22. Oswald GA, Corcoran S, Yudkin JS (1984) Prevalence and risks of hyperglycaemia and undiagnosed diabetes in patients with acute myocardial infarction. Lancet i: 1264–1267
23. Jarrett RJ, Keen H (1975) Diabetes and atherosclerosis. In: Keen H, Jarrett RJ (eds)

Complication of diabetes. Edward Arnold, London, pp 179–203
24. Fuller JH, Shipley MJ, Rose G, Jarrett RJ, Keen H (1983) Mortality from coronary heart disease and stroke in relation to degree of glycaemia: the Whitehall Study. Br Med J 287: 867–870
25. Jarrett RJ (1984) Type 2 (non-insulin-dependent) diabetes mellitus and coronary heart disease—chicken, egg or neither? Diabetologia 26: 99–102
26. Micossi P, Gallus G, Valsania P, Garancini P, Radaelli G, Pozza G (1987) First degree family history of diabetes and risk factors for cardiovascular disease in non diabetic subjects: a metabolic survey. Eur J Epidemiol 3: 46–53
27. Epstein FH, Francis T Jr, Hayner NS, Johnson BC, Kjelsberg MO, Napier JA, Ostrander LD Jr, Payne MW, Dodge HJ (1965) Prevalence of chronic disease and distribution of selected physiologic variables in a total community—Tecumseh, Michigan. Am J Epidemiol 81: 307–312
28. Pell S, D'Alonzo CA (1972) Factors associated with long-term survival of diabetics. J Am Med Assoc 214: 1833–1843
29. Pell S, D'Alonzo CA (1967) Some aspects of hypertension in diabetes mellitus. J Am Med Assoc 202: 104–110
30. Janka HU (1985) Macrovascular changes: atherosclerosis as related to diabetes mellitus. In: Krall LP, Alberti KGMM, Serrano-Rios M (eds) World book of diabetes in practice, vol 2. Elsevier, Amsterdam, New York, Oxford, pp 162–168
31. Pyke DA (1968) Arterial disease and diabetes. In: Oakley WG, Pyke DA, Taylor KW (eds) Clinical diabetes and its biochemical basis. Blackwell, Oxford, p 530
32. Freedman P, Moulton R, Spencer AG (1958) Hypertension and diabetes mellitus. Q J Med 27: 293–305
33. Vande Molen R, Brewer G, Honeyman MS, Morrison J, Hoobler SW (1970) A study of hypertension in twins. Am Heart J 79: 454–460
34. Keys A, Aravanis C, Blackburn H, Van Buchem FSF, Buzina R, Djordjevic BS, Fidanza F, Karvonen MJ, Menotti A, Puddu V, Taylor HL (1972) Coronary heart disease—overweight and obesity as risk factors. Ann Intern Med 77: 15–27
35. Dyer AR, Stamler J, Berkson DM, Lindberg HA (1975) Relationship of relative weight and body mass index to 14-year mortality in the Chicago People's Gas Company Study. J Chron Dis 28: 109–123
36. Jarrett RJ, Shipley MJ, Rose G (1982) Weight and mortality in the Whitehall Study. Br Med J 285: 535–537
37. Hubert HB, Feinlieb M, McNamara PM, Castelli WP (1982) Obesity as an independent risk factor for cardiovascular disease. In: Shekelle RB (ed) CVD epidemiology newsletter, No. 31 of Council of Epidemiology of American Heart Association. American Heart Association, New York
38. Brunzel JD, Chait A, Bierman EL (1985) Plasma lipoproteins in human diabetes mellitus. In: Alberti KGMM, Krall LP (eds) The diabetes annual/1. Elsevier Science Publishers, Amsterdam, New York, Oxford, pp 463–479
39. Ganda OP (1980) Pathogenesis of macrovascular disease in the human diabetic. Diabetes 29: 931–942
40. Barrett-Connor E, Witzum JL, Holdbrook MA (1983) A community study of high density lipoproteins in adult non-insulin-dependent diabetics. Am J Epidemiol 117: 186–192
41. West KM, Ahuja MMS, Bennett PH, Czyzyk A, Mateo de Acosta O, Fuller JH, Grab B, Grabauskas V, Jarrett RJ, Kosaka K, Keen H, Krolewski AS, Miki E, Schliack V, Teuscher A, Watkins PJ, Stober JA (1983) The role of circulating glucose and triglyceride concentrations and their interactions with other 'risk factors' as determinants of arterial disease in nine diabetic population samples from the WHO

multinational study. Diabetes Care 6: 361–369

42. Nikkilä EA (1981) High density lipoproteins in diabetes. Diabetes 30 (Suppl 2): 82–87
43. Beltz WF, Kesaniemi YA, Howard BV, Grundy SM (1985) Development of an integrated model for analysis of the kinetics of apolipoprotein B in plasma lipoprotein VLDL, IDL and LDL. J Clin Invest 76: 575–585
44. Borch-Johansen K, Kreiner S, Deckert T (1986) Mortality of Type 1 (insulin-dependent) diabetes mellitus in Denmark: a study of relative mortality in 2930 Danish Type 1 diabetic patients diagnosed from 1933 to 1972. Diabetologia 29: 767–772
45. Dorman JS, LaPorte RE, Kuller LH, Cruickshanks KJ, Orchard TJ, Wagener DK, Becker DJ, Cavender DE, Drash AL (1984) The Pittsburgh insulin-dependent disbetes (IDDM) morbidity and mortality study. Mortality results. Diabetes 33: 271–276
46. Deckert T, Poulsen JE, Larsen M (1978) Prognosis of diabetics with diabetes onset before the age of thirty-one. I. Survival, causes of death, and complications. Diabetologia 14: 363–370
47. Christlieb AR, Warram JH, Krolewski AS, Busick EJ, Ganda OMP, Asmal AC, Soeldner JS, Bradley RF (1981) Hypertension: the major risk factor in juvenile-onset insulin-dependent diabetics. Diabetes 30 (Suppl 2): 90–96
48. Krolewski AS, Warram JH, Christlieb AR, Busick EJ, Kahn CR (1985) The changing natural history of nephropathy in Type 1 diabetes. Am J Med 78: 785–794
49. Viberti GC, Jarrett RJ, Mahmud U, Hill RD, Argyropoulos A, Keen H (1982) Microalbuminuria as a predictor of clinical nephropathy in insulin-dependent diabetes mellitus. Lancet i: 1430–1432
50. Mogensen CE, Christensen CK (1984) Predicting diabetic nephropathy in insulin-dependent patients. N Engl J Med 311: 89–93
51. Mathiesen ER, Oxemboll K, Johansen PA, Svendsen PA, Deckert T (1984) Incipient nephropathy in Type 1 (insulin-dependent) diabetes. Diabetologia 26: 406–410
52. Mogensen CE (1984) Microalbuminuria predicts clinical proteinuria and early mortality in maturity-onset diabetes. N Engl J Med 310: 356–360
53. Jarrett RJ, Viberti GC, Argyropoulos A, Hill RD, Mahmud U, Murells TJ (1983) Microalbuminuria predicts mortality in non-insulin-dependent diabetes. Diabetic Med 1: 17–19
54. Hypertension Detection and Followup Cooperative Group (1979) Five year findings of the hypertension and followup program: reduction in mortality of persons with high blood pressure, including mild hypertension. J Am Med Assoc 242: 2562–2571
55. Wiseman M, Viberti G, Mackintosh D, Jarrett EJ, Keen H (1984) Glycaemia, arterial pressure and microalbuminuria in Type 1 (insulin-dependent) diabetes mellitus. Diabetologia 26: 401–405

Diabetic Complications: Early Diagnosis and Treatment
Edited by D. Andreani, G. Crepaldi, U. Di Mario and G. Pozza


CHAPTER 3

# *Serum Lipoproteins and Atherosclerosis in Type 1 and Type 2 Diabetes*

M.-R. TASKINEN*, T. KUUSI and E. A. NIKKILÄ**
*Second* and Third Departments of Medicine, University of Helsinki, Finland*

Premature atherosclerosis is one of the most common complications of diabetes. There is ample evidence that the incidence and prevalence of all major manifestations of atherosclerosis, coronary heart disease (CHD), cerebrovascular disease and peripheral vascular disease, are markedly higher in diabetic than in non-diabetic subjects (1). The pathogenesis of premature atherosclerosis in diabetes is not clear but it is apparent that common risk factors for atherosclerosis are operative also in diabetes. Since plasma lipid abnormalities are frequent in diabetes the increased risk of atherosclerosis has been often attributed to changes in lipoprotein profile. However, recent studies on individual lipoproteins (VLDL, LDL, HDL and its subfractions) have shown that their concentrations in diabetes are highly variable. Firstly, the lipoprotein profile is totally different in the two types of diabetes. It is atherogenic in Type 2 diabetes, whereas Type 1 patients with good or moderate glycemic control have normal or even anti-atherogenic lipid profiles (2). Furthermore, in the majority of studies the subjects have not been adequately classified into Type 1 or Type 2 patients (1). In addition, the concentration and metabolism of plasma lipoproteins in diabetes are influenced by several factors: the degree of glycemic control, the mode of treatment and other metabolic changes (i.e. insulin resistance and concentrations of plasma free fatty acids and insulin antagonist hormones). Finally, genetic and environmental factors which influence plasma lipoproteins in the non-diabetic population are also operative in diabetes. Therefore it is not surprising that available data on plasma lipoproteins and their impact on atherosclerosis in diabetes are ambiguous.

** This work is dedicated to Esko Nikkilä. It was begun by him and was completed by his co-workers after his death in September 1986.

## LIPOPROTEIN DISTURBANCES IN TYPE 1 DIABETES

In Type 1 diabetes the plasma lipoprotein profile is influenced by ambient levels of plasma insulin achieved by insulin therapy which can vary from conventional therapy with one or two injections per day to insulin delivery by an implanted insulin pump. In conventional therapy the concentration of insulin in peripheral blood is higher than in portal blood which contrasts with the situation in non-diabetic subjects. This is also true for patients receiving subcutaneous insulin infusion.

In insulin deficiency the lipoprotein profile is characterized by a rise of VLDL, normal or subnormal LDL and a fall of HDL (2). The elevation of VLDL is caused by its increased production, as well as by impaired clearance, in the presence of low lipoprotein lipase (LPL) activity. In untreated Type 1 diabetic subjects there is an inverse correlation between the VLDL concentration and adipose tissue LPL activity (3). It is well established that LPL is an insulin-dependent enzyme (4). In accordance, we have shown that after the institution of insulin therapy LPL activity in tissues is restored to normal in parallel with a fall in VLDL triglyceride (3). In insulin deficiency the changes in both LDL and HDL evidently reflect disturbances in the early phase of the lipoprotein cascade, but it cannot be excluded that insulin deficiency also has direct effect on LDL or HDL metabolism. The changes in LDL and HDL are also reversible by insulin therapy but their responses are slower than that of VLDL. Since a true insulin deficiency is uncommon and present only in untreated or inadequately treated Type 1 patients, the observed changes in lipoproteins cannot contribute significantly to the increment of risk for atherosclerosis.

Table 1. Serum lipoproteins and apoproteins in insulin-treated Type 1 diabetics

| | Good glycemic control | Poor glycemic control |
|---|---|---|
| VLDL | Normal or subnormal | Increased |
| IDL | Normal | Increased |
| LDL | Subnormal | Normal or increased |
| HDL | Normal or increased | Reduced |
| Apoprotein B | Decreased | Increased |
| Apoprotein AI | Normal or increased | Decreased |
| Apoprotein AII | Normal | Normal or subnormal |

The lipoprotein profile in chronically insulin-treated Type 1 patients with good or moderate glycemic control is not atherogenic but, in contrast, non-atherogenic (Table 1). The concentration of VLDL is normal or even subnormal but it correlates positively with the degree of glycemic control (2). The elevation of serum triglyceride levels becomes clearly apparent if the glycemic control is suboptimal and it is more pronounced in women than in men (5). Both the production rate and fractional catabolic rate of VLDL seem to be normal or near normal in patients with good control (2, 6). It is noteworthy that the institution of rigorous glycemic control by insulin pump or artificial beta cell is followed by a further lowering of VLDL due to a fall in VLDL production (6, 7).

LDL cholesterol in Type 1 diabetic patients with moderate or good glycemic control seems to be within the normal range or even reduced (2). We have recently surveyed plasma lipoproteins in 42 male and 49 female insulin-treated Type 1 diabetic subjects and in age, sex and relative body weight matched control subjects. Interestingly, LDL cholesterol was significantly reduced in diabetic patients of both sexes compared to non-diabetic subjects (2.75 ± 0.11 vs 3.42 ± 0.13 mmol/l, $p<0.001$ for men and 2.79 ± 0.11 vs 3.12 ± 0.10 mmol/l, $p<0.05$ for women) (8). Moreover, Winocour et al. (9) have reported that serum LDL cholesterol levels tend to be lower in Type 1 diabetic patients than in control subjects. In addition, Type 1 diabetic men show also lower apoprotein B levels than control subjects (9, 10). There is evidence to suggest that the composition of LDL is abnormal, since it is enriched in cholesterol (10). This implies that the cholesterol/apoprotein B ratio is increased in Type 1 diabetic patients compared to non-diabetic subjects.

It is also worth noting that both LDL cholesterol and particularly apoprotein B levels are closely related to the degree of glycemic control (10). Again, the elevation of LDL becomes evident when the glycemic control is suboptimal. In accordance, intensive insulin therapy is followed by a fall in LDL cholesterol and apoprotein B (10, 11). To date the metabolism of LDL in Type 1 diabetes is not well established. In order to assess LDL metabolism more precisely we have recently studied LDL apoprotein B kinetics in Type 1 diabetic patients. Both the LDL apoprotein B transport rate and the fractional catabolic rate (FCR) were normal in patients with fair to good control. However, the FCR of LDL apoprotein B showed an inverse correlation with $HbA_1$ (Taskinen and Kesäniemi, unpublished data). This is consistent with the finding that the binding properties of Type 1 LDL particles improve when hyperglycemia is corrected by insulin therapy (12). Furthermore, there are data to indicate that insulin enhances in vivo LDL catabolism (12).

Several studies have shown that the HDL cholesterol levels in insulin-treated patients are either normal or increased (13). The elevation of HDL cholesterol in Type 1 patients receiving conventional insulin therapy was first documented by Nikkilä and Hormila in 1978 (14). This unexpected finding evoked a major interest in HDL in Type 1 diabetes. Apoprotein AI has been reported to be decreased (15, 16), normal (10) or increased (17), whereas apoprotein AII remains within the normal range. The available data on HDL subfractions are inconsistent but the majority of studies have indicated that $HDL_2$ is relatively further increased than $HDL_3$ (2). We recently reported that in insulin-treated men with fair or good control the concentrations of $HDL_2$ triglyceride, cholesterol and phospholipids are higher than in non-diabetic subjects, whereas the levels of $HDL_3$ cholesterol and phospholipids are reduced (8). Diabetic women tended to have parallel alterations in HDL subfractions to men but the changes were less pronounced. There is also some evidence to indicate that the composition of HDL particles may be abnormal; they are enriched in triglyceride and poor in apoprotein AI (17). Further studies on AI/AII and AI particle distribution are needed to provide information on the physiological relevance of the changes in HDL subfractions.

In insulin-treated diabetic patients both $HDL_2$ cholesterol and $HDL_2$ phospholipids correlate positively with postheparin plasma LPL activity (4). This suggests that in Type 1 diabetic patients on conventional therapy LPL activity is an important determinant of HDL ($HDL_2$) concentration (2, 4). In fact this finding confirmed the original observation of Nikkilä and Hormila (14) on the interrelationship between HDL and postheparin plasma LPL activity in Type 1 diabetes. High LPL activity in chronically insulin-treated diabetic patients would increase the flux of triglyceride-rich particles, and consequently the formation of HDL ($HDL_2$). Since LPL is an insulin-dependent enzyme, it is plausible that peripheral hyperinsulinism in conventionally treated patients induces LPL activity. Indeed, LPL activity is often high in chronically insulin-treated patients (4, 13, 14, 18). However, there is no correlation between LPL activity and either insulin dose or plasma free insulin values (Taskinen et al., unpublished data). Obviously some contradictory factors obscure the picture. Interestingly, it has been recently reported that HDL is inversely related to insulin resistance (19). On the other hand, the impact of glycemic control on HDL levels is not clear. First of all, in the majority of studies there is no correlation between the indices of glycemic control and HDL levels (2, 13). Although short-term intensive insulin therapy has not been reported to increase HDL levels (6), stringent glycemic control achieved and maintained by pump therapy for several months is followed by a definite rise in HDL which is due to elevation of both $HDL_2$ and $HDL_3$ (20–22). This occurs despite the lower dose of insulin on pump therapy than on conventional therapy. It is notable that pump therapy improves insulin sensitivity and this may account for the rise in HDL. Obviously further information is required on the kinetic behaviour of HDL and apoproteins AI and AII in order to understand the changes of HDL in Type 1 diabetes.

## LIPOPROTEIN DISTURBANCES AND ATHEROSCLEROSIS IN TYPE 1 DIABETES

Since the average lipoprotein profile in Type 1 diabetic patients with fair to good glycemic control is not particularly atherogenic, the increment of CHD risk is not easily explained by changes in lipoproteins. This does not necessarily indicate that Type 1 patients with CHD do not have disturbances in lipoprotein metabolism. However, to date there are surprisingly few data on serum lipids and lipoproteins in Type 1 diabetic patients with documented CHD. As noted previously, the two types of diabetes have not been adequately separated in cross-sectional studies addressing the risk factors of CHD in middle-aged diabetic patients, and therefore the available data are primarily confined to Type 2 diabetes. Moreover, Type 1 patients with CHD commonly also have diabetic nephropathy or renal diseases which are associated with an atherogenic lipoprotein profile (2). Finally, to date there are no prospective studies on the predictive values of serum lipoproteins as a risk factor of CHD in Type 1 diabetes.

Recently we examined serum lipids and lipoproteins in a series of Type 1 diabetic patients who had survived myocardial infarction or had a well-documented history of coronary symptoms (Taskinen et al., unpublished data). Serum total and VLDL triglyceride levels were significantly higher in both diabetic men and women with CHD than in those without CHD or in non-diabetic controls without CHD (Table 2). On the other hand, both LDL and HDL cholesterol were similar in diabetic patients with and without CHD. Furthermore, LDL and HDL levels in diabetic patients with CHD did not differ from those observed in non-diabetic CHD-free controls matched for sex, age and relative body weight with the diabetic groups. It is noteworthy that diabetic patients had normal renal function and the degree of glycemic control was comparable in the diabetic groups with and without CHD. In an earlier study on insulin-treated middle-aged diabetic patients LDL and HDL cholesterol were also similar in men with and without CHD (23). Furthermore, in diabetic women the level of LDL cholesterol did not permit the identification of CHD, but HDL cholesterol was lower in diabetic women with CHD than in those without CHD. Again total serum and VLDL triglyceride levels tended to be higher in diabetic patients with CHD than in those without. Laakso et al. (24) have also reported that Type 1 patients of both sexes with CHD have higher total serum and VLDL triglyceride levels than Type 1 patients without CHD. In addition, HDL cholesterol was reduced in Type 1 patients regardless of sex. Moreover, the elevation of LDL cholesterol was a marker for CHD in men but not in women. It should be noted, however, that both LDL and HDL cholesterol levels in Type 1 diabetic women with CHD were not different from those in non-diabetic women without CHD (24). Although the elevation of triglyceride-rich particles seems to be a fairly consistent phenomenon in Type 1 patients with CHD the molecular mechanism through which excess VLDL promotes atherogenesis is not clear. Interestingly, VLDL from Type 1 patients has been reported to stimulate cholesteryl ester synthesis in human macrophages more than normal VLDL and thus promote foam cell formation (25). The predictive value of VLDL triglyceride as a risk factor for CHD in Type 1 diabetes requires, however, prospective long-term studies.

In contrast, the data on HDL and LDL as discriminators of CHD in Type 1 diabetes are not entirely consistent. Obviously the concentrations of LDL and HDL cholesterol do not distinguish CHD as well in Type 1 diabetes as in the non-diabetic population. This may be due to the fact that they are not major risk factors for CHD in Type 1 diabetes. Alternatively, LDL and HDL in Type 1 diabetes may contain structural changes which predispose to atherosclerosis. Preliminary data indicate that HDL particles in Type 1 diabetes show changes in phospholipid composition and triglyceride content which may impair reverse cholesterol transport (26). Non-enzymatic glycosylation of the major apoproteins AI, AII, B and E is known to occur also in vivo and this alters essentially the function of lipoproteins and may render them potentially atherogenic (27).

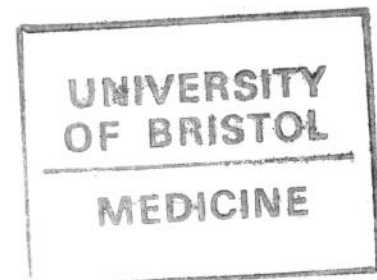

Table 2. Serum lipoproteins in Type 1 diabetics with and without coronary heart disease (CHD)

| | Type 1 diabetic men | | Non-diabetic men | Type 1 diabetic women | | Non-diabetic women |
|---|---|---|---|---|---|---|
| | +CHD ($n$ = 16) | −CHD ($n$ = 18) | −CHD ($n$ = 38) | +CHD ($n$ = 7) | −CHD ($n$ = 11) | −CHD ($n$ = 50) |
| Total triglyceride (mg/dl) | 132 ± 15*** | 107 ± 9 | 113 ± 6 | 158 ± 13*** | 125 ± 19 | 106 ± 4 |
| VLDL triglyceride (mg/dl) | 69.2 ± 11.9* | 53.2 ± 6.5 | 60.0 ± 4.6 | 79.5 ± 11.4** | 57.5 ± 11.6 | 45 ± 3 |
| Total cholesterol (mg/dl) | 227 ± 10 | 218 ± 9 | 223 ± 7 | 241 ± 17* | 213 ± 18 | 233 ± 5 |
| LDL cholesterol (mg/dl) | 163 ± 8 | 152 ± 14 | 164 ± 5 | 165 ± 14 | 143 ± 17 | 164 ± 5* |
| HDL cholesterol (mg/dl) | 51 ± 3 | 54 ± 2 | 49 ± 2 | 53 ± 6 | 54 ± 4 | 57 ± 2 |

The results are means ± SEM.
*$p < 0.05$, **$p < 0.01$, ***$p < 0.001$ for difference from values in diabetics without CHD.

## SERUM LIPOPROTEINS IN TYPE 2 DIABETES

The lipoprotein disturbances in Type 2 diabetes are much more frequent than in Type 1 diabetes. The lipoprotein profile is characterized by the elevation of serum total and VLDL triglyceride, normal LDL cholesterol and by the lowering of HDL cholesterol (2). In terms of epidemiology these changes of lipoprotein pattern are considered to be atherogenic. It is noteworthy that the lipoprotein abnormalities are present at the time of diagnosis of diabetes as well as in cross-sectional studies where the duration of diabetes and the mode of treatment are variable. Since Type 2 diabetes is commonly associated with obesity and genetic hyperlipidemia, it is not easy to separate the impact of diabetes on serum lipoproteins. Moreover, insulin resistance of variable degree is always present in Type 2 diabetes and this can also influence lipoprotein metabolism.

Hypertriglyceridemia is the most common lipoprotein abnormality in Type 2 diabetes. In addition to the elevation of VLDL concentrations there are also structural changes in VLDL particles which are enriched in triglyceride but poor in apoprotein B (2). This means that the particle size is increased. It is well established that VLDL production is generally increased in Type 2 diabetes (19). This is particularly clear in patients with co-existing hyperlipidemia and/or obesity. However, there are multiple disturbances of VLDL metabolism in Type 2 diabetes (28). Firstly, the overproduction of VLDL triglyceride seems to be more marked than that of VLDL apoprotein B and this may explain the altered particle structure (28). Furthermore, the triglyceride-rich VLDL is less readily converted to LDL than normal VLDL (29). Consequently the direct removal of VLDL apoprotein B is increased and this may be potentially an atherogenic event (29).

The possible contribution of defective VLDL removal to the elevation of serum triglyceride in Type 2 diabetes is less clear. There is a subgroup of hyperlipidemic Type 2 patients who have decreased fractional catabolic rate of VLDL and this abnormality is explicable by a concomitant reduction in LPL activity (2, 19). Similarly in untreated Type 2 diabetic patients the LPL activity in adipose tissue and in postheparin plasma is often subnormal in comparison to weight-matched controls (4). This finding is consistent with the decreased clearance of VLDL observed in some but not all studies (19). Pima Indians represent a unique group where low LPL activity and concomitantly decreased removal of VLDL exist even in normolipidemic or mild hyperlipidemic Type 2 diabetic subjects (19). In conclusion, subnormal LPL activity may become critical when the overproduction of VLDL is persistent and consequently the compensatory capacity of the removal system is exceeded.

Successful correction of hyperglycemia with caloric restriction, oral agents or insulin therapy lowers VLDL triglyceride levels by decreasing VLDL production and by enhancing VLDL removal (2). The fact that the response is similar regardless of the mode of therapy suggests that the reversal of diabetic metabolism is of primary importance. The overproduction of VLDL has been linked to hyperinsulinism in Type 2 diabetes (2, 19). The fall of VLDL production during insulin therapy is not compatible with this concept. The correction of hyperglycemia is associated with changes in free fatty acid metabolism and insulin resistance which may contribute to the lowering of VLDL production. The elevation of VLDL triglyceride levels in Type 2 patients treated by oral agents probably indicates that the average diabetic control is not stringent enough to normalize VLDL metabolism.

In the majority of studies the concentration of LDL cholesterol is virtually similar in Type 2 diabetic patients and in matched control groups. Futhermore, the level of LDL cholesterol is not related to the mode of therapy or to the degree of glycemic control (30). In contrast, the average concentration of LDL triglyceride is increased (2, 19). This can be partly attributed to the inclusion of IDL in the LDL fraction due to inadequate separation techniques, but a true rise of LDL triglyceride occurs at least in Type 2 patients with poor control (Taskinen et al., unpublished data). Despite minimal changes in LDL concentration there are several abnormalities in LDL metabolism. In Type 2 patients with moderate to severe hyperglycemia the catabolism of LDL is impaired (29, 31). This may reflect the altered LDL composition and be accounted for by decreased binding of LDL to receptors. Furthermore, the glycosylation of LDL protein may impair the catabolism by the LDL receptor pathway. However, the physiological relevance of apoprotein B glycosylation to the metabolism of LDL requires kinetic studies with LDL from patients with good and poor glycemic control and the estimation of glycosylation levels. The catabolic defect in LDL metabolism is not compatible with the finding that LDL cholesterol levels are generally normal. The observation that the direct removal of VLDL is increased in Type 2 diabetes provides a logical explanation for this controversy (29).

Low HDL cholesterol is as common a finding in Type 2 diabetes as is the elevation of serum triglyceride levels. The fall of HDL is attributed to that of the $HDL_2$ level, whereas the concentration of $HDL_3$ is comparable to that in respective control groups (30). It should be noted that there is a similar inverse correlation between HDL cholesterol and VLDL triglyceride in Type 2 diabetes and in non-diabetic subjects. In Type 2 diabetes, HDL particles also show structural alterations, since they are enriched in triglyceride but poor in apoprotein AI (2, 19). There is also an increase in HDL cholesteryl esters, whereas VLDL and LDL are enriched in free cholesterol. These changes indicate a defect of the cholesteryl ester transfer system (32). It is of particular interest that the reduction of HDL is apparent in untreated patients as well as in diabetic patients treated with diet, oral agents or with conventional insulin therapy. In addition the concentration of HDL is not closely dependent on glycemic control even though low HDL is a consistent finding in patients with poor glycemic control (2). The basic mechanism behind the lowering of HDL in Type 2 diabetes is not clear. Subnormal LPL activity and high hepatic lipase activity, commonly present in Type 2 diabetes, may contribute to the reduction of HDL (4, 13). Interestingly, the concentration of HDL cholesterol is not influenced by intensified insulin therapy which results in near normal glycemic control (33). Nevertheless, intensive insulin therapy induces marked changes in the distribution of HDL subfractions; $HDL_2$ increases but $HDL_3$ decreases concomitantly with an induction of adipose tissue LPL acitivity (Taskinen et al., unpublished data). It is worth noting that insulin therapy is followed only by a minor increase in apoprotein AI and this may explain why the total concentration of HDL remains unchanged (Taskinen et al. unpublished data). The data suggest that other metabolic factors, in addition to hyperglycemia and ambient insulin levels, influence HDL metabolism in Type 2 diabetes.

The characteristics of the lipoprotein profile in Type 2 diabetes, notably low HDL and increased VLDL levels, are considered to be atherogenic. In accordance with this fact epidemiological data suggest that low HDL values are indeed associated with CHD in Type 2 patients (1). Furthermore, Laakso et al. (34) have shown that Type 2 patients with CHD have significantly lower HDL and $HDL_2$ cholesterol levels than diabetic patients without CHD. This indicates that the low HDL in Type 2 diabetes is further reduced by the presence of CHD. The inverse relation between HDL concentration and CHD was apparent in both sexes and it was independent of age, smoking, obesity, duration of diabetes, as well as of the degree of glycemic control. However, prospective studies are required to verify that low HDL and $HDL_2$ cholesterol levels are also predictors of CHD in Type 2 diabetes. Similarly, the relevance of increased VLDL levels to atherogenesis remains to be established by prospective studies.

## REFERENCES

1. Pyörälä K, Laakso M, Uusitupa M (1987) Diabetes and atherosclerosis: an epidemiologic view. Diabetes/Metab Rev (in press)
2. Nikkilä EA (1984) Plasma lipid and lipoprotein abnormalities in diabetes. In: Jarrett (ed) Diabetes and heart disease. Elsevier Science Publishers, Amsterdam, pp 133–167
3. Taskinen M-R, Nikkilä EA (1979) Lipoprotein lipase activity of adipose tissue and skeletal muscle in insulin-deficient human diabetes. Relation to high-density and very-low-density lipoproteins and response to treatment. Diabetologia 17: 351–356
4. Taskinen M-R (1987) Lipoprotein lipase in diabetes. Diabetes/Metab Rev (in press)
5. Walden CE, Knopp RH, Wahl PW, Beach KW, Strandness E (1984) Sex differences in the effect of diabetes mellitus on lipoprotein triglyceride and cholesterol concentration. N Engl J Med 311: 953–959
6. Pietri AO, Dunn FL, Grundy SM, Raskin P (1983) The effect of continuous subcutaneous insulin infusion on very-low-density lipoprotein triglyceride metabolism in type 1 diabetes mellitus. Diabetes 32: 75–81
7. Vlachokosta FV, Asmal AC, Ganda OP, Aoki TT (1983) The effect of strict control with the artificial $\beta$-cell on plasma lipid levels in insulin-dependent diabetes. Diabetes Care 6: 351–355
8. Taskinen M-R, Kuusi T, Nikkilä EA (1985) Regulation of HDL and its subfractions in chronically insulin treated patients with type 1 diabetes. In: Crepaldi G et al. (eds) Diabetes, obesity and hyperlipidemias. Elsevier Science Publishers, Amsterdam, pp 251–259
9. Winocour PH, Durrington PN, Ishola M, Anderson DC (1986) Lipoprotein abnormalities in insulin-dependent diabetes mellitus. Lancet i: 1176–1178
10. Gonen B, White N, Schonfeld G, Skor D, Miller P, Santiago J (1985) Plasma levels of apoprotein B in patients with diabetes mellitus: the effect of glycemic control. Metabolism 34: 675–679

11. Lopes-Virella MF, Wohltmann HJ, Mayfield RK, Loadholt CB, Colwell JA (1983) Effect of metabolic control on lipid, lipoprotein, and apolipoprotein levels in 55 insulin-dependent diabetic patients. A longitudinal study. Diabetes 32: 20–25
12. Brunzell JD, Chait A, Bierman EL (1985) Plasma lipoproteins in human diabetes mellitus. In: Alberti KGMM, Krall LP (eds) The diabetes annual. Elsevier Science Publishers, Amsterdam, pp 463–479
13. Nikkilä EA (1981) High density lipoproteins in diabetes. Diabetes 30: 82–87
14. Nikkilä EA, Hormila P (1978) Serum lipids and lipoproteins in insulin-treated diabetes. Demonstration of increased high density lipoprotein concentrations. Diabetes 27: 1078–1086
15. Schernthaner G, Kostner GM, Kieplinger H, Prager R, Mühlhauser I (1983) Apolipoproteins (A-I, A-II, B), Lp(a) lipoprotein and lecithin : cholesterol acyltransferase activity in diabetes mellitus. Atherosclerosis 49: 277–293
16. Briones ER, Mao SJT, Palumbo PJ, O'Fallon WM, Chenoweth W, Kottke BA (1984) Analysis of plasma lipids and apolipoproteins in insulin-dependent and non-insulin-dependent diabetics. Metabolism 33: 42–49
17. Eckel RH, Albers JJ, Cheung MC, Wahl PW, Lindgren FT, Bierman EL (1981) High density lipoprotein composition in insulin-dependent diabetes mellitus. Diabetes 30: 132–138
18. Agardh C-D, Santor G, Nilsson-Ehle P (1983) Plasma high density lipoproteins and lipolytic enzyme activities in diabetic patients. Acta Med Scand 213: 123–128
19. Howard BV (1987) Lipoprotein metabolism in diabetes mellitus. J Lipid Res (in press)
20. Dunn FL, Pietri A, Raskin P (1981) Plasma lipid and lipoprotein levels with continuous subcutaneous insulin infusion in type 1 diabetes mellitus. Ann Intern Med 95: 426–431
21. Falko JM, O'Dorisio TM, Cataland S (1982) Improvement of high-density lipoprotein-cholesterol levels. J Am Med Assoc 247: 37–39
22. Nikkilä EA, Helve E (1986) Antiatherogenic changes in lipoprotein induced by continous insulin infusion (CSII) therapy. Diabetologia 29: 576A
23. Hormila P (1985) Ischemic heart disease and its risk factors in insulin-dependent diabetes. Academic dissertation, University of Helsinki
24. Laakso M, Pyörälä K, Sarlund H, Voutilainen E (1986) Lipid and lipoprotein abnormalities associated with coronary heart disease in patients with insulin-dependent diabetes mellitus. Arteriosclerosis 6: 679–684
25. Lyons TJ, Klein RL, Baynes J, Lopes-Virella MF (1986) VLDL and LDL from diabetic patients stimulate increased cholesteryl ester (CE) synthesis in human monocyte derived macrophages. Diabetes 35 (Suppl 1): 67A
26. Bagdade JD, Subbaiah PV (1986) Atherosclerosis in the type 1 diabetic female: does her HDL protect or predispose? Diabetes 35 (Suppl 1): 67A
27. Curtiss LK, Witztum JL (1985) Plasma apolipoproteins AI, AII, B, CI and E are glucosylated in hyperglycemic diabetic subjects. Diabetes 34: 454–461
28. Taskinen M-R, Beltz WF, Harper I, Fields RM, Schonfeld G, Grundy SM, Howard BV (1986) Effects of NIDDM on very-low-density lipoprotein triglyceride and apolipoprotein B metabolism. Studies before and after sulfonylurea therapy. Diabetes 35: 1268–1277
29. Howard BV, Abbott WGH, Beltz WF, Harper I,Fields RM, Grundy SM, Taskinen M-R (1987) Integrated study of low density lipoprotein metabolism and very low density lipoprotein metabolism in non insulin dependent diabetes. Metabolism (in press)
30. Laakso M, Voutilainen E, Sarlund H, Aro A, Pyörälä K, Penttilä I (1985) Serum lipids and lipoproteins in middle-aged non-insulin-dependent diabetics. Atherosclerosis 56: 271–281
31. Kissebah AH, Alfarsi S, Evans DJ, Adams PW (1983) Plasma low density lipoprotein

transport kinetics in non-insulin-dependent diabetes mellitus. J Clin Invest 71: 655–667

32. Fielding CJ, Reaven GM, Liu G, Fielding PE (1984) Increased free cholesterol in plasma low and very low density lipoproteins in non-insulin-dependent diabetes mellitus: Its role in the inhibition of cholesteryl ester transfer. Proc Natl Acad Sci USA 81: 2512–2516
33. Hollenbeck CB, Ida Chen Y-D, Greenfield MS, Lardinois CK, Reaven GM (1986) Reduced plasma high density lipoprotein-cholesterol concentrations need not increase when hyperglycemia is controlled with insulin in non–insulin-dependent diabetes mellitus. J Clin Endocrinol Metab 62: 605–608
34. Laako M, Voutilainen E, Pyörälä K, Sarlund H (1985) Association of low HDL and $HDL_2$ cholesterol with coronary heart disease in non-insulin-dependent diabetics. Arteriosclerosis 5: 653–658

Diabetic Complications: Early Diagnosis and Treatment
Edited by D. Andreani, G. Crepaldi, U. Di Mario and G. Pozza


# CHAPTER 4

# *Diabetic Cardiopathy*

R. Nosadini, C. Vigorito* and G. Crepaldi
*Istituto di Medicina Interna, University of Padua; *Istituto di Medicina Interna, University of Naples, Italy*

Since the discovery of insulin, cardiac diseases have replaced the metabolic coma as the main cause of death in insulin-dependent diabetes mellitus (IDDM) (1). The traditional view was that diabetic heart disease was simply the result of accelerated atherosclerosis in the coronary arteries. In fact large epidemiological studies demonstrated that atherosclerotic changes are found more frequently among diabetic than non-diabetic subjects (1). On the other hand, some years ago the results of the Framingham study showed that diabetes and heart disease were associated in a large number of patients even if there was no clinical evidence of ischemia or coronary atherosclerotic structural changes (2). These findings were summarized by W. Kannel as follows: 'Diabetes promotes coronary disease in some unique fashion outside the usual atherogenic mechanism of hyperlipidemia and hypertension' (2).

More recently Ledet et al. (3) hypothesized the existence of a cardiac disease peculiar to diabetes as a result and combination of microangiopathy, macroangiopathy, neuropathy and metabolic dysfunction; they suggested the term 'diabetic cardiopathy' rather than 'diabetic cardiomyopathy' which gives the idea only of non-vascular heart disease.

In the last few years new information on heart function in diabetes mellitus has been provided by clinical studies using non-invasive techniques, by histological studies of hearts from old and young subjects, and by research into the autonomic nervous system. The purpose of this brief report is to review the relations of myocardial function to the clinical features of diabetes irrespective of the presence of coronary artery disease.

## CARDIAC DYSFUNCTION IN DIABETES MELLITUS WITHOUT CLINICAL EVIDENCE OF ISCHEMIA

Non-invasive studies using systolic time intervals and echocardiography have investigated the relationship between glucose metabolism and myocardial contractility in diabetes. More particularly, the ratio between the pre-ejection period (PEP) and the left ventricular ejection time (LVET) has been used by Shapiro et al. (4) to find evidence of incipient congestive heart failure in a large population of Type 1 diabetic patients without clinical symptoms of impaired coronary blood flow. In this group of patients the ratio PEP/LVET was significantly increased compared to that of normal subjects, but it fell to within the normal range of values after 2–4 months of therapy achieving a significant decrease in blood glucose concentrations. These findings in maturity-onset diabetes were confirmed by Friedman et al. (5) in Type 1 insulin-dependent diabetic patients in whom a significant correlation was shown between the PEP/LVET ratio and glycosylated hemoglobin patterns. Although these clinical studies did not investigate directly the patency of coronary arteries, they provide strong evidence to support the hypothesis that the degree of metabolic control influences the function of the myocardial cells in diabetes mellitus. From a clinical point of view it is well-known that the acute metabolic status of diabetic patients admitted with myocardial infarction influences the short- and long-term prognosis since congestive heart failure is more frequent in those patients with high blood glucose concentrations (2). In most of the reports in the literature on this topic the mortality after infarction in diabetic patients shows a two-fold increase. Elevated blood glucose levels are frequently associated with myocardial infarction of a large area and usually it is suggested that hyperglycemia at admittance most probably indicates the pre-existence of diabetes mellitus. On the other hand, the incidence of cardiogenic shock and the mortality rate are also related to the patterns of blood glucose and glycosylated hemoglobin Alc showed by the patient when admitted to the intensive care coronary unit. Thus several epidemiological, clinical and prospective studies tend to support the conclusion that the main clinical cardiac complication in diabetes, with or without myocardial infarction, consists of decreased contractility of the left ventricle (6).

Autonomic neuropathy is also frequently found in diabetes and it may account for the possibility of sudden unexpected death, above all after general anesthesia (7).

An abnormally long QT interval has also been found by several authors in diabetic subjects. The pathogenesis of this electrocardiographic abnormality needs further investigation, but it is well known that a prolonged QT interval may account for an increased frequency of ventricular arrhythmias (6) and indicates the presence of abnormal myocardial depolarization. Both parasympathetic and sympathetic autonomic reflex pathways can be seriously impaired in insulin-dependent diabetes (7). A constant impaired capacity of heart muscle to adjust heart ejection fraction to changes in heart volume, secondary to standing up, deep breathing and sustained hand-grip, thereby speeding-up or decreasing the heart rate, accounts for the proneness of diabetic subjects to cardiac failure. Namely, since cardiac denervation does not allow changes in heart rate, the only mechanism of accommodation which these subjects can utilize to increase left ventricular output is a prolongation of diastolic release to allow a greater blood left ventricular filling according to Starling's curve, which in turn results in cardiac hypertrophy.

An increased incidence of atrioventricular and intraventricular conduction disturbances complicating myocardial infarcts has been also reported in diabetic patients (6).

Generalized thickening and proliferation of the capillary basement membranes is found in diabetes (8) and capillary microaneurysms in the heart have been described (9). The microvascular abnormalities are, however, not pathognomonic for diabetes mellitus and could be related to other structural lesions, such as diffuse interstitial fibrosis. Ledet et al. (3) described three types of connective tissue accumulation: interstitial, perivascular and focal scar-like accumulations. All three types seem to occur more commonly and more extensively in the hearts of young diabetic patients (3). In old diabetic patients Ledet found an increased amount of fat and calcium in the extramural coronary arteries than in a non-diabetic control group (3). An increased fibrosis of heart tissue at several levels (myocell, capillaries and arteries) could theoretically account for both an impaired contractility of the myocardium and a major proneness towards electrocardiographic abnormalities.

Necroscopy and biopsy studies indicate that diabetic patients frequently have abnormalities of coronary microcirculation and myocardium: endothelial proliferation, perivascular fibrosis, glycoprotein deposition and interstitial myocardial fibrosis can be extensive and are independent of coronary atherosclerosis and also of systemic hypertension (4, 6). Capillary microaneurysms have been found in silicone rubber injected preparations of diabetic myocardium, suggesting that the vascular abnormalities are similar to those in the retina.

## A METABOLIC BASIS FOR CARDIAC DYSFUNCTION IN DIABETES

A metabolic basis for heart failure in diabetes has been recently hypothesized by Teagtmeyer and Passmore (10). Diabetic subjects with poor metabolic control often show elevated circulating free fatty acid (FFA) and ketone body concentrations. However, ketone bodies, though readily oxidized, do not sustain the full work-load of the heart. With glucose as substrate, acetyl-CoA is utilized as fast as it is produced from pyruvate in the perfused isolated heart and rapid flux through the tricarboxylic acid cycle prevents the accumulation of metabolites. With ketone bodies as substrate, there is an accumulation of acetyl-CoA, citrate, 2-oxoglutarate and glutamate due to an impaired flux of tricarboxylic acid in the Krebs cycle. Impaired activity of the Krebs cycle could account for a lower availability of ATP in the hearts of diabetic subjects with poor metabolic control. The accumulation of acetyl-CoA leads to inhibition of pyruvate dehydrogenase and the accumulation of citrate leads to inhibition of phosphofructokinase. The net result of these metabolic abnormalities is an increased intracellular content of triglycerides, FFA, and glycogen.

In the attempt to investigate the role of metabolic abnormalities in the development of IDDM heart disease, we measured the arterial–venous differences of carbohydrate, lipid and amino acid intermediary metabolites in a group of diabetic and non-diabetic subjects. Two groups of normal and insulin-dependent Type 1 subjects underwent diagnostic catheterization for evaluation of cardiac function because of valvular heart or coronary artery disease. The severity of heart failure was quantitated according to the criteria of the New York Heart Association and all subjects were class I or II patients. The two groups were well matched for sex, age, weight and height. The diabetic subjects were Type 1 insulin-dependent, C peptide free patients. Insulin therapy was abruptly withdrawn 12 hours before the metabolic study. Three blood samples were drawn simultaneously from the aorta and the coronary sinus using a catheter devised also to allow the measurement of coronary blood flow in order to determine plasma glucose, plasma FFA, and blood acetoacetate, 3-hydroxybutyrate and lactate concentrations. Further details have been given elsewhere (11). The net balance of the substrate in the heart tissue was calculated using the product of arterial−venous differences of each individual metabolite by coronary sinus blood flow. The production and utilization rate of lactate and ketone bodies was calculated on the basis of arterial−venous differences of tracer and tracee during a priming constant infusion of [$^{14}$C] lactate and D-[$^{3}$H]-3-hydroxybutyrate.

Plasma glucose concentrations after an overnight fast were 5.11 ± 0.20 (mmol/l (mean ± SEM) in non-diabetic subjects and 18.06 ± 1.22 ($p<0.01$) in diabetic patients. Blood concentrations of ketone bodies were 0.360 ± 0.054 (mmol/l in non-diabetic subjects and 2.733 ± 0.150 ($p<0.01$) in diabetic patients.

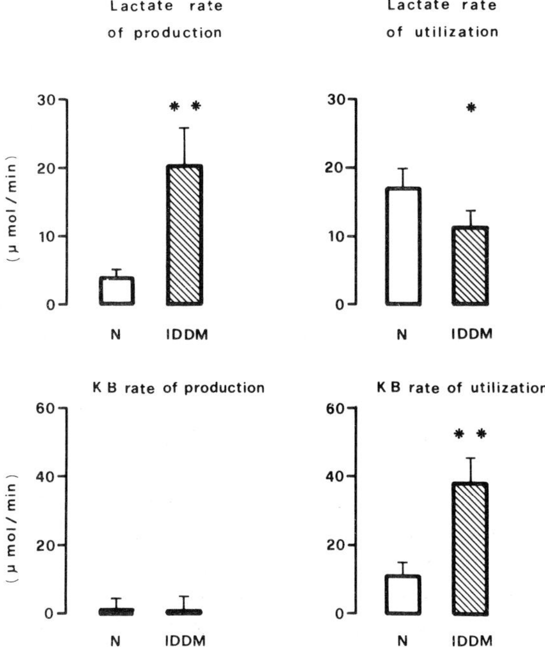


Figure 1. Rate of production and utilization of lactate and ketone bodies (KB) in control (N) and diabetic (IDDM) subjects (white and dashed columns respectively). *$p<0.01$ (mean ± SEM).

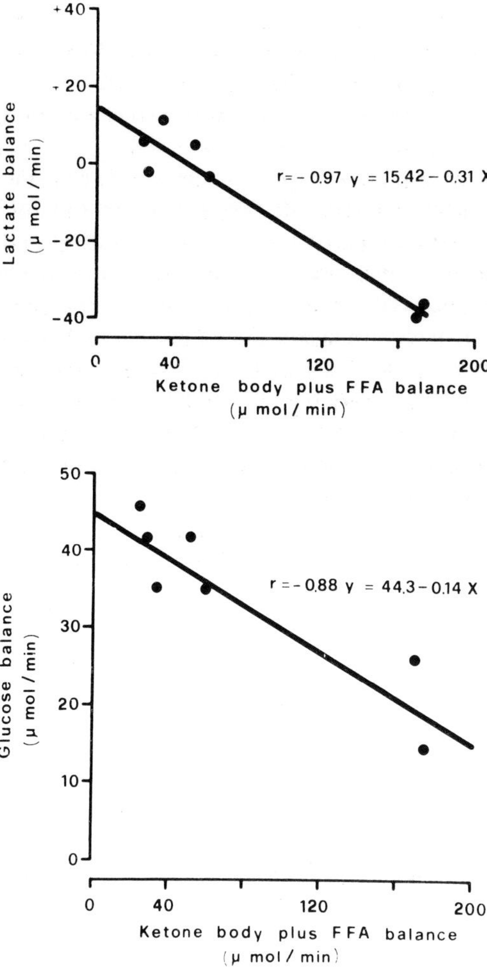


Figure 2. Correlation between lactate and glucose net balance across myocardium and that of ketone body plus FFA in IDDM subjects.

In IDDM patients despite hyperglycemia myocardial glucose uptake was slightly reduced. The kinetics of lactate and ketone bodies across myocardium in non-diabetic and diabetic (IDDM) subjects are shown in Figure 1. Lactate was simultaneously produced and taken up by the myocardium in control subjects and in diabetic patients. However, in the control group lactate uptake exceeded its production, whereas in diabetic patients lactate production was the predominant process. Consequently, the myocardial lactate balance was a net uptake in the control subjects (12.7 ± 2.7 μmol/min) and a net production in diabetic patients (7.9 ± 2.1 μmol/min, $p<0.01$). Myocardial uptake of ketone bodies was significantly higher in diabetic patients than in control subjects (39 ± 6 μmol/min vs 11 ± 3 μmol/min, $p < 0.01$). Thus, a greater utilization of ketone and a reduction of lactate uptake does occur in the diabetic heart in spite of intact coronary arteries. The net balance of glucose and lactate across the myocardium was significantly and inversely related to ketone body plus FFA balance in IDDM patients (Figure 2).

These data are compatible with the hypothesis of a metabolic basis for the cardiac dysfunction in diabetes, suggesting that an excessive delivery of lipid substrates to the heart can impair the carbohydrate utilization rate in the Krebs cycle of IDDM patients, possibly leading to a reduced ATP production. Moreover, lactate release at rest cannot be considered an index of myocardial ischemia in insulin-deficient subjects at variance with normal subjects, since the impaired lactate metabolism is related to a purely metabolic abnormality rather than to an impaired oxygen supply. From a more general point of view these findings suggest that strict metabolic control could be important in IDDM subjects not only to achieve satisfactory normal glucose and lipid patterns, but also to obtain a normal left ventricular pump capacity.

## REFERENCES

1. Marks HH, Krall LP (1971) Onset, course prognosis and mortality in diabetes mellitus. In: Marble A, White P, Bradley RF, Krall LP (eds) Joslin's Diabetes Mellitus. Lea & Febiger, Philadelphia, pp 209–254
2. Kannel WB, Hjortland M, Castelli WP (1974) Role of diabetes in congestive heart failure: The Framingham Study. Am J Cardiol 34: 29–34
3. Ledet T, Neubauer B, Christensen NJ, Lundbaek K (1979) Diabetic cardiopathy. Diabetologia 16: 207–209
4. Shapiro LM, Leatherdale BA, Mackinnon J, Fletcher RF (1981) Left ventricular function in diabetes mellitus. II. Relation between clinical features and left ventricular function. Br Heart J 45: 129–132
5. Friedman HS, Sacerdote A, Baudu I, Jubay F, Herrera A, Vasavava B, Bleicher S (1984) Abnormalities of the cardiovascular response to cold pressor test in type 1 diabetes. Correlation with blood glucose control Arch Intern Med 144: 43–47
6. Gotzsche O (1986) Myocardial cell dysfunction in diabetes mellitus: a review of clinical and experimental studies. Diabetes 35: 1158–1162
7. Ewing D, Clarke B (1986) Autonomic neuropathy: its diagnosis and prognosis. Clin Endocrinol Metab 15: 855–888
8. Williamson JR, Kilo C (1976) Basement membrane thickening and diabetic microangiopathy. Diabetes 25: 925–927
9. Factor SM, Okum EM, Minase T (1980) Capillary microaneurysms in the human diabetic heart. N Engl J Med 302: 384–388
10. Teagtmeyer H, Passmore J (1985) Defective energy metabolism of the heart in diabetes. Lancet i: 139–141
11. Nosadini R, Avogaro A, Saccà L, Vigorito C, De Kreutzenberg S, Cobelli C, Toffolo G, Trevisan R, Tessari P, Tiengo A, Crepaldi G (1985) Ketone body metabolism in normal and diabetic human skeletal muscle. Am J Physiol 249: E131–E136

Diabetic Complications: Early Diagnosis and Treatment
Edited by D. Andreani, G. Crepaldi, U. Di Mario and G. Pozza


CHAPTER 5

# *Hypertension and Diabetes: A Poorly Understood Relationship*

K. Pyörälä, M. Uusitupa and M. Laakso
*Department of Medicine, University of Kuopio, Finland*

Several studies have shown that the prevalence of hypertension is higher in diabetic patients than in non-diabetic subjects. In population-based prospective studies the relationship of hypertension to cardiovascular morbidity and mortality has been shown to be similar in both diabetic and non-diabetic subjects, but, because of the independent effect of diabetes on cardiovascular risk, at every level of blood pressure cardiovascular morbidity and mortality are higher in diabetic patients than in non-diabetic subjects (1–3). Because of the increased prevalence of hypertension in diabetic patients, the excess morbidity and mortality attributable to hypertension are greater in the diabetic population than among non-diabetic subjects. In addition to its impact on the excessive occurrence of atherosclerotic vascular disease in diabetic subjects, hypertension is an important cause of left ventricular failure in diabetic subjects and it promotes the progress of diabetic nephropathy. Furthermore, there is also evidence which indicates that the incidence of diabetic retinopathy is higher in diabetic subjects with elevated blood pressure than in normotensive diabetic subjects (4).

Although a large body of information exists on the occurrence of hypertension in diabetes, the underlying mechanisms remain so far poorly understood. This review deals with the following aspects of hypertension in diabetes:

1. Blood pressure level and the prevalence of hypertension.
2. Factors associated with the increased occurrence of hypertension in diabetes.

## BLOOD PRESSURE LEVEL AND THE PREVALENCE OF HYPERTENSION

### Insulin-Dependent Diabetes

Only a few studies are available on blood pressure levels or the prevalence of hypertension in patients with insulin-dependent diabetes (IDDM) as compared to non-diabetic control subjects. Moss (5) reported elevated systolic blood pressure levels in both diabetic boys and girls after the age of 13 years and speculated that this increase was due to subclinical renal disease. The correlation between actual blood pressure levels and the duration of diabetes, however, remained low. Karlefors (6) studied blood pressure levels at rest and during bicycle ergometer tests in 84 diabetic and 76 non-diabetic men aged 17–44 years. The diabetic subjects were grouped according to the duration of the disease and the degree of retinopathy. There were no differences in blood pressure levels between control subjects and diabetic patients with 0–4 years' duration of the disease. Diabetic subjects with 5–14 years' duration of the disease tended to show higher blood pressure levels during exercise than control subjects, while diabetic subjects with a duration of the disease of 15 or more years had higher blood pressure even at rest than control subjects. Diabetic subjects with advanced degrees of retinopathy showed elevated blood pressure levels even at rest and marked rises of blood pressure during exercise, indicating an association between hypertension and diabetic microangiopathy in these patients, most of whom had IDDM. Studies by Christlieb et al. (7) on cohorts of diabetic patients treated at the Joslin Clinic showed that in both sexes, at any age after 24 years, the prevalence of hypertension was higher in patients with IDDM than in the general population, using the Framingham Study population or the population of the US Survey of Hypertension as a reference. Only in the age group 25–34 years did the duration of diabetes increase the risk of hypertension. In the Finnish Social Insurance Institution's Study (8) the prevalence of hypertension, at any age after 19 years, was higher in diabetic than in non-diabetic subjects. The excess of hypertension among diabetic subjects was particularly marked in those under the age of 40 years, most of whom had IDDM.

In studies performed at the Joslin Clinic, patients with juvenile-onset IDDM who later died from renal failure usually developed both hypertension and proteinuria approximately at the same time between the age of 20 and 30 years, thus indicating that hypertension is of renal origin in these cases (7). Recent studies indicate, however, that blood pressure levels may be elevated in patients with IDDM even before the onset of clinical proteinuria. Microalbuminuria (urinary albumin excretion rate 30–200 $\mu$g/min), which is a characteristic finding in early diabetic nephropathy, may be associated with an increase in blood pressure in young adult patients with IDDM (9–11).

Three recent studies have dealt with blood pressure levels in young subjects with IDDM and in control groups. Cruickshanks et al. (12) reported higher systolic and diastolic blood pressure levels in 149 diabetic patients, aged 9–16, compared to 45 unaffected siblings; Kaas-Ibsen et al. (13), on the other hand, could not find any difference in systolic blood pressure levels between diabetic and non-diabetic girls, whereas the diastolic blood pressure level tended to be even lower in diabetic girls. Tarn and Drury (14) examined blood pressure levels in 97 male and 66 female patients with IDDM, aged 4–32 years, and in 137 male and 95 female non-diabetic siblings. There were no significant differences in systolic blood pressure levels between diabetic and non-diabetic siblings of either sex, but phase IV diastolic blood pressure was significantly higher in male diabetic subjects. The mean difference in diastolic blood pressure between male diabetic and non-diabetic subjects was 2.8 mmHg. Altogether 19% of male patients with IDDM had 'relative hypertension' (mean blood pressure above the 90th percentile for age, derived from values of siblings for each sex separately) compared to 9% of non-diabetic siblings. For females the respective figures were 14% and 13%. Age did not account for the rise in diastolic blood pressure in male diabetic subjects; nor was it solely explained by early diabetic nephropathy. The duration of diabetes showed no significant effect on blood pressure in either sex.

### Non-Insulin-Dependent Diabetes

Several studies on representative groups of middle-aged diabetic subjects, most of them evidently affected by non-insulin-dependent diabetes (NIDDM), and comparable groups of non-diabetic subjects have shown either higher mean values for systolic or diastolic blood pressure or a higher prevalence of hypertension in the diabetic group compared to non-diabetic subjects (8, 15–22). In the Bedford Survey and the Whitehall Study, subjects with newly diagnosed diabetes and subjects with impaired glucose tolerance had significantly higher systolic and diastolic blood pressure levels in comparison to normoglycemic subjects, but in the Whitehall Study, however, the mean values for systolic and diastolic blood pressure in subjects with previously known diabetes were similar to those observed in normoglycemic subjects (23). Similarly, in the Israel Ischemic Heart Disease Study, men with newly diagnosed diabetes revealed elevated mean values of systolic blood pressure, whereas subjects with previously diagnosed diabetes had similar blood pressure levels to normoglycemic subjects (24). On the other hand, in our own studies on newly diagnosed and previously known middle-aged diabetic subjects of both sexes with NIDDM and on comparable non-diabetic subjects, the prevalence of hypertension was equally increased in both newly diagnosed and known diabetic subjects and was 1.5–2 times higher than in non-diabetic control subjects (25, 26). Recently we re-examined diabetic subjects with newly diagnosed NIDDM and non-diabetic control subjects 5 years after the first examination and observed that the incidence of hypertension was about 1.5 times higher in diabetic than in non-diabetic subjects (27).

Several population-based studies on normoglycemic subjects and on subjects with various degrees of glucose intolerance have shown a positive correlation between fasting or post-load blood glucose and blood pressure levels (21–23, 28, 29). Obesity and age do not entirely explain this association. Several studies have shown that the prevalence of hypertension is higher in subjects with impaired glucose tolerance than in normoglycemic subjects (22, 30–33).

## FACTORS ASSOCIATED WITH THE INCREASED OCCURRENCE OF HYPERTENSION IN DIABETES

Diabetic nephropathy is the main cause of elevated blood pressure in IDDM, whereas essential hypertension is the most common type of hypertension in subjects with

NIDDM. In the following section the factors underlying the susceptibility to an elevation of blood pressure in diabetes will be discussed.

### Diabetic Nephropathy

As mentioned earlier, blood pressure in patients with IDDM may rise at an early stage of diabetic nephropathy characterized by microalbuminuria (9–11). Yet young patients with IDDM may have higher diastolic blood pressure levels even without evidence of renal damage, and thus other mechanisms may be involved in the rise of blood pressure in IDDM (14). Likewise, although diabetic nephropathy may account for elevated blood pressure in some patients with NIDDM, other factors play a major role in the pathogenesis of hypertension in these patients.

### Sodium Metabolism

Several recent studies indicate that body exchangeable sodium may be increased in diabetic subjects irrespective of age or the presence of diabetic nephropathy or retinopathy. Furthermore, in diabetic subjects with hypertension or diabetic nephropathy a positive correlation occurs between blood pressure level and the total exchangeable sodium (34, 35). Weidmann et al. (34) have reviewed the mechanisms which may result in sodium retention in diabetes. Most of these mechanisms are still hypothetical or are associated with diabetic nephropathy. The following factors may cause a shift of sodium and water from the intravascular to the extravascular space; hypoalbuminemia, an increase in microvascular permeability, and changes in the collagen composition which enhances the avidity of tissues for sodium. Insulin resistance or hyperinsulinemia may lead to intracellular sodium retention. Among the renal factors which may contribute to sodium retention are renal insufficiency per se, hypovolemia due to the shift of sodium and water from the intravascular to the extravascular space, renal vasculopathy, and the lack of renal vasodilator prostaglandins or kinins.

According to recent studies, circulating plasma volume appears to be normal or even decreased in hypertensive patients with IDDM or NIDDM (34, 35).

### Catecholamines

Catecholamines may be involved in the elevation of blood pressure. There are no consistent differences in epinephrine or norepinephrine concentrations between adequately treated diabetic patients and normal subjects (34, 36, 37). However, it has been shown that the pressor effect of norepinephrine may be exaggerated in both types of diabetes regardless of age, type of treatment, or the presence or absence of diabetic microvascular complications, neuropathy or high blood pressure (34).

### The Renin–Angiotensin–Aldosterone System

Plasma renin activity has been reported to be normal or low in patients with diabetic nephropathy, whereas it is usually normal in diabetes without complications (34, 37), even though there are also reports on elevated renin activity in diabetic subjects without complications (38) and in patients with proliferative retinopathy (39). It should be emphasized, however, that renin activity is dependent on many factors, including blood pressure and serum sodium concentration. The differences between these may explain, at least in part, the divergent results concerning renin activity. Serum aldosterone and angiotensin levels are generally within the normal range in metabolically stable diabetic patients (34), but patients with IDDM may have an increased vasopressor responsiveness to angiotensin II (40).

### Blood Glucose

As mentioned previously, there is a positive relationship between blood glucose and blood pressure levels in non-diabetic subjects. In diabetic subjects, on the other hand, there is no consistent association between metabolic control and blood pressure (12, 14), and the causal role of hyperglycemia in the elevation of blood pressure remains speculative.

### Insulin

Several studies suggest that there may be a link between high plasma insulin levels and blood pressure. This relationship has been reported in non-diabetic subjects, in subjects with impaired glucose tolerance (22, 41–44), and in patients with NIDDM (45, 46). Furthermore, the relationship between insulin and blood pressure has been shown to be independent of obesity (22, 46). In experimental studies insulin has been shown to affect sodium transport, and in man it increases sodium tubular reabsorption (47). This effect is independent of the changes in blood glucose, glomerular filtration rate or plasma aldosterone concentration. An increase in sodium tubular reabsorption results in an increase in exchangeable sodium in the body and consequently it may lead to the elevation of blood pressure. On the other hand, high plasma insulin or insulin resistance may increase intracellular sodium concentration in resistance arterioles making them hyperresponsive to sympathetic stimulation (47).

### Obesity

Most patients with NIDDM and subjects with impaired glucose tolerance are obese, and, since obesity is strongly associated with hypertension, this could largely explain the increased prevalence of hypertension in NIDDM and in subjects with impaired glucose tolerance. Several studies have shown, however, that the higher prevalence of hypertension or elevated blood pressure levels among patients with NIDDM or impaired glucose tolerance cannot be accounted for by obesity alone (48).

### Physical Activity

A high level of physical activity may decrease blood pressure in non-diabetic subjects

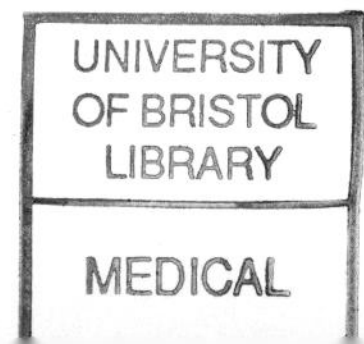

(49), and it is conceivable that the same could also be true in diabetic subjects, in particular in patients with NIDDM. No consistent differences have been found between diabetic and non-diabetic subjects regarding the level of physical activity (48, 50), but subjects with impaired glucose tolerance have been reported to be more often inactive than normoglycemic subjects (33).

### Other Factors

In diabetic subjects with advanced vascular complications blood viscosity is increased. This has been suggested to result in a rise in blood pressure levels, but direct evidence for the impact of blood viscosity is lacking. Elderly subjects and patients with a long duration of diabetes may have diminished arterial compliance which may lead to systolic hypertension (7, 36, 37).

## CONCLUSIONS

(1) The prevalence of hypertension is higher in patients with IDDM and NIDDM than in comparable non-diabetic subjects.

(2) Diabetic nephropathy is the most important cause of hypertension in patients with IDDM and recent studies indicate that blood pressure levels may be elevated already at an early phase of diabetic nephropathy characterized by microalbuminuria. Furthermore, young patients with IDDM may show a slight rise in the average diastolic blood pressure even without signs of renal damage, but the underlying mechanisms of this early increase in blood pressure levels remain obscure.

(3) Hypertension in NIDDM is clinically similar to essential hypertension in non-diabetic subjects, and the increased occurrence of hypertension in this type of diabetes is largely explained by the high frequency of obesity in NIDDM. In addition, other factors may also be involved in the pathogenesis of hypertension in NIDDM, e.g. the interaction of hyperinsulinemia or insulin resistance with blood pressure homeostasis.

## REFERENCES

1. Kannel WB, McGee DL (1979) Diabetes and cardiovascular risk factors: the Framingham study. Circulation 59: 8–13
2. Aromaa A, Reunanen A, Pyörälä K (1985) Hypertension and mortality in diabetic and non-diabetic Finnish men. J Hypertension 2 (Suppl 3): 205–207
3. Jarrett RJ, Shipley MJ (1985) Mortality and associated risk factors in diabetics. Acta Endocrinol 110 (Suppl 272): 21–26
4. Knowler WC, Bennett PH, Ballantine EJ (1980) Increased incidence of retinopathy in diabetics with elevated blood pressure. N Engl J Med 302: 645–650
5. Moss AJ (1962) Blood pressure in children with diabetes. Pediatrics 30: 932–936
6. Karlefors T (1967) Circulatory studies during exercise with particular reference to diabetics. Acta Med Scand 180 (Suppl 449): 1–87

7. Christlieb AR, Warram JH, Krolewski AS, Busick EJ, Ganda OP, Asmal AC, Soeldner JS (1981) Hypertension: the major risk factor in juvenile-onset insulin-dependent diabetics. Diabetes 30 (Suppl 2): 90–96
8. Aromaa A (1981) Epidemiology and public health impact of high blood pressure in Finland (in Finnish, with English summary). Kansanterveystieteen julkaisuja, AL:17, Helsinki
9. Wiseman M, Viberti G, MacKintosh D, Jarrett RJ, Keen H (1984) Glycaemia, arterial pressure and microalbuminuria in Type 1 (insulin-dependent) diabetes mellitus. Diabetologia 26: 401–405
10. Mathiesen ER, Oxenboll B, Johansen K, Svendsen PAa, Deckert T (1984) Incipient nephropathy in Type 1 (insulin-dependent) diabetes. Diabetologia 26: 404–410
11. Mogensen CE, Christensen CK (1984) Predicting diabetic nephropathy in insulin-dependent patients. N Engl J Med 311: 89–93
12. Cruickshanks KJ, Orchard TJ, Becker DJ (1985) The cardiovascular risk profile of adolescents with insulin-dependent diabetes mellitus. Diabetes Care 8: 118–124
13. Kaas-Ibsen K, Rotne H, Hougaard P (1983) Blood pressure in children with diabetes mellitus. Acta Paediatr Scand 72: 191–196
14. Tarn AC, Drury PL (1986) Blood pressure in children, adolescents and young adults with Type 1 (insulin-dependent) diabetes. Diabetologia 29: 275–281
15. Ostrander LD, Francis T, Hayner NS, Kjelsberg MO, Epstein FH (1965) The relationship of cardiovascular disease to hyperglycaemia. Ann Intern Med 62: 1188–1198
16. Pell S, D'Alonzo CA (1967) Some aspects of hypertension in diabetes mellitus. J Am Med Assoc 202: 104–110
17. Garcia MJ, McNamara PM, Gordon T, Kannel WB (1974) Morbidity and mortality in diabetics in the Framingham population. Sixteen year follow-up study. Diabetes 23: 105–111
18. Ingelfinger JA, Bennett PH, Liebow IM, Miller M (1976) Coronary heart disease in the Pima Indians. Electrocardiographic findings and postmortem evidence of myocardial infarction in a population with a high prevalence of diabetes mellitus. Diabetes 25: 561–565
19. Heyden S, Heiss G, Bartel AG, Hames CG (1980) Sex differences in coronary mortality among diabetics in Evans county, Georgia. J Chron Dis 33: 265–273
20. Dupree E, Meyer MB (1980) Role of risk factors in complications of diabetes mellitus. Am J Epidemiol 112: 100-112
21. Barrett-Connor E, Criqui MH, Klauber MR, Holdbrook M (1981) Diabetes and hypertension in a community of older adults. Am J Epidemiol 113: 276–284
22. Modan M, Halkin H, Almog S, Lusky A, Eshkol A, Shefi M, Shitrit A, Fuchs Z (1985) Hyperinsulinemia. A link between hypertension, obesity and glucose intolerance. J Clin Invest 75: 809–817
23. Jarrett RJ, Keen H, McCartney M, Fuller HJ, Hamilton PJS, Reid DD, Rose G (1978). Glucose tolerance and blood pressure in two population samples: their relation to diabetes mellitus and hypertension. Int J Epidemiol 63: 54–64
24. Herman JB, Modalie KG, Goldbourt U (1977) Differences in cardiovascular morbidity and mortality between previously known and newly diagnosed adult diabetics. Diabetologia 13: 229–234
25. Uusitupa M, Siitonen O, Aro A, Pyörälä K (1985) Prevalence of coronary heart disease, left ventricular failure and hypertension in middle-aged newly diagnosed Type 2 (non-insulin-dependent) diabetic subjects. Diabetologia 28: 22–27
26. Laakso M (1986) Atherosclerotic vascular disease and its risk factors in non-insulin-dependent diabetics in East Finland. Academic dissertation. University of Kuopio, Department of Medicine, Kuopio

27. Uusitupa M, Niskanen L, Siitonen O, Pyörälä K (1987) Hyperinsulinemia and hypertension in patients with newly diagnosed non-insulin-dependent diabetes. Diabete Metab (in press)
28. Stamler R, Stamler J (eds) (1979) Asymptomatic hyperglycemia and coronary heart disease. A series of papers by the international collaborative group based on studies in fifteen populations. J Chron Dis 32: 638–837
29. Persky V, Dyer A, Stamler J, Shekelle RB, Schoenberger J, Wannamaker J, Upton M (1979) The relationship between postload plasma glucose and blood pressure at different resting heart rates. J Chron Dis 32: 263–268
30. Jarrett RJ, McCartney P, Keen H: The Bedford Study (1982) Ten year mortality rates in newly diagnosed diabetics, borderline diabetics and normoglycaemic controls and risk indices for coronary heart disease in borderline diabetics. Diabetologia 22: 79–84
31. Yano K, Kagan A, McGee D, Rhoads GG (1982) Glucose intolerance and nine-year mortality in Japanese men in Hawaii. Am J Med 72: 71–80
32. Barrett-Connor E, Wingard DL, Criqui MH, Suarez L (1984) Is borderline fasting hyperglycemia a risk factor for cardiovascular death? J Chron Dis 37: 773–779
33. Cederholm J, Wibell L (1985) Glucose intolerance in middle-aged subjects—a cause of hypertension. Acta Med Scand 217: 363–371
34. Weidmann P, Beretta-Piccoli C, Trost BN (1985) Pressor factors and responsiveness in hypertension accompanying diabetes mellitus. Hypertension II (Suppl II): II-33–II-42
35. O'Hare JA, Ferriss JB, Brady D, Twomey B, O'Sullivan DJ (1985) Exchangeable sodium and renin in hypertensive diabetic patients with and without nephropathy. Hypertension 7 (Suppl II): II-43–II-48
36. Drury PL (1983) Diabetes and arterial hypertension. Diabetologia 24: 1–9
37. Cristlieb AR (1982) The hypertensions of diabetes. Diabetes Care 5: 50–58
38. Burden AC, Thurston H (1979) Plasma renin activity in diabetes mellitus. Clin Sci 56: 255–259
39. Drury PL, Bodansky HJ (1985) The relationship of the renin-angiotensin system in Type 1 diabetes to microvascular disease. Hypertension 7 (Suppl II): II-84–II-89
40. Drury PL, Smith GM, Ferriss JB (1984) Increased vasopressor responsiveness to angiotensin II in type 1 (insulin-dependent) diabetic patients without complications. Diabetologia 27: 174–179
41. Welborn TA, Breckenridge A, Rubenstein AH, Dolley CT, Fraser TR (1966) Serum insulin in essential hypertension and peripheral vascular disease. Lancet i: 1336–1337
42. Pyörälä K, Savolainen E, Kaukola S, Haapakoski J (1985) Plasma insulin as coronary heart disease risk factor: relationship to other risk factors and predictive value during 9 1/2-year follow-up of the Helsinki policemen study population. Acta Med Scand 701: (Suppl): 38–52
43. Singer P, Gödicke W, Voight S, Hadju I, Weiss M (1985) Postprandial hyperinsulinemia in patients with mild essential hypertension. Hypertension 7: 182–186
44. Christlieb AR, Krolewski AS, Warram JH, Soeldner JS (1985) Is insulin the link between hypertension and obesity? Hypertension 7 (Suppl II): II-54–II-57
45. Lowenthal LM, Pim B, Hillson RM, Dhar H, Hockaday TDR (1985) Blood pressure at diagnosis of type 2 diabetes correlated with plasma insulin concentration but not during the next 5 yr. Diabetes Res 2: 65–69
46. Uusitupa M, Siitonen O, Pyörälä K, Mustonen J, Voutilainen E, Hersio K, Penttilä I (1987) Relationship of blood pressure and left ventricular mass to serum insulin levels in newly diagnosed non-insulin-dependent (Type 2) diabetic patients and in non-diabetic subjects. Diabetes Res (in press)
47. DeFronzo RA (1981) The effect of insulin on renal sodium metabolism. A review with clinical implications. Diabetologia 21: 165–171

48. Pyörälä K, Laakso M, Uusitupa M (1987) Diabetes and atherosclerosis: an epidemiologic view. Diabetes/Metab Rev (in press)
49. Nelson L, Jennings GL, Esler MD, Korner PI (1986) Effect of changing levels of physical activity on blood pressure and haemodynamics in essential hypertension. Lancet ii: 473–476
50. Jarrett RJ, Shipley MJ, Hunt R (1986) Physical activity, glucose tolerance and diabetes mellitus: the Whitehall study. Diabetic Med 3: 549–551

# Retinopathy

Diabetic Complications: Early Diagnosis and Treatment
Edited by D. Andreani, G. Crepaldi, U. Di Mario and G. Pozza


CHAPTER 6

# *Pathogenic Mechanisms in the Development of Diabetic Retinopathy*

E. M. Kohner
*Royal Postgraduate Medical School, Hammersmith Hospital, London, UK*

Diabetic retinopathy is the most common microvascular complication of diabetes. In the Wisconsin epidemiological study (1, 2) 97% of those diagnosed before the age of 30 years had some retinopathy after 15–20 years' duration of diabetes. In those diagnosed after the age of 30 years the presence of retinopathy was lower, only about 60%, but still a very common condition.

Microaneurysms are the hallmark of diabetic retinopathy in its early stages, but these never occur unless some capillaries are occluded. Capillary occlusion can be well demonstrated on fluorescein angiograms. Even before capillaries occlude there are histological changes. The earliest of these is the basement membrane thickening noted in most capillary beds, but possibly not of great importance in the retina. Loss of pericytes also occurs early, and this may be a more important feature, as pericytes may well have a regulatory influence on endothelial cells.

It has been established by comparison of fluorescein angiograms with digest preparations of the retina that, while endothelial cells are intact, capillaries are perfused (3). Capillary occlusion is thus secondary to endothelial cell damage. The other features of retinopathy all follow this capillary occlusion which may lead to localized dilatation of neighbouring vessels, microaneurysms, or generalized dilatation associated with leakage. Where large areas of the capillary bed are occluded the disease process extends to the neighbouring arterioles and veins. Only when these larger vessels are occluded do new vessels develop.

What are the pathogenic mechanisms involved in the evolution of retinopathy? Both systemic and local factors play a role. This overview will briefly state the present 'state of the art' on possible pathogenic mechanisms.

## GENETIC FACTORS

That genetic factors may be of importance was suggested by the role which they play in both insulin-dependent diabetes (IDD) and non-insulin-dependent diabetes (NIDD). Cudworth examined the association between proliferative retinopathy and HLA grouping (4) and he also reviewed the world literature in 1982 and could find no relationship (5). More recently, a large case-control study was reported from the Joslin Clinic by Baker et al. (6). These authors found that both proliferative and non-proliferative retinopathy was increased for phenotypes HLA DR 4/0, 5/0 and X/X compared with HLA non-susceptible individuals, HLA DR 3/4, 3/X and 4/X. This genetic susceptibility was, however, abolished in the presence of myopia (defined as a refractive error of −2.00 D). This work to some extent supports that of Dornan et al. (7) although their patients were highly selected and other HLA groups were important.

Another recent report from Birmingham (8) suggests that the genetic components C4 and B3 were associated with diabetic microangiopathy; furthermore, the authors infer an immunological basis to the condition. However, this latter study did not differentiate between the different groups of retinopathy.

A genetic component is likely to play a role in NIDD: Leslie and Pyke (9) have demonstrated that, of 37 identical diabetic twins with NIDD, 35 pairs were in the same retinal category.

Thus genetic influence cannot be ruled out, though it has not been proven, nor has it been shown why and how the genetic influences act.

## BLOOD FLOW AND AUTOREGULATION

Since ischemia is one of the major factors leading to the proliferative changes, and possibly also to the exudative changes, in diabetic retinopathy, a reduction in blood flow in early diabetes and early retinopathy would be expected. However, previous studies in humans using mean transit time measurement (10) and the blue light entoptic phenomenon (11) suggested that blood flow in early retinopathy is increased. This work was supported by experimental work, the best of which was that by Atherton et al. (12) which suggested that a sudden rise in blood glucose could increase blood flow and maintain it at high levels for long periods of time. This increased blood flow was thought by McMillan (13) to be of sufficient severity to damage endothelial cells, thus leading later to reduced blood flow and vascular occlusion. This theory was shattered by the recent work by Riva's group, who developed the laser doppler velocimeter for the measurement of retinal blood flow (14). This group found reduced flow velocity in diabetic patients even when there was only background retinopathy and flow velocity was even further reduced with the increasing severity of retinopathy. This reduction was maintained even after photocoagulation, presumably because of reduced viable retinal tissue. So while there is agreement on altered flow in diabetes, the magnitude and nature of this alteration has not been fully established.

Not only is there a change in flow velocity and volume flow in diabetes, but autoregulation is also altered. Thus, Fallon et al. found that in normal subjects breathing 60% oxygen markedly reduced flow velocity (by 46% of that found with breathing room air), and breathing 10% oxygen increased flow velocity by 36% (15). In diabetic patients with proliferative retinopathy the response to hypoxia was almost completely abolished (3%), while the response to hyperoxia was still maintained, suggesting hypoxia to be already present. Grunwald et al. (16) found reduced response to breathing 100% oxygen in all types of diabetic retinopathy, but noted that the reduced response was markedly restored by panretinal photocoagulation.

These abnormalities of autoregulation accompany diabetic retinopathy, as do the flow changes. The author thinks that they are a marker, not a predisposing pathogenic mechanism, of retinopathy.

## VISCOSITY AND COAGULATION

There are innumerable communications which indicate abnormal viscosity and abnormally coaguable blood in diabetes. Abnormal viscosity in those with proliferative retinopathy was found by Torpe et al. (17) and was also noted by the Hammersmith group, although in the latter it was only the 'corrected' viscosity which was abnormal (unpublished observation). Little (18) reviewed the subject and felt that the increased viscosity in diabetes predisposed to stagnation of flow and increased coagulation. Abnormalities of platelets and other coagulation factors have been reported by many authors and have been reviewed by Colwell (19). Koneti-Rao and co-workers found plasma cofactor activity (which correlates with platelet hyperaggregation) to be higher in both adult diabetic subjects and diabetic children than in control groups (20). Increased platelet volume, suggesting increased platelet turnover, was found by Cagliero et al. (21), but Porta et al. (22) found no correlation between different parameters of platelet function, platelet survival and diabetic retinopathy. Dornan's studies also suggested elevated levels of factor VIII and all its components in diabetes, and this correlated with the severity of retinopathy (23).

All platelet studies suffer from their in vitro measurement, mostly in 'platelet rich plasma', which isolates platelets from their natural environment. In particular, the action of PG12, which has a very short half-life, cannot really be measured in this environment.

Studies with anti-platelet agents would be of interest. In the study of aspirin alone, aspirin and dipyridamole and placebo in early diabetic retinopathy, the results showed a statistical significance in favour of anti-platelet agents. However, the differences, although statistically significant, were not clinically important (24) and therefore definite conclusions could not be drawn.

The present state of knowledge does not therefore allow us to state with certainty that abnormal viscosity or abnormal aggregation of platelets is important. Indeed, it is likely that the platelet abnormalities are secondary to endothelial cell damage and that they represent a reparative process, rather than initiate damage themselves.

## ENDOTHELIAL CELLS

Since endothelial cell loss is a prerequisite for the development of clinically significant diabetic retinopathy, it is reasonable to suggest that endothelial cells are diseased in diabetes.

### Pericytes

The earliest change, pericyte loss, has been demonstrated in experimental animals (25). Pericyte loss could be prevented by an islet cell transplant in diabetic mice, provided the transplant was performed early in the course of the disease; it could not be prevented when diabetes was present for over 4 months (26). Retinal endothelial cell growth and multiplication can be enhanced by growing the cells in a pericyte-conditioned medium (Wong, personal communication). The presence of pericytes is essential for the integrity of endothelial cells; the nature of their regulatory function has not been clearly established, but there is now little doubt about their importance.

### Glucose Transport

Diabetic animals were shown to have increased glucose transport across the blood–retina barrier (27). Endothelial cells contain free glucose even when the glucose concentration of the medium is normal. Free glucose increases strikingly when the glucose concentration in the medium is raised, and this could damage the cells. Although King et al. (28) found endothelial cells reasonably resistant to glucose, Tripathi and Tripathi (29) found that retinal endothelial cells from human cadavers were slightly damaged when cultured in 200 mg% glucose, and that the damage was irreversible when the glucose content was over 400 mg%.

There is now ample evidence that both retinal tissue and retinal microvessels possess insulin receptors. These differ from receptors in other tissues. The role of insulin receptors is not established as it is thought that the retina, like the brain, does not require insulin for glucose transport. At the Hammersmith Hospital a recent study of transport of [$^{14}$C]-3-*O*-methyl-D-glucose across the blood–brain barrier using positron emission tomography failed to demonstrate any defect of hexose transport in diabetic subjects (30). This suggests that either the retinal vessels differ from brain vessels in this respect or that they are more sensitive to raised glucose levels.

### The Role of Sorbitol Accumulation

Glucose damage could of course be due to the accumulation of sorbitol in cells. That sorbitol might be of importance was proposed in a study by Engerman and Kern (31) which demonstrated that non-diabetic dogs fed on a high galactose diet developed a retinopathy which was indistinguishable from diabetic retinopathy. In the dog, galactose is metabolized in the cells to dulcitol through the activity of the enzyme aldose reductase, which is also the enzyme responsible for the conversion of glucose to sorbitol. The polyols are not readily metabolized and they do not penetrate cell membranes easily. They may therefore reach high levels within cells and cause damage by hypertonicity. This, however, is unlikely. It is more plausible that the sorbitol levels interfere with myoinositol concentration and thus cell function and structure is damaged. The problem is the uncertainty of the presence of aldose reductase in the endothelial cells (32). Kinoshita's group—the foremost workers in the field—demonstrated dulcitol accumulation in endothelial cells cultured in galactose (33). They also showed that the aldose reductase inhibitor, Sorbinil, prevented basement membrane thickening in galactose-fed rats. Kennedy et al. (34) were not convinced that sorbitol accumulation was in any way responsible for the retinopathy of diabetic subjects, but this was as expected, since they were not convinced that there was any sorbitol accumulation in the endothelial cells.

The fact that the aldose reductase inhibitor Sorbinil, now in use in the US in a clinical trial of early diabetic retinopathy, has not shown any significant result over a period of 3 years suggests that, if it has an effect, it is not a very marked one.

Sorbitol accumulation could be one but by no means the only factor in the development of diabetic retinopathy.

## GROWTH HORMONE

Growth hormone (GH) hypersecretion was found in diabetic subjects over 24-hour periods, and excessive GH is produced in diabetic patients in response to a number of stimuli; this does not occur in normal subjects (35). The importance of GH was proposed by Lundbaek (36) and has since found some support, although its role is still not proven. Evidence for the role of GH starts with the effect of pituitary ablation.

### Pituitary Ablation in the Treatment of Diabetic Retinopathy

Pituitary ablation was the only method of treatment for diabetic retinopathy before photocoagulation became available. It was an effective method of treatment for new vessels, especially in florid diabetic retinopathy (37). A long-term follow-up of the patients was recently carried out (38). It showed that following the operation there was a marked reduction in mortality, at 5 years only 17.6% and at 10 years 51%, in spite of 13% of all deaths being due to consequences of the operation, such as steroid deficiency and hypoglycemia. Most remarkable was the low rate of renal death in this largely young IDD population, suggesting the influence on microvascular effect also outside the eye. Ophthalmological follow-up of 100 consecutive patients treated between 1965 and 1975 showed marked improvement of new vessels; these improved according to the Hammersmith grading of disc vessels (39) from 2.7 ± 1.6 at entry, to 0.8 ± 1.2 after 5 years and no new vessels at all after 10 years. There was a similar improvement in peripheral new vessels. The initial improvement was certainly related to the completeness of the pituitary ablation, and after 10 years none of the patients had any GH reserve, presumably because of the continued fibrosis of the gland.

### Why is there Hypersecretion of GH in Diabetes?

It is important to note that of all the hormones secreted by the pituitary only GH is elevated in diabetic patients. Therefore it is reasonable to suggest that the pituitary abnormality does not lie in the gland itself, but rather in the controlling mechanisms of GH secretion. It is possible that the high glucose levels act on the hypothalamic glucose-sensitive cells; certainly, improved glucose control reduces abnormal GH secretion in diabetes.

The availability of growth hormone releasing factor (GRF) led to further work in the field. It was demonstrated that although in normal subjects hyperglycemia leads to GRF-mediated GH secretion (39), this suppression does not always occur in diabetes (40). This suggests that the GH suppressive mechanism initiated by hyperglycemia in normal man is defective in diabetic subjects. This mechanism is mediated by hypothalamic somatostatin. It is therefore possible that either somatostatin release is defective in diabetic subjects, or that the pituitary becomes resistant to its action. The problem is that chronic overproduction of somatostatin would be expected to be present in acromegaly, yet in this condition exogenous somatostatin is effective. As already shown (31) there does not seem to be any abnormal permeability to glucose in the brain, so this mechanism cannot be blamed.

A further cause for GH overproduction exists at tissue level. Insulin-like growth factor 1 (IGF-1) is a GH-dependent growth factor. There appears to be a negative correlation between serum levels of IGF-1 and glycemic control as assessed by $HbA_1$ levels (41); this is also demonstrated by our own observations. This finding has been confirmed in children, where those with good glycemic control have been shown to have a greater IGF-1 response to the exogenous GH administration than those with poor control (42). Thus, a GH resistance may exist at peripheral level leading to the elevation of GH levels by a negative feedback mechanism.

Finally, the long-acting somatostatin analogue SMS 201-995, which is effective in suppressing GH production in acromegalic patients and normal subjects, was not found to be effective in suppressing excessive GH production in diabetic subjects with active neovascularization who were resistant or at least not fully responsive to photocoagulation (manuscript in preparation).

## GROWTH FACTORS

Ischemia plays a major part in the development of proliferative retinopathy. The ischemic retina is said to produce a 'vasoproliferative factor' which stimulates the growth of new vessels. This could be interpreted as a tissue growth factor of importance in the development of proliferative lesions. That such a factor exists is further demonstrated by the fact that panretinal photocoagulation causes regression of the new vessels, probably by abolishing this vasoproliferative factor.

The nature and number of tissue growth factors are not known at present, but it is likely that they will be identical or similar to the ones already found and sequenced, such as insulin-like growth factors, fibroblast growth factor, platelet-derived growth factor and nerve growth factor. Of all these insulin-like growth factor 1 (IFG-1) has received most attention because it was the first for which valid assays were available.

While in the diabetic population no rise in IGF-1 was found by the majority of investigators, Merimee et al. suggested that patients with rapidly advancing aggressive proliferative retinopathy had higher than normal levels (43). Our own group has found that there is a significant correlation between IGF-1 and the activity of diabetic retinopathy, but even in active proliferative retinopathy levels are not significantly different from normal. With regression of new vessels after photocoagulation, the IGF-1 levels fall further, suggesting that even modest elevation is a transient feature in retinopathy. Thus it is not possible to ascribe a definite role to IFG-1 in the pathogenesis of proliferative retinopathy. However, raised levels may exist in the eye and this local concentration is not necessarily reflected by levels in the blood. Grant et al. (44) found elevated levels of IGF-1 in the vitreous of diabetic patients who had undergone vitrectomies; these were not found in non-diabetic subjects.

The other growth factor which may be important is fibroblast growth factor (FGF), the basic form of which has been isolated from various tissues such as pituitary, retina and brain. FGF causes an increase in extracellular matrix and proliferation of both vascular and fibrous tissue. Because of its presence in the pituitary it is an attractive contender for the role of being responsible for improvement in retinopathy after pituitary ablation. Its presence in the retina and in the vitreous of patients with proliferative retinopathy (45) may also be of importance but this has not yet been fully established. The active interest in tissue growth factors will soon establish their precise roles, even if at present the evidence for their importance is slim.

It appears that there are several pathogenic mechanisms at play in the development of retinopathy and a unique role for any of them is missing. The likelihood is that the interplay of many factors results in those forms of retinopathy which most severely threaten the sight.

## REFERENCES

1. Klein R, Klein BE, Moss SE, Davis MD, DeMets DL (1984) The Wisconsin epidemiological study of diabetic retinopathy. II. Prevalence and risk of diabetic retinopathy when age at diagnosis is less than 30 years. Arch Ophthalmol 102: 520–526
2. Klein R, Klein BE, Moss SE, Davis MD, DeMets DL (1984) The Wisconsin epidemiological study of diabetic retinopathy. III. Prevalence and risk of diabetic retinopathy when age at diagnosis is over 30 years. Arch Ophthalmol 102: 527–532
3. Kohner EM, Henkind P (1970) Comparison of fluorescein study and retinal digest

preparation in a diabetic patient. Am J Opthalmol 69: 403–414
4. Bodansky HJ, Wolf E, Cudworth AG, Dean BM, Nineham LJ, Botazzo GF, Matthews P, Kurtz AB, Kohner EM (1982) Genetic and immunological factors in microvascular disease of type 1 insulin dependent diabetes. Diabetes 31: 70–74
5. Cudworth AG, Bodansky HJ (1982) Genetic and immunological factors in diabetic complications. In: Keen H, Jarrett J (eds) Complications of diabetes. London, Edward Arnold, Chapter 1
6. Baker RR, Rand LI, Krolewski AS (1984) Myopia and proliferative retinopathy in insulin dependent diabetes. Invest Ophthalmol Vis Sci 25: 128–132
7. Dornan TL, Ting H, McPherson CK, Peckar CO, Mann JI, Turner RC, Morris PJ (1982) Genetic susceptibility to the development of retinopathy in insulin dependent diabetics. Diabetes 31: 226–230
8. Mijovic C, Fletcher J, Bradwell AR, Harvey T, Barnet AH (1985) Relation of gene expression of the fourth component of complement to insulin dependent diabetes and its microangiopathic complications. Br Med J 291: 9–11
9. Leslie RDJ, Pyke DA (1982) Diabetic retinopathy in identical twins. Diabetes 31: 19–21
10. Kohner EM, Hamilton AM, Saunders SJ, Sutcliffe BH, Bulpitt CJ (1975) The retinal blood flow in diabetes. Diabetologia 11: 27–33
11. Fallon TJ, Chowienczyk P, Kohner EM (1986) Measurement of retinal blood flow in diabetes by the blue light entoptic phenomenon. Br J Ophthalmol 70: 43–48
12. Atherton A, Hill DW, Keen H, Young S, Edwards EJ (1980) The effect of acute hyperglycaemia on the retinal circulation of the normal cat. Diabetologia 18: 233–237
13. McMillan DE (1978) Rheological and related factors in diabetic retinopathy. Ophthalmol Clin 4: 35
14. Riva CE, Feke GT (1981) Laser doppler velocimetry in the measurement of retinal blood flow. In: Goldman L (ed) The biomedical laser. Springer Verlag, New York, p 135
15. Fallon TJ, Maxwell D, Kohner EM (1985) Retinal vascular autoregulation in conditions of hyperoxia and hypoxia using the blue light entoptic phenomenon. Ophthalmology 92: 701–705
16. Grunwald JE, Riva CE, Bruckner AJ, Sinclair SJ, Petrig BV (1984) Altered vascular response to 100% oxygen breathing in diabetes mellitus. Ophthalmology 91: 1447–1452
17. Torpe GE, Lowe GDO, Ghafour IM, Foulds WS, Forbes CP (1983) Blood viscosity in proliferative diabetic retinopathy and complicated retinal vein thrombosis. Trans Ophthalmol Soc UK 103: 108–110
18. Little HL (1983) The role of blood elements in the pathogenesis of diabetic retinopathy. In: Little HL, Jack RL, Paiz A, Forsham PH (eds) Diabetic retinopathy. Thieme-Stratton, New York, Chapter 13
19. Colwell JA (1983) Platelets and diabetic retinopathy. In: Little HL, Jack RL, Paiz A, Forsham PH (eds) Diabetic retinopathy. Thieme-Stratton, New York, Chapter 10
20. Koneti-Rao A, Goldberg DE, Walsh PN (1984) Platelet coagulant activities in diabetes mellitus. J Lab Clin Med 103: 82–92
21. Cagliero E, Porta M, Cousins S, Kohner Em (1981) Increased platelet volume, an index of accelerated platelet turnover in diabetic retinopathy. Diabetologia 20: 667–670
22. Porta M, O'Brien ME, Kohner EM (1981) Platelet abnormalities related to diabetic retinopathy. Horm Metab Res Suppl II: 50–54
23. Dornan TL, Rhymes IL, Cederholm-Williams SA, Rizza CR, Pepys MB (1983) Plasma haemostatic factors and diabetic retinopathy. Eur J Clin Invest 13: 231–235
24. The DAMAD Study Group (1987) The effect of aspirin and dipyridamole in early diabetic retinopathy (in press)
25. Sima AAF, Garcia-Salinas R, Basu PK (1983) The BB Wistar rat: an experimental model for diabetic retinopathy. Metab Clin Exp (Suppl) 32: 136–140

26. Naeser P, Anderson D (1983) Effect of pancreatic islet cell transplantation on the morphology of retinal capillaries in alloxan diabetic mice. Acta Ophthalmol 61: 30–36
27. Ennis SR, Johnson JE, Pautler EL (1982) In situ kinetics of glucose transport across the blood retinal barrier in normal rats and rats with streptozotocin induced diabetes. Invest Ophthalmol Vis Sci 23: 447–452
28. King GL, Buzney SM, Kahn CR, Heru N, Buchwald SH, McDonald SG, Rand LI (1985) Differential responsiveness to insulin of endothelial and support cells from micro and macrovessels. J Clin Invest 71: 974–979
29. Tripathi BJ, Tripathi RC (1982) Human retinal vessels in tissue culture. Ophthalmology 89: 858–861
30. Brooks DJ, Gibbs JSR, Sharp P, Harold S, Turton DR, Luthia SK, Kohner EM, Bloom SR, Jones T (1986) Regional cerebral glucose transport in insulin dependent diabetic patients studied, using $^{14}$C-3-*O*-methyl glucose and positron emission tomography. J Cerebral Bloodflow Metab 6: 240–244
31. Engerman RC, Kern TS (1984) Experimental galactosaemia produces diabetes like retinopathy. Diabetes 33: 92–97
32. Russel P, Merola LO, Yajima Y, Kinoshita JM (1982) Aldose reductase activity in cultured human retinal cell line. Exp Eye Res 35: 331–337
33. Robinson WG, Kador PF, Kinoshita JH (1983) Retinal capillaries: basement membrane thickening by galactosaemia prevented by aldose reductase inhibitor. Science 221: 1177–1179
34. Kennedy A, Frank RN, Varma SD (1983) Aldose reductase activity in retinal and cereberal microvessels and cultured vascular cells. Invest Ophthalmol Vis Sci 24: 1250–1256
35. Lundbaek K, Christensen NJ, Jensen VA (1970) Diabetes, diabetic angiopathy and growth hormone. Lancet ii: 131–133
36. Lundbaek K, Nalmios R, Anderson HC (1969) Hypoplypectomy for diabetic angiopathy: a controlled clinical trial. Excerpta Medica International Congress Series No 172. Excerpta Medica, Amsterdam, pp 127–139
37. Kohner EM, Hamilton AM, Joplin GF, Fraser TR (1976) Florid diabetic retinopathy and its response to treatment by photocoagulation or pituitary ablation. Diabetes 25: 104–110
38. Sharp P, Fallon TJ, et al. (1987) Long term follow up of pituitary ablation. (in press)
39. Kohner EM, Panisset A, Cheng H, Fraser TR (1971) Diabetic retinopathy: new vessels arising from the optic disc. I. Grading system and natural history. Diabetes 20: 816–823
40. Sharp P, Foley K, Kohner EM (1984) Evidence for central abnormality in the regulation of growth hormone secretion in insulin dependent diabetes. Diabetic Med 1: 205–208
41. Winter RS, Phillips LS, Klein MN, Traisman HS, Greeh OC (1979) Somatomedin activity and diabetic control in insulin dependent diabetic children. Diabetes 28: 952–956
42. Blethen SL, Sargeant DT, Whitlow MG, Santiago JV (1981) Effect of pubertal stage and recent blood glucose control on plasma somatomedin C in children with insulin dependent diabetes mellitus. Diabetes 30: 868–872
43. Merimee TJ, Zapf J, Froesch ER (1983) Insulin like growth factors: studies in diabetics with and without retinopathy. N Engl J Med 527: 309–312
44. Grant N, Russell B, Fitzgerald C, Merimee TJ (1986) Insulin like growth factors in the vitreous: studies in control and diabetic subjects with neovascularisation. Diabetes 35: 416–422
45. Baird A, Culler F, Jones KC, Guillemin R (1985) Angiogenic factor in human occular fluid. Lancet ii: 563

Diabetic Complications: Early Diagnosis and Treatment
Edited by D. Andreani, G. Crepaldi, U. Di Mario and G. Pozza


CHAPTER 7

# *Blood Glucose Control and Diabetic Retinopathy*

T. Segato and E. Midena
*Diabetic Retinopathy and Retinal Vascular Clinic, Institute of Ophthalmology, University of Padua, Italy*

The pathogenesis of diabetic retinopathy remains an area of active research. Many factors, genetic and environmental, are thought to influence the onset and progression of retinopathy (1–4), but evidence from experimental, epidemiological and clinical studies suggests an important role for hyperglycemia in the development of this late complication of diabetes. Current pathogenetic hypotheses involving hyperglycemia as the causative factor of diabetic retinopathy, and the clinical trials both performed and in progress concerning the relationship between blood glucose control and retinopathy will be outlined in this chapter. The aim is to provide a wide basis of information from which to formulate an individual opinion regarding this stimulating aspect of diabetic patient management.

## HYPERGLYCEMIA AS A CAUSE OF DIABETIC RETINOPATHY

Animal studies, particularly those performed on dogs, indicate a direct causal relationship between hyperglycemia and the onset and progression of early retinal lesions characteristic of diabetic retinopathy (5–7). Other animal models, as for example rodents, may also be useful to confirm these observations (8, 9).

Several investigators have identified the selective loss of retinal capillary pericytes as the earliest histological lesion of diabetic retinopathy (10–12). Recently, Akagi et al. demonstrated the selective presence of aldose reductase on human and animal retinal pericytes (13, 14). These observations sustain the role of aldose reductase in the pathogenesis of early retinal diabetic lesions and directly indicate hyperglycemia, through the sorbitol pathway, as a causative factor of retinal alterations.

Hyperglycemia is also considered to be responsible for the alterations in the blood–retina barrier as is documented by vitreous fluorophotometry (15). Using this technique, Waltman et al. reported that increased permeability of the blood–retina barrier is an early change—in diabetic animals—that can be reversed by insulin treatment (16). To date there is no general agreement about the site, or sites, of alteration in the blood–retina barrier responsible for abnormal fluorophotometric results in diabetic patients. It has yet to be discovered both how this dysfunction occurs in diabetes and how the alterations in the blood–retina barrier and the histopathological lesions of diabetic retinopathy are associated. However, vitreous fluorophotometry is a valuable diagnostic method to follow up diabetic patients who undergo different therapeutic strategies (17).

Previous and current experimental and clinical studies recently allowed Frank to put forward a comprehensive hypothesis regarding the pathogenesis of diabetic complications, particularly retinopathy (18). He hypothesized that all late complications of diabetes are caused by the effects of chronic hyperglycemia on different metabolic pathways. The rapid development of diabetic complications in subjects under apparently good glucose control, and their marked delay in individuals with poor control, relates to the variation, for genetic or other reasons, in the activity of these pathways. This attractive hypothesis needs a careful and exact demonstration during all of its stages. But it clearly points to the fundamental role of blood glucose as the key factor in the development of diabetic retinopathy.

## EPIDEMIOLOGICAL AND RETROSPECTIVE STUDIES

Tchobroutsky, in his review on the relationship between diabetic control and the development of microvascular complications, maintained that bad metabolic control is associated with more and severer forms of diabetic complications (19). But he failed to find definitive evidence that good metabolic control determines a lower frequency of onset and the regression of established diabetic retinopathy.

A direct relationship between retinopathy and glycemic control in insulin-dependent diabetic patients seems to be well demonstrated by retrospective and epidemiological studies (20–24). This relationship has also been confirmed in non-insulin-dependent diabetic patients (25–28). Ishihara et al. recently also reported that the blood glucose level at the initial hospital visit is also a simple but reliable predictor of the subsequent development of retinopathy in non-insulin-dependent diabetic patients (29).

In our epidemiological study on the prevalence of diabetic retinopathy in the Italian Veneto region, we observed a progressive increase in the frequency of retinopathy which was directly related to the deterioration of metabolic control. This was determined by means of three parameters: fasting and postprandial glycemia and glycosylated hemoglobin (30).

However, it is not correct to infer from these retrospective and epidemiological studies that the risk of developing diabetic retinopathy can be reduced by therapeutic intervention to lower hyperglycemia. Such an inference assumes that the correlational association actually describes a causal or reversible relationship. The statement that a causal relationship exists between a reduction of hyperglycemia and a decreased risk of developing retinopathy requires controlled experimentation.

However, until a few years ago, it was not possible to obtain a long-term normalization, or even near normalization, of blood glucose levels in large groups of diabetic patients (30). This fact limited the possibility of performing accurate controlled experiments.

The development of blood glucose self-monitoring and the introduction of multiple injections of insulin and continuous subcutaneous insulin infusion (CSII) enabled insulin-dependent diabetic patients to maintain near normal metabolic control (31, 32). Since then a growing number of studies have been performed with CSII-treated diabetic patients to evaluate the effect of good metabolic control on diabetic retinopathy.

## CONTINUOUS SUBCUTANEOUS INSULIN INFUSION: FIRST STUDIES

In 1979, Irsigler et al. published the first report on diabetic retinopathy and CSII (33). The authors demonstrated the remission of proliferative retinopathy in a young diabetic female after a few months of CSII therapy. We have also reported the regression of proliferative retinopathy after 9 months of strict diabetic control, obtained through the use of CSII (34). These and other exciting results (35) were not borne out by the systematic study of a large number of patients (36). During the latter study, most of the patients' eyes deteriorated: preproliferative retinopathy progressed to the proliferative form and photocoagulation was necessary in all eyes affected by proliferative retinopathy. Moreover, Daneman et al. observed a rapid progression of retinopathy in four children affected by Mauriac's syndrome following the improvement of metabolic control by means of CSII; severe proliferative retinopathy appeared in three of them (37). Subsequently, similar cases were sporadically reported (38, 39) (Table 1).

Numerous factors are considered to be related to the above-described progression of retinopathy: an increase in somatomedin levels from subnormal to normal values; a reduction in retinal blood flow, secondary to an increase in tissue oxygenation, with a deterioration of established retinal ischemia; the metabolic effect of hypoglycemia, which is often present when strict glycemic control is rapidly obtained.

Afterwards, Tamborlane and Puklin et al. studied 17 diabetic patients with different degrees of retinopathy using between 1 and 2 years of insulin pump treatment (40, 41). They concluded that CSII does not reverse established microvascular complications, despite a sustained improvement in metabolic control. Zaluski et al. drew the same conclusions (42). Kelly et al. (43) tested 10 diabetic patients and observed no beneficial effect on the severity of retinopathy when metabolic control was improved over a 6-month period of CSII therapy. In this study the number of patients is small and the time of observation too short to allow the researchers to detect deterioration or improvement in retinal conditions. In 1982 a study was performed using vitreous fluorophotometry as an indicator of the modification of retinopathy (44). The authors observed a decrease of fluorophotometric values in most of their

Table 1. The role of blood glucose control on diabetic retinopathy: the first studies

| Authors | Year | Diabetics | Treatment | Observation period | Results |
|---|---|---|---|---|---|
| Irsigler et al. (33) | 1979 | 1 | CSII | 4 months | Remission of proliferative retinopathy |
| White et al. (35) | 1981 | 1 | CSII + CIT | 18 months | Remission of macular edema; some areas of retinal revascularization |
| Daneman et al. (37) | 1981 | 4* | CIT | 9 months | Progression of retinopathy; three developed proliferative retinopathy |
| Segato et al. (34) | 1982 | 5 | CSII | 9 months | Stabilization of previously laser-treated eyes; regression of proliferative retinopathy in two eyes (of different patients) |
| Lawson et al. (36) | 1982 | 12 | CSII | 4–19 months | No improvement (sometimes deterioration) of proliferative and preproliferative retinopathy despite good glucose control |
| Lorenzi et al. (38) | 1983 | 1 | CIT | 13 months | Deterioration of background to proliferative retinopathy despite good glucose control |
| Ballegooie et al. (39) | 1984 | 19 | CSII | 12–14 months | Progression of retinopathy (proliferative) in the preproliferative group; slight deterioration in the background retinopathy group |

CSII = continuous subcutaneous insulin infusion, CIT = conventional insulin therapy.
* Affected by Mauriac's syndrome.

CSII-treated patients, but the results were considered to be of uncertain clinical significance. Friberg and collaborators studied 57 insulin-dependent diabetic patients (33 CSII and 24 CIT) without randomization for an average of more than 30 months (45). Three of the patients in the CSII group revealed early proliferative retinopathy at baseline. The authors found that the CSII group had better control and a significantly less rapid progression of retinopathy—measured using two methods—compared to the group treated with conventional insulin therapy (CIT). Bell et al. evaluated 17 patients and concluded that improved blood glucose control did not appear to halt the progression of background diabetic retinopathy (46) (Table 2).

These preliminary studies were not randomized and patients were not recruited according to precise ophthalmological criteria. By consequence, different and hardly comparable results were obtained. Moreover, the risk of provoking a progression of retinopathy and other dangerous and unexpected effects has induced most ophthalmologists to concentrate their attention on the earlier phases of retinopathy (47).

## CONTINUOUS SUBCUTANEOUS INSULIN INFUSION: CURRENT TRIALS

Before the introduction of CSII the only randomized study on the relationship between hyperglycemia and diabetic complications was a 4-year French study, in which the evaluation of microaneurysms was used to determine progression or regression of retinopathy (48). The authors showed that insulin-dependent diabetic patients treated with divided insulin injections had a slower rate of progression of microaneurysms compared to diabetic patients receiving a single daily insulin injection. This work was subsequently questioned on account of several methodological biases.

After the introduction of CSII, the first prospective, randomized and controlled clinical trial to be developed was the Steno Study (49). It was originally designed as a 1-year study, but the results of the 2-year follow-up have recently been reported (50). The Kroc, Oslo, Aarhus and Italian CNR Studies are the other prospective trials now in progress for the comparison of CSII- and CIT-treated patients (51–54). All these studies, with the exception of Aarhus, recruited—at baseline—insulin-dependent diabetic patients affected by background retinopathy. In the Aarhus Study 10 of the 24 patients revealed no sign of diabetic retinopathy on baseline fundus examination (6 CSII, 4 CIT) (53). All patients in the CNR Study were affected by mild to advanced background retinopathy with angiographically confirmed retinal ischemic areas (54). A large variety of fundus aspects were present in the patients involved in the other trials. The Kroc and Oslo Studies, after 8 and 12 months respectively, have reported that nearly normal blood glucose levels do not retard progression of retinopathy, and may—at least initially—worsen established diabetic retinopathy (51, 52). The deterioration is generally represented by the appearance of cottonwool spots. The Steno Study researchers concluded, after 2 years, that the retinal situation

Table 2. CSII vs CIT: the first studies concerning diabetic retinopathy

| Authors | Year | Diabetics | Treatment | Observation period | Results |
|---|---|---|---|---|---|
| White et al. (44) | 1982 | 36 | 11 intensively treated<br>25 conventional therapy | 9 months | Fluorophotometry values decrease following intensive therapy; retinal lesions do not improve |
| Tamborlane et al. (40) | 1982 | 17 | CSII | 12–24 months | Pump treatment does not reverse diabetic retinopathy; the 10 eyes without retinopathy remain without |
| Kelly et al. (43) | 1984 | 10 | 6 months CIT, then<br>6 months CSII | 12 months | Intensive therapy neither reverses retinopathy nor prevents its development |
| Zaluski et al. (42) | 1985 | 24 | CSII | 13–41 months | Stabilization of background non-ischemic retinopathy; no effect on ischemic retinopathy |
| Friberg et al. (45) | 1985 | 57 | 33 CSII, 24 CIT | 31 months (mean) | Less progression of retinopathy in CSII-treated diabetics |
| Bell et al. (46) | 1985 | 17 | 9 CSII, 8 CIT | 30 weeks | No difference in the course of retinopathy in the two groups; no signs of regression |

CSII = continuous subcutaneous insulin infusion, CIT = conventional insulin therapy.

demonstrated a slight tendency towards more frequent improvement with CSII therapy than CIT (50). The same authors had previously reported the deterioration of retinopathy after 6 and 12 months of follow-up (49). The initial worsening of retinopathy appears to be due to abrupt metabolic correction, sometimes associated with frequent episodes of hypoglycemia (51). The CNR Study was not able to show any difference between the CSII and CIT groups with regard to the evolution of retinopathy. However, our CSII and CIT patients have similar glucose control (54). Danish researchers from the Aarhus Study found no statistically significant difference in the progression rate of retinopathy after one year (53). They consider that the results obtained are due to the different stages of retinopathy at the start of pump therapy in comparison to the other studies (Table 3).

This consideration leads to the important assumption that diabetic retinopathy may be influenced by glucose control only in its early and mild phases. The so-called 'point of no return' may be represented as the limit beyond which any intervention aimed at improving metabolic control no longer affects diabetic retinopathy. But even this statement needs to be accurately demonstrated.

Published results have shown that, at present, no conclusive considerations are possible. Perhaps the Diabetes Control and Complications Trial (DCCT) alone will prove capable of giving us a definitive answer to the question: 'Is blood glucose control effective in preventing or delaying the onset and progression of diabetic retinopathy?' (55)

The ultimate objective of the DCCT is 'to assess whether a program of therapy aimed at near normalization of blood glucose levels results in a significant difference in the rate of progression of microvascular complications, particularly retinopathy, when compared with a program of standard therapy aimed at the maintenance of clinical well-being' (55). The feasibility phase has been concluded and the full-scale clinical trial is beginning. It will involve 1400 insulin-dependent diabetic patients: 700 for the primary prevention study (no retinopathy and microalbuminuria at baseline), and 700 for the secondary intervention study (some retinopathy, and possibly microalbuminuria). All subjects will be followed for at least 5 years, some up to 10 years.

## COMMENTS

Diabetic retinopathy is one of the most important causes of blindness in Western countries. Up until now no drug therapy has been available to treat this disease and photocoagulation is the only effective therapy for proliferative diabetic retinopathy and diabetic maculopathy.

Hyperglycemia seems to play a key role in the pathogenesis of diabetic retinopathy. Therefore it is reasonable to assume that accurate blood glucose control may positively influence the appearance and progression of this late complication of diabetes. As was outlined in previous paragraphs, no clear demonstration of this assumption is available at present, and even if we may assume that near normal blood

Table 3. CSII vs CIT: current randomized clinical trials

| Authors | Year | Diabetics | Treatment | Observation period | Results |
|---|---|---|---|---|---|
| Steno Study Group (50) | 1985 | 30 | 15 CSII, 15 CIT | 2 years | More frequent improvement of retinal morphology in the CSII group |
| Kroc Study (51) | 1984 | 70 | 35 CSII, 35 CIT | 8 months | Nearly normal blood glucose (CSII) does not retard progression of established retinopathy |
| Beck-Nielsen et al. (53) | 1985 | 24 | 12 CSII, 12 CIT | 1 year | CSII treatment is unable to stop the progression of retinopathy, but it does not induce cotton-wool spots or proliferation in minor or no background retinopathy |
| Oslo Study (52) | 1985 | 45 | 15 CSII, 15 MI, 15 CIT | 1 year | Progressive deterioration in the CIT group; no significant changes in the MI and CSII groups |
| Italian CNR Study (54) | 1987 | 38 | 19 CSII, 19 CIT | 2 years | No differences in the evolution of retinopathy in the two groups |

CSII = continuous subcutaneous insulin infusion, MI = multiple injections, CIT = conventional insulin therapy.

glucose control is a fundamental goal of diabetes management, it is to be hoped that a definitive answer regarding the exact relationship between hyperglycemia and diabetic retinopathy will be obtained in the near future.

## REFERENCES

1. Leslie RDG, Pyke DA (1982) Diabetic retinopathy in identical twins. Diabetes 31: 19–21
2. Dornan TL, Ting A, McPherson CO, Mann JI, Turner RC, Morris PJ (1982) Genetic susceptibility to the development of retinopathy in insulin-dependent diabetics. Diabetes 31: 226–231
3. Siperstein MD, Unger RH, Madison LL (1978) Studies of muscle capillary basement membranes in normal subjects, diabetic and prediabetic patients. J Clin Invest 47: 1973–1999
4. Frank RN (1986) Diabetic retinopathy: current concepts of evaluation and treatment. Clin Endocrinol Metab 15: 933–1003
5. Engerman RL, Bloodworth JMB Jr, Nelson S (1977) Relationship of microvascular disease in diabetes to metabolic control. Diabetes 26: 760–769
6. Engerman RL, Kern TS (1984) Experimental galactosemia produces diabetic-like retinopathy. Diabetes 33: 97–100
7. Engerman RL, Kern TS (1986) Hyperglycemia as a cause of diabetic retinopathy. Metabolism 35 (Suppl 1): 20–23
8. Sima AAF, Chakrabarti S, Garcia-Salinas R, Basn PK (1985) The BB-rat an authentic model of human diabetic retinopathy. Curr Eye Res 4: 1087–1092
9. Midena E, Segato T, Radin S, Di Giorgio G, Piermarocchi S, Meneghini F (1986) Diabetic retinopathy in db/db mice. Diabetologia 29: 571A
10. Cogan DG, Toussaint D, Kuwabara T (1961) Retinal vascular patterns. IV. Diabetic retinopathy. Arch Ophthalmol 66: 366–378
11. Speiser P, Gittelsohn AM, Patz A (1968) Studies on diabetic retinopathy. III. Influence of diabetes on intramural pericytes. Arch Ophthalmol 80: 332–337
12. Addison DJ, Garner A, Ashton N (1970) Degeneration of intramural pericytes in diabetic retinopathy. Br Med J i: 264–266
13. Akagi Y, Kador PF, Kuwabara T, Kinoshita JH (1983) Aldose reductase localization in human retinal mural cells. Invest Ophthalmol Vis Sci 24: 1516–1519
14. Akagi Y, Terubayashi H, Miller J, Kador PF, Kinoshita JH (1986) Aldose reductase localization in dog retinal mural cells. Curr Eye Res 5: 883–886
15. Cunha-Vaz JG (1983) Studies on the pathophysiology of diabetic retinopathy. The blood retinal barrier in diabetes. Diabetes 32 (Suppl 2): 20–27
16. Waltman SR, Krupin T, Hanish S, Oesterich C, Becker B (1978) Alteration of the blood-retinal barrier in experimental diabetes mellitus. Arch Ophthalmol 96: 878–883
17. Waltman SR (1984) Sequential vitrous fluorophotometry in diabetes mellitus: a five year prospective study. Trans Am Ophthalmol Soc 82: 827–848
18. Frank RN (1984) On the pathogenesis of diabetic retinopathy. Ophthalmology 91: 626–634
19. Tchobroutsky G (1978) Relation of diabetic control to development of microvascular complications. Diabetologia 15: 143–152
20. Pirart J (1978) Diabetes mellitus and its degenerative complications: a prospective study of 4400 patients observed between 1947 and 1973. Diabetes Care 1: 168–188
21. West KM, Ahuja MMS, Bennet PH, Grab B, Grabouska V, Mateo-de-Acosta O, Fuller JH, Jarret RJ, Keen H, Kosaka K, Krolevski AS, Miki E, Schliach V, Teuscher A (1982)

Interrelationship of microangiopathy, plasma glucose and other risk factors in 3583 diabetic patients: a multinational study. Diabetologia 22: 412–420

22. Constable IJ, Knuiman MW, Welborn TA, Cooper RL, Stanton KM, McConn VJ, Grose GC (1984) Assessing the risk of diabetic retinopathy. Am J Ophthalmol 97: 53–61
23. Doft BH, Kingsley LA, Orchard TJ, Kuller L, Drash A, Becker D (1984) The association between long-term diabetic control and early retinopathy. Ophthalmology 91: 763–769
24. Klein R, Klein BEK, Moss SE, Davis MD, De Mets DC (1984) The Wisconsin Epidemiologic Study of Diabetic retinopathy. LL. Arch Ophthalmol 102: 520–526
25. Klein R, Klein BEK, Moss SE, Davis MD, De Mets DC (1984) The Wisconsin Epidemiologic Study of diabetic retinopathy. III. Arch Ophthalmol 102: 527–532
26. Ishihara M, Yukimura Y, Yamada T, Ohto K, Yoshizawa K (1984) Diabetic complications and their relationship to risk factors in a Japanese care. Diabetes Care 7: 533–538
27. Nathan DM, Singer DE, Godine JE, Hodgson L, Harrington C, Perlmuter LC (1986) Retinopathy in older type II diabetics. Association with glucose control. Diabetes 35: 797–801
28. Monson JP, Koios G, Toms GC, Kopelman PG, Boucher BJ, Evans SJW, Alexander WL (1986) Relationship between retinopathy and glycaemia control in insulin-dependent and non-insulin-dependent diabetes. J R Soc Med 79: 274–276
29. Ishihara M, Yukimura Y, Yamada T, Ohto K, Yoshizawa K (1986) BG level and body weight at initial hospital visit correlate well with subsequent development of diabetic retinopathy. Diabetes Care 9: 104–105
30. Segato T, Midena E, Piermarocchi S, Fedele D, Schievano C, Grigoletto F, Crepaldi G (1985) The Veneto multicentric epidemiologic study of diabetic retinopathy. Second NEI symposium on eye disease epidemiology. NIH, Bethesda 1985, A-4
31. Mecklenburg RS, Benson JW, Bacher (1982) Clinical use of insulin infusion in 100 patients with type 1 diabetes. N Engl J Med 307: 513–518
32. Schiffrin A, Belmonte MM (1982) Comparison between continuous subcutaneous insulin infusion and multiple injection of insulin. Diabetes 31: 255–264
33. Irsigler K, Kritz H, Najemnik C, Freyler H (1979) Reversal of florid diabetic retinopathy. Lancet ii: 1068
34. Segato T, Midena E, Piermarocchi S, Crepaldi G, Tiengo A (1982) The effect of continuous subcutaneous insulin infusion treatment on proliferative diabetic retinopathy. Am J Ophthalmol 94: 685–686
35. White MC, Kohner EM, Pickup JC, Keen H (1981) Reversal of diabetic retinopathy by continuous subcutaneous insulin infusion: a case report. Br J Ophthalmol 65: 307–311
36. Lawson PM, Champion MC, Conny C, Kingsley R, White MC, Duprè J, Kohner EM (1984) Continuous subcutaneous insulin infusion (CSII) does not prevent progression of proliferative retinopathy. Br J Ophthalmol 66: 762–766
37. Daneman D, Drash AL, Lobes LA, Becker DJ, Baher LM, Travis LB (1981) Progressive retinopathy with improved control in diabetic dwarfism (Mauriac's Syndrome). Diabetic Care 4: 362–365
38. Lorenzi M, Goldbaum MH, Spencer EM, Cheney C (1983) Improved diabetic control and retinopathy. N Engl J Med 308: 1600
39. Ballegooie E, Hooymans JMM, Timmerman Z, Reitsma WD, Sluiter WJ, Schweitzer NM, Doorenbos H (1984) Rapid deterioration of diabetic retinopathy during treatment with continuous subcutaneous insulin infusion. Diabetic Care 7: 236–242
40. Tamborlane WV, Puklin JE, Bergman M, Verdonk C, Rudolf MC, Felig P, Gennel M, Sherwin R (1982) Long-term improvement of metabolic control with the insulin pump does not reverse diabetic microangiopathy. Diabetes Care 5 (Suppl 1): 58–64
41. Puklin JE, Tamborlane WV, Felig P, Gennel M, Sherwin RS (1982) Influence of long-

term insulin infusion pump treatment of type 1 diabetes on diabetic retinopathy. Ophthalmology 89: 735–747
42. Zaluski S, Millet P, Selam JL (1985) Améliorations de la retinopathie du diabetique traité par pompe à l'insuline intrapéritoneale. J Fr Opthalmol 8: 449–454
43. Kelly TM, Sanborn GE, Haug PJ, Edwards CQ (1982) Effect of insulin infusion pumps use in diabetic retinopathy. Arch Ophthalmol 102: 1156–1159
44. White NH, Waltman SR, Krupin T, Santiago JV (1982) Reversal of abnormalities in ocular fluorophotometry in insulin-dependent diabetes after five to nine months of improved metabolic control. Diabetes 31: 80–85
45. Friberg TR, Rosenstock J, Sanborn G, Vaghefi A, Raskin P (1985) The effect of long-term near normal glycemic control on mild diabetic retinopathy. Ophthalmology 92: 1055–1058
46. Bell PM, Hayes JR, Hadden DR, Archer DB (1985) The effect of plasma glucose control by continuous subcutaneous insulin infusion on conventional therapy on retinal morphology and urinary albumin excretion. Diabete Metab 11: 254–261
47. Unger RH (1982) Meticulous control of diabetes: benefits, risks, and precautions. Diabetes 31: 479–483
48. Eschwege E, Job D, Guyot-Argenton C, Aubry JP, Tchobroutsky G (1979) Delayed progression of diabetic retinopathy by divided insulin administration: a further follow-up. Diabetologia 16: 13–15
49. Steno Study Group (1982) Effect of six months of strict metabolic control on eye and kidney function in insulin-dependent diabetics with background retinopathy. Lancet i: 121–124
50. Lauritzen T, Frost-Larsen K, Larsen HW, Deckert T and the Steno Study Group (1985) Two-year experience with continuous subcutaneous insulin infusion in relation to retinopathy and neuropathy. Diabetes 34 (Suppl 3) 74–79
51. The Kroc Collaborative Study Group (1984) Blood glucose control and the evolution of diabetic retinopathy and albuminuria. N Engl J Med 311: 365–372
52. Brinchmann-Hansen O, Dahl-Jorgensen K, Hanssen KF, Sandvik L, and the Oslo Study Group (1985) Effects of intensified insulin treatment on various lesions of diabetic retinopathy. Am J Ophthalmol 100: 644–653
53. Beck-Nielsen H, Ricklsen B, Mogensen CE, Olsen T, Ehlers N, Nielsen CB, Charles P (1985) Effect of insulin pump treatment for one year on renal function and retinal morphology in patients with IDDM. Diabetes Care 8: 585–589
54. Crepaldi G (1986) Metabolic control and diabetic retinopathy. Italian National Research Study. One year report. Diabetologia 29: 530 A
55. The DCCT Research Group (1986) The Diabetic Control and Complications Trial (DCCT). Design and methodologic considerations for the feasibility phase. Diabetes 35: 530–545

Diabetic Complications: Early Diagnosis and Treatment
Edited by D. Andreani, G. Crepaldi, U. Di Mario and G. Pozza


CHAPTER 8

# *Methods to Quantify Diabetic Retinopathy: Structural and Functional*

G. H. BRESNICK
*Department of Ophthalmology, University of Wisconsin, Madison, Wisconsin, USA*

The ability to quantify the severity of diabetic retinopathy in a reliable and reproducible fashion is essential to performing accurate studies of the epidemiology, natural course, and therapeutic response of the disease. Measures of the severity of retinopathy can be divided into *morphologic* (i.e. structural changes in the retinal blood vessels and surrounding retinal tissue) and *functional*. The latter can be subdivided further into functional abnormalities of the retinal vessels and functional derangement of the visual process.

In the morphologic area, significant advances in classifying diabetic retinopathy and grading its severity according to a standard fundus photography protocol have emerged in the past 15 years (1–3). This has provided a 'common language' that has facilitated pooling of data from multicenter collaborative clinical trials (4, 5), comparison of results from different clinical trials performed at different times, and completion of large-scale epidemiologic surveys (6, 7). More recent has been the development of a standard protocol and grading system for classifying diabetic retinopathy according to fluorescein angiographic findings (3).

A wide variety of visual function abnormalities have been found in diabetic retinopathy. These visual functions, which include visual acuity, color vision, perimetry and contrast sensitivity, lend themselves well to quantification. In addition, electrophysiology, especially electroretinography (ERG), has been found useful both as a measure of the severity of retinal functional abnormality, as well as a predictor of the progression of retinopathy (8, 9).

In the area of vascular physiology, permeability abnormalities of the blood–retina barrier have been quantified with a technique called vitreous fluorophotometry (10). In addition, hemodynamic abnormalities have been described using laser doppler velocimetry (11, 12) and other methods to measure blood flow (13). These techniques will be discussed elsewhere in this volume.

## MORPHOLOGIC ABNORMALITIES

### Background

Diabetic retinopathy is usually classified into a non-proliferative and proliferative stage. Non-proliferative retinopathy (NPDR) refers to the *intraretinal* abnormalities, including microaneurysms, dilated retinal capillaries, retinal hemorrhages, cotton-wool spots (ischemic infarcts), hard exudates and retinal edema. These morphologic changes can be understood in terms of two basic underlying pathophysiologic processes: retinal vessel closure and abnormal retinal vessel permeability.

Retinal capillary closure occurs at a relatively early stage of retinopathy, and microaneurysms (saccular capillary dilations) tend to develop adjacent to areas of capillary non-perfusion. Thus microaneurysm formation may be a response to local tissue hypoxia. Similarly, dilated intraretinal capillary segments occur in areas of capillary non-perfusion. These abnormally tortuous vessels have been termed intraretinal microvascular abnormalities (IRMA) and may represent both dilation of pre-existing retinal capillaries as well as intraretinal new vessel formation. A more profound degree of retinal ischemia occurs when precapillary arterioles close and produce ischemic infarcts of the nerve fiber layer of the retina (cottonwool spots), and in some cases hemorrhagic infarcts (large, dark blot hemorrhages). Focally dilated beaded veins may develop adjacent to such areas of arteriolar closure and cottonwool spot formation.

Permeability abnormalities of the retinal vessels can lead to retinal edema (thickening of the retina with extracellular fluid) and to hard exudate formation (extracellular lipoprotein deposition) in the plexiform layers of the retina. If the edema or exudate is located in the central retina, macular edema with decreased visual acuity and other abnormal central visual functions develop.

Proliferative diabetic retinopathy (PDR) consists of proliferation of fibrovascular and glial tissue in front of the retina, a process thought to be a response to underlying retinal ischemia. Preretinal new vessels can cause preretinal and vitreous hemorrhage. In addition, the fibrous and glial tissue may shrink and cause elevation of the new vessels, detachment of the vitreous, tractional detachment of the retina or distortion and displacement of the retina due to dragging.

### Classification of Diabetic Retinopathy by Color Fundus Photographic Criteria

A detailed classification of diabetic retinopathy was originally developed for a collaborative clinical trial of photocoagulation for diabetic retinopathy, known as the Diabetic Retinopathy Study (DRS) (2). The classification was modified from an earlier classification proposed at an international symposium on diabetic retinopathy, the Airlie House Symposium held in 1969 (1). Seven standard photographic fields were defined and a grading system was based on the quantitative evaluation of certain lesions in stereo color fundus photographs of the seven fields. A further modification of this system has been developed for a subsequent collaborative trial, the Early Treatment Diabetic Retinopathy Study (ETDRS); this system allows a finer grading scale for certain types of lesions (3).

The ETDRS system grades the severity of the following retinal lesions in comparison with a set of standard photographs: microaneurysms, retinal hemorrhages, IRMA, hard exudates, soft exudates, venous abnormalities (beading, focal narrowing, venous loops and reduplications), venous sheathing, and arteriovenous nicking. In addition, the following proliferative abnormalities are graded: new vessels (NV) (subdivided into NV on the optic disc (NVD) and NV elsewhere), fibrous proliferation, retinal elevation, and preretinal and vitreous hemorrhage. In the central photographic field, the macula is evaluated for the extent of edema and hard exudate formation. Other macular abnormalities such as distortion from tension lines, pigmentary changes, dragging of the macular, and macular scar formation are also evaluated.

The details of this rather complex grading system can be obtained through the ETDRS Coordinating Center (3). A method of summarizing the overall severity of diabetic retinopathy into seven levels based on a compilation of the severity of individual lesions has been described, and has proven useful in epidemiologic and other descriptive studies (6, 7). This has been published for the earlier DRS grading system (14). An abbreviated form is shown in Table 1.

Table 1. Definition of retinopathy levels (14)

| | |
|---|---|
| Level 1: | No retinopathy |
| Level 2: | Microaneurysms (one or more) only |
| Level 3: | Microaneurysms and one or more of the following: retinal hemorrhages, but total of hemorrhages and microaneurysms (H/Ma) less than Standard Photo 2A*; hard exudates (HE) $<$ Standard Photo 3*; soft exudates (SE) questionably present; intraretinal microvascular abnormalities (IRMA) questionably present; venous beading (VB) questionably present or venous focal narrowing or loops definitely present |
| Level 4: | Microaneurysms and one or more of the following, but definition of Level 5 not met: H/Ma $\geqslant$ Standard Photo 2A; HE $\geqslant$ Standard Photo 3*; SE definitely present; IRMA definitely present; VB definitely present |
| Level 5: | In fields 4 to 7 only, any three of the following: H/MA $\geqslant$ Standard Photo 2A* in at least one field; SE definitely present in $\geqslant$ 2 fields; VB definitely present in $\geqslant$ 2 fields; or IRMA Present in 4 fields and $\geqslant$ Standard Photo 8A* in $\geqslant$ 2 fields |
| Level 6: | New vessels and/or fibrous proliferations (disc or elsewhere) less than DRS High Risk Characteristics (4) |
| Level 7: | New vessels and/or fibrous proliferations equal to or greater than DRS High Risk Characteristics (4) |

* The Standard Photos refer to a set of Standard Photographs used at the University of Wisconsin Fundus Photograph Reading Center, 610 N. Walnut St., PO Box 5240, Madison, Wisconsin 53705, USA.

### Classification of Diabetic Retinopathy by Fluorescein Angiographic Criteria

A standardized fluorescein angiographic protocol and grading system has also been developed for the ETDRS (3). The photographic fields comprise early phase photographs of a 30 degree field centered temporal to the center of the macula and a later phase field centered nasal to the disc. (Details are found in the ETDRS manual (3).)

The severity of individual lesions is again graded in comparison with a set of standard angiographic phtographs. The most important lesions are graded as follows: capillary non-perfusion, fluorescein leakage, and arteriolar changes (narrowing, occlusion and staining). A quantification of the approximate retinal area of non-perfusion and leakage based on this grading system has been used in a study relating angiographic abnormalities to color vision findings in diabetic retinopathy (15). A summary method to classify eyes into levels according to the severity of angiographic lesions is expected from ETDRS in the near future.

Fluorescein angiography that includes more of the peripheral fundus has been shown to detect capillary non-perfusion that would have been underestimated with conventional posterior angiographic fields alone (16, 17). By using wide-angle photography (45° to 60°) over multiple fields, a composite montage covering up to 130° of the fundus is obtained. The fundus is subdivided into sectors by radial lines and concentric circles such that 418 fundus segments are individually graded. Each segment is graded for severity of non-perfusion. A topographical map of the fundus by severity of non-perfusion can then be plotted using a computer-graphics program. Applying this technique the authors have found midperipheral capillary non-perfusion with relatively little posterior pole non-perfusion in approximately 60% of the eyes examined. ('Midperipheral' was defined as a zone less than 5 disc diameters from the optic disc, but beyond the usual central fields.) Eyes with midperipheral or a combination of midperipheral and central (generalized) capillary non-perfusion were at high risk to develop neovascularization. The distribution and severity of non-perfusion thus carries important prognostic significance. Good quality angiography in these more peripheral areas is easier to achieve in patients with darkly pigmented fundi (as in this study from Japan); it is difficult to achieve in lightly pigmented individuals. Nonetheless, it should be recognized that studies utilizing angiography not including the midperipheral area are likely to underestimate substantially the degree of non-perfusion.

## VISUAL FUNCTIONAL ABNORMALITIES

Quantification of visual functional abnormalities in diabetic retinopathy is important for several reasons:

1. To evaluate the extent of visual disability caused by the vascular lesions.
2. To look for functional abnormalities that might predict the future progression of vascular retinopathy.

3. To detect early functional changes that might precede clinically visible retinopathy.

It may be useful to consider diabetic retinopathy as a neurosensory disorder as well as a vasculopathy; indeed, some of the visual functional abnormalities may be due directly to the systemic metabolic consequences of diabetes mellitus in addition to being caused by the vascular lesions themselves (9, 18). This is especially the case with the earliest stages of retinopathy in which sensory deficits have been demonstrated prior to the onset of ophthalmoscopically detectable retinopathy.

## Visual Psychophysical Tests

Visual psychophysics is the study of the subjective visual response to a light stimulus. Visual acuity, color vision and perimetry are typical clinical psychophysical tests. Sophisticated techniques have been developed to quantify the stimuli and responses and to reduce their variability; this recommends the tests for inclusion in studies requiring repeated measurements over time. Less complex techniques can provide semiquantitative data that is also useful in certain clinical settings.

### *Color Vision*

Diabetic patients show a color vision defect that increases with the severity of retinopathy, particularly in relation to the degree of macular edema. The color deficiency begins as a disorder of the blue–yellow component of color vision, but includes the red–green system as retinopathy worsens (19). A relatively easy method for detecting the color deficits is a color arrangement test, the Farnsworth D-15 test, which consists of 15 movable caps with different colored paper discs that are to be arranged according to hue. The subject's cap sequence is plotted on a score sheet and errors in arrangement may assume a characteristic distribution for blue–yellow (tritan) as opposed to red–green (protan, deutan) color defects (Figure 1). The test can be made more sensitive for mild color defects by using relatively desaturated colored caps (20). A scoring system has been developed that allows an error score to be calculated according to the degree of cap displacement (21).

A more detailed and time-consuming color test, the Farnsworth–Munsell 100 hue test, uses 85 colored caps, arranged in four boxes, to encompass the visible spectrum with much smaller wavelength steps between caps than in the D-15 test. This tests hue discrimination to a finer degree than the D-15, and also shows characteristic error 'axes' for tritan, protan and deutan defects. A quantitative error score is calculated and the distribution of errors can be plotted on a color-circle graph (Figure 2).

Screening tests for color deficiency, such as pseudoisochromatic plates, can detect color deficits in diabetic patients, but the results are only semiquantitative. The American Optical Hardy–Rand–Rittle (AO-HRR) test can detect tritan defects (but the test is out of print) as can the newer Standard Pseudo-Isochromatic Plate Test

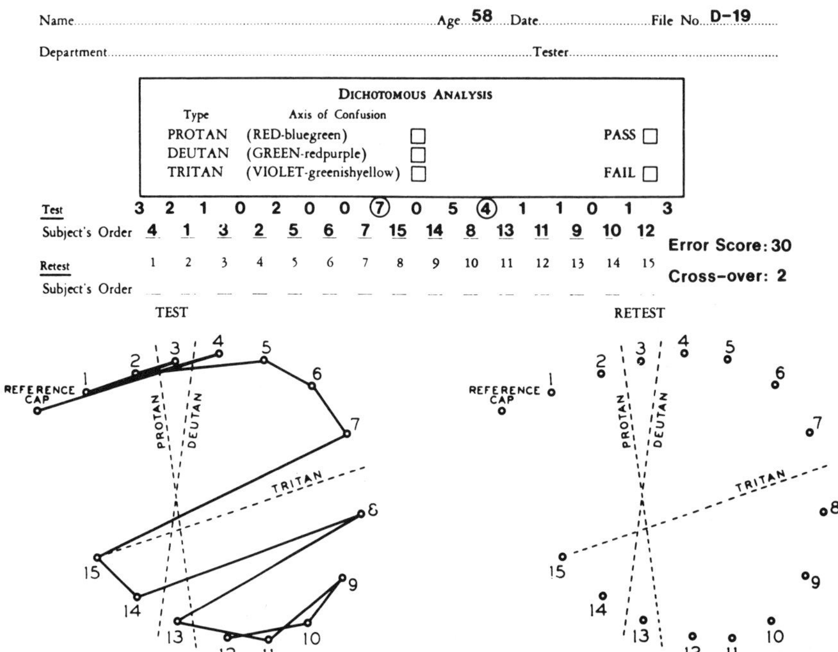


Figure 1. Desaturated Farnsworth D-15 test in a 58-year-old male diabetic patient with proliferative diabetic retinopathy and macular edema. The cap sequence is indicated by connecting the numbers with lines in the order that the patient placed the caps. Cross-over errors resulted in a tritan (blue–yellow) axis. Reproduced with permission from Bresnick GH, Crawford J, Groo A (1984) In: Verriest G (ed) Colour deficiencies VII. Dr W Junk, The Hague, pp 393–405.

(22). The classical Ishihara Pseudo-Isochromatic Plate Test will detect protan/deutan, but not tritan defects. It should be noted that all the color tests mentioned above require special lighting that simulates daylight conditions for accurate results. Special filters for incandescent lights and special fluorescent lights are commercially available for this purpose.

The major findings of color deficiency in diabetic patients using the above and other tests can be summarized as follows:

(1) The extent of color defect correlates with the severity of diabetic retinopathy. Some increases in hue discrimination abnormality occur with progression from non-proliferative to proliferative retinopathy, but the greatest deficits are found in eyes with macular edema (15, 23).

(2) Color deficiency can be demonstrated in some eyes before clinically visible retinopathy appears (19, 24). Reduced sensitivity of the short wavelength sensitive

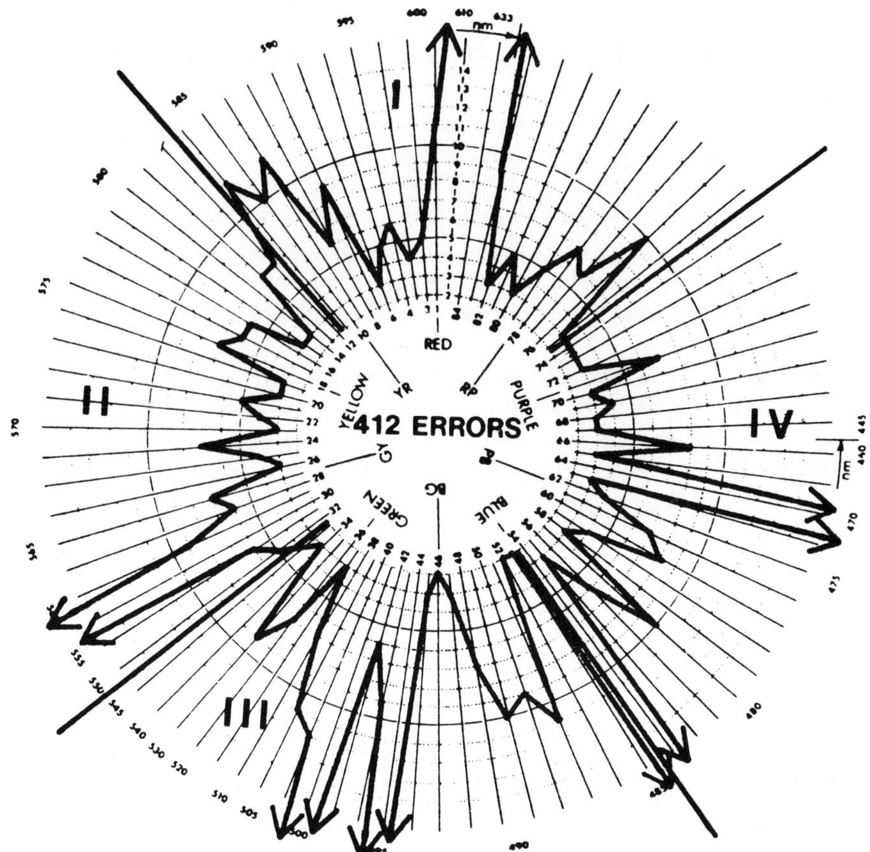


Figure 2. Farnsworth 100 hue test in a 68-year-old male diabetic patient with non-proliferative diabetic retinopathy and macular edema. The error score of 412 is well beyond the normal upper limit (271) for his age. The predominant error axis is vertical, which coincides with a tritan (blue–yellow) axis. Reproduced with permission from Bresnick et al. (1985) Arch Ophthalmol 103: 1317–1324. Copyright 1985, American Medical Association.

(SWS), or blue-cone system is the earliest defect detectable (25). The response of the blue-cone system can be isolated by using a blue test spot on a bright yellow background; the yellow light suppresses the red- and green-cone system, while the dim blue test spot is first detected by the blue-cone system. A simplified version of this test has been developed, and it can detect early color abnormalities in diabetic patients with little or no retinopathy (26, 27).

(3) Colour deficiency may have some predictive value for progression of retinopathy. In a long-term follow-up study of diabetic patients without retinopathy, an abnormal blue–green anomaloscope equation was shown to be a risk factor for the subsequent development of retinopathy (28). (The anomaloscope is a device that measures the

relative mixture of two colored lights used to make a match to a third standard light.) More such longitudinal studies are needed to determine the predictive value of color testing.

(4) If the color deficiency is severe it may interfere with the ability of diabetic patients to perform accurately color-dependent urinary or blood glucose tests (29–31). Since color vision generally deteriorates in dim lighting, some of the difficulty in urinary glucose testing can be overcome with bright lighting (30). Diabetic patients with macular edema, especially older patients who may also have crystalline lens changes that further interfere with color vision, should be monitored for color vision deficiency and for their ability to perform these tests, before using the self-monitored test to adjust insulin dosage.

Since a number of factors such as age, lens changes, and medications can affect color vision, these must be taken into consideration before attributing color deficits to diabetic retinopathy. Age-corrected norms are available for the Farnsworth–Munsell 100 hue test (32). The contribution of the lens (especially yellowing of the nucleus with age) to a color deficit is difficult to measure, but can be estimated by slit-lamp biomicroscopy.

### *Visual Acuity and 'Spatial Vision'*

The ability to read a standard visual acuity chart is still the clinical mainstay for measuring central retinal and higher order visual function. Improvements have been made in the standard Snellen Visual Acuity Charts that make quantification of visual acuity for the purpose of clinical studies more accurate (33). The chart used by the ETDRS has 5 letters on every line, a regular progression of letter size on each successive line, and spacing between adjacent lines that is proportional to the letter size of the line. One advantage of such a chart is that a worsening in acuity of 3 lines (15 letters), regardless of the starting acuity, represents a doubling of the visual angle, and conversely an improvement in acuity of 3 lines is a halving of the visual angle. One can also give the patient credit for every letter read correctly, and calculate a visual acuity score that lends itself to statistical analysis. Such an approach was used in an ETDRS report demonstrating that focal argon laser photocoagulation has a beneficial effect on clinically significant macular edema (5).

Related to visual acuity is the measurement of spatial contrast sensitivity: for example, the determination of the sensitivity of the visual system to alternate grey and white stripes of different spatial frequencies. In the usual test, vertical stripes varying in contrast between dark and light stripes in a sinusoidal fashion are displayed on a video terminal, the least contrast at which the dark and light stripes can be distinguished being called the threshold. When the threshold for different widths of stripes (different spatial frequencies) is determined in the normal observer a parabolic function with maximum sensitivity at about 3 cycles per degree, and a decrease in sensitivity at higher and lower spatial frequencies are found (34) (Figure 3). Contrast sensitivity at different spatial frequencies is a more sensitive test to detect early defects in spatial vision than is conventional visual acuity testing which uses maximum contrast letters. A recent study (34) demonstrated reduced contrast sensitivity at high spatial frequencies (i.e. narrow, closely packed stripes) to be an early functional deficit in non-insulin-dependent diabetic patients with no retinopathy, and reduced contrast sensitivity across all spatial frequencies in non-insulin-dependent diabetic patients with non-proliferative retinopathy (NPDR); standard visual acuity test results were normal in most of these patients (Figure 2). Similar findings have been reported in several other studies (35–37).

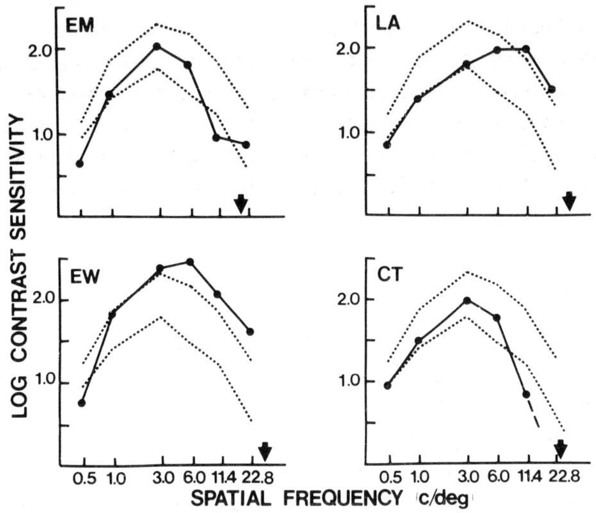


Figure 3. Monocular contrast sensitivity functions in two patients with non-insulin-dependent diabetes mellitus (NIDDM) without retinopathy (patients LA and CT) and two patients with NIDDM and background retinopathy (patients EM and EW). For each patient, upper broken line indicates mean contrast sensitivity of age-matched normal subjects; lower broken line, 95% confidence limit; arrow, spatial frequency equivalent of each patient's Snellen acuity. Reproduced with permission from Sokol et al. (1985) Arch Ophthalmol 103: 51–54. Copyright 1985, American Medical Association.

### *Dark Adaptation*

Delayed adaptation of the cone system following exposure to a bright light using a technique called nyctometry has been reported in diabetic patients. Abnormality in the test helped select patients with NPDR at high risk to develop PDR (38). Improved nyctometry results also followed the institution of strict diabetes control with continuous subcutaneous insulin infusion even at a time when retinal vascular lesions showed a slight worsening (39). Thus the measure of visual function (nyctometry) and the measure of vascular retinopathy (retina microaneurysms, hemorrhages, and cottonwool spots) can sometimes give conflicting information (see also ERG oscillatory potentials described below).

### *Perimetry*

The measurement of the visual field has also been used to quantify functional deficits in diabetic retinopathy. This has become clinically more feasible with the development of commercially available automated perimeters. With these instruments the 'increment threshold' can be determined fairly rapidly at a number of loci in the visual field with a computerized control of the location and brightness of the test spot. (The term 'increment threshold' refers to the minimal amount of light needed in a test spot just to detect the spot against a diffuse light background.) The strategy of the automated perimeter is to present test spots that are slightly above expected threshold at various loci in the visual field, then to reduce the brightness until it is not seen, and finally to increase the brightness until it is just seen again (threshold). The sequence of location of test spots is varied in an irregular fashion.

Using automated perimetry several groups have demonstrated elevated perimetric thresholds that correlate with sites of angiographic abnormalities (capillary non-perfusion and fluorescein leakage) in the corresponding retinal location (40, 41). Since good quality angiography in the midperipheral fundus can be difficult to achieve, perimetry may offer a non-invasive alternative to evaluating both the posterior and the midperipheral fundus in diabetic patients. It may also be possible to use automated perimetry to study the blue-cone system in diabetes (see color vision discussion above) by employing a blue test target on a bright yellow background (42), rather than the conventional white test spot on a white background. If one of the earliest visual functional deficits occurs in the blue-cone system in diabetes, 'blue-cone perimetry' should be a sensitive way to detect this abnormality.

## Electrophysiologic Tests

The electroretinogram (ERG) is a recording of the electrical response of the retina to a light stimulus. It is measured clinically at the cornea using corneal contact lens electrodes. The normal ERG shows an initial negative a-wave, derived from the photoreceptor cells (rods and cones), followed by a positive b-wave, which originates in the inner nuclear layer of the retina, probably from the Müller (glial) cells, but requires intact bipolar cells for its generation. Since the inner retina is supplied by the retinal circulation and the outer retina (photoreceptors) is indirectly nourished by the choroidal circulation across the retinal pigment epithelium, it is not surprising that retinal vascular disorders such as diabetic retinopathy affect the b-wave in preference to the a-wave. Reduced b-wave amplitudes are found in the more advanced proliferative stages of diabetic retinopathy (43, 44), but usually not in the non-proliferative phase.

More sensitive than b-wave amplitude changes is reduction in the amplitudes of the oscillatory potentials (OP) of the ERG, which is found in some eyes with NPDR; more severe reduction or absence of OP is found in most eyes with PDR. OP are small wavelets on the ascending limb of the b-wave with a more rapid frequency (100–160 Hz) than the slower a- and b-waves (less that 25 Hz) (Figure 4). OP are also sensitive to circulatory abnormalities of the retina in conditions other than diabetic retinopathy, such as retinal vein occlusion and carotid artery stenosis with reduced retinal perfusion (45).

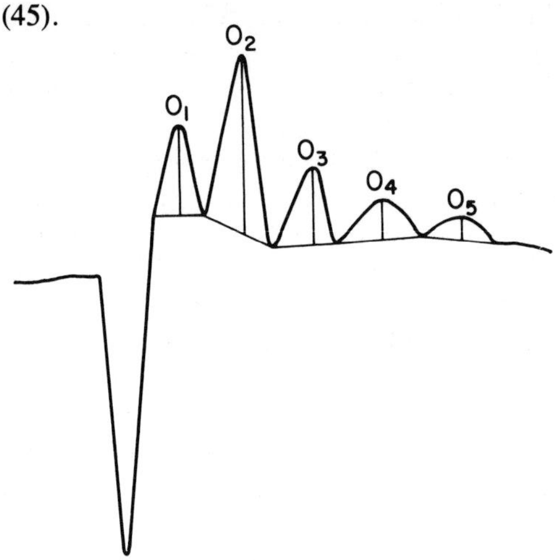

Figure 4. Diagram of measurement technique for oscillatory potential (OP) amplitudes. Amplitude of the OP nodes ($O_1$, $O_2$, $O_3$, $O_4$, $O_5$) is determined by connecting adjacent troughs and measuring height from OP peak to line so drawn. Summed OP amplitude is calculated by adding individual OP amplitudes. Reproduced with permission, from Bresnick et al. (1984) Arch Ophthalmol 102: 1307–1311. Copyright 1984, American Medical Association.

Of greater interest is the finding that reduced OP amplitudes can identify eyes with NPDR that are at high risk to develop PDR (46–48) (Figure 5). The reduction in amplitude of OP correlates with the extent of capillary non-perfusion and fluorescein leakage on angiography. It is likely, therefore, that the value of OP in predicting progression of retinopathy to PDR rests in the ability of the ERG to detect capillary non-perfusion and/or leakage. (Retinal ischemia is thought to be the stimulus for new vessel growth in diabetic retinopathy and other proliferative retinopathies.)

Since ERG measures the mass response of the retina to light, it is able to detect diffuse retinal disease, and is therefore an effective non-invasive tool to quantify the extent of retinal vascular abnormality, and perhaps also to detect abnormalities of the retina due to the metabolic consequences of diabetes. The finding of improved oscillatory potential amplitudes following tightening of diabetes control with continuous subcutaneous insulin infusion, at a time when focal vascular lesions showed some worsening, suggests again that the overall function of the retina was improving diffusely, although local areas of the retina may have temporarily deteriorated (49–51).

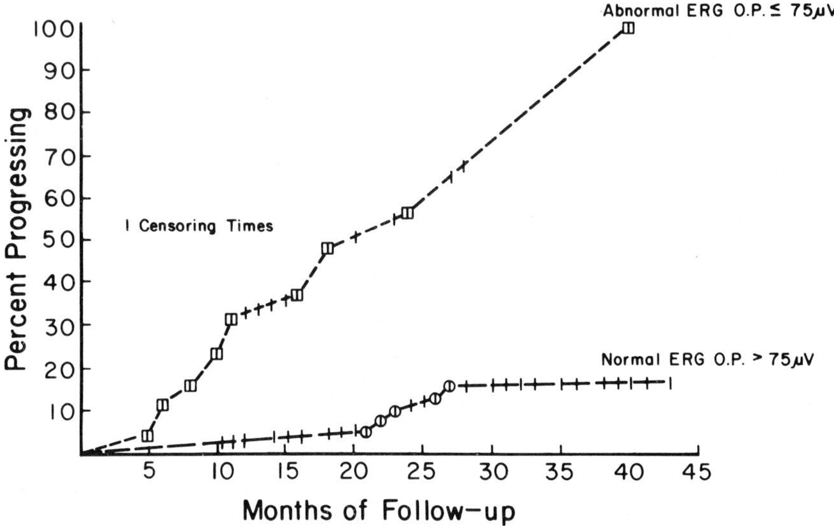


Figure 5. Cumulative percentage of eyes progressing to severe proliferative diabetic retinopathy (PDR) (DRS high risk characteristics), comparing eyes with abnormal and normal oscillatory potential (OP) amplitudes. ERG indicates electroretinographic. Values above a cut-point of 75 $\mu$V were considered normal; values at or below 75 $\mu$V were considered abnormal. The rate of developing PDR was much higher in eyes with abnormal OP amplitudes. Reproduced with permission, from Bresnick et al. (1984) Arch Ophthalmol 102: 1307–1311. Copyright 1984, American Medical Association.

## SUMMARY

In summary, diabetic retinopathy can be classified and quantified both by morphologic and by functional measurements. The use of standardized methods of measurement facilitates the pooling of data from multicenter collaborative trials. In the earlier stages of retinopathy or even before clinically detectable morphologic changes, abnormalities in visual function can be detected and measured. These functional abnormalities may be useful parameters to follow as indicators of the response to systemic therapy for diabetes and its complications. The functional abnormalities have also been shown to predict in some instances the future progression of morphologic retinal disease.

## REFERENCES

1. Davis MD, Norton EWD, Myers FL (1968) Airlie classification of diabetic retinopathy. In: Goldberg MF, Fine SL (eds) Symposium on the treatment of diabetic retinopathy. Public Health Service Publication No. 1890, Washington, DC

2. Diabetic Retinopathy Study Research Group (1981) Report 7. A modification of the Airlie House Classification of diabetic retinopathy. Invest Ophthalmol Vis Sci 21: 210–226
3. Early Treatment Diabetic Retinopathy Study—Manual of operations. University of Maryland School of Medicine, Department of Epidemiology and Preventative Medicine, Division of Clinical Investigation, 600 Wyndhurst Ave., Baltimore, MD 21210, USA
4. Diabetic Retinopathy Research Group (1978) Photocoagulation treatment for proliferative diabetic retinopathy: the second report of Diabetic Retinopathy Study findings. Ophthalmology 85: 82–106
5. The Early Treatment Diabetic Retinopathy Study Research Group (1985) Photocoagulation for diabetic macular edema. Early Treatment Diabetic Retinopathy Study Report 1. Arch Ophthalmology 103: 1796–1806
6. Klein R, Klein BEK, Moss SE, et al. (1984) The Wisconsin Epidemiologic Study of Diabetic Retinopathy. II. Prevalence and risk of diabetic retinopathy when age at diagnosis is less than 30 years. Arch Ophthalmol 102: 520–526
7. Klein R, Klein BEK, Moss SE, et al. (1984) The Wisconsin Epidemiologic Study of Diabetic Retinopathy. III. Prevalence and risk of diabetic retinopathy when age at diagnosis is 30 or more years. Arch Ophthalmol 102: 527–532
8. Bresnick GH (1985) Electroretinography and color vision in diabetes mellitus. Presented at 12th Congress of the International Diabetes Foundation, 'Microvascular and neurological complications of diabetes' Granada, Spain (in press)
9. Bresnick GH (1986) Diabetic retinopathy viewed as a neurosensory disorder. Arch Ophthalmol 104: 989–990
10. Cunha-Vaz JG, Fonseca JR, Abreu JF, Ruas JF (1979) Detection of early retinal changes in diabetes by vitreous fluorophotometry. Diabetes 28: 16–19
11. Riva CE, Grunwald JE, Sinclair SH, et al. (1985) Blood velocity and volumetric flow rate in human retinal vessels. Invest Ophthalmol Vis Sci 26: 1124–1132
12. Grunwald JE, Riva CE, Sinclair SH (1986) Laser doppler velocimetry study of retinal circulation in diabetes mellitus. Arch Ophthalmol 104: 991–996
13. Kohner EM, Hamilton AM, Saunders SJ, et al. (1975) The retinal blood flow in diabetes. Diabetologia 11: 27–33
14. Klein BEK, Davis MD, Segal P, et al. (1984) Diabetic retinopathy: assessment of severity and progression. Ophthalmology 91: 10–17
15. Bresnick GH, Condit RS, Palta M, et al. (1985) Association of hue discrimination loss and diabetic retinopathy. Arch Ophthalmol 103: 1317–1324
16. Shimizu K, Kobayashi Y, Muraoka K (1981) Midperipheral fundus involvement in diabetic retinopathy. Ophthalmology 88: 601–612
17. Niki T, Muraoka K, Shimizu K (1984) Ophthalmology 91: 1431–1439
18. Bresnick GH. Diabetic retinopathy considered as a neurosensory disorder. Results of electroretinography. Front Diabetes 8 (in press)
19. Lakowski R, Aspinall PA, Kinnear PR (1973) Association between color vision losses and diabetes mellitus. Ophthalmol Res 4: 145–149
20. Lanthony P (1978) The desaturated panel D-15. Doc Ophthalmol 46: 185–189
21. Bowman KJ (1982) A method for quantitative scoring of the Farnsworth Panel D-15. Acta Ophtalmol 60: 907–916
22. Tanabe S, Hukami K, Ichikawa H (1984) New pseudoisochromatic plates for acquired color vison defects. Doc Ophthalmol 39: 199–205
23. Begg IS, Lakowski R (1980) A comparison of color vision with other methods of clinical assessment in diabetics with macular edema. In: Verriest G (ed) Color vision deficiencies V, Adam Hilger, Bristol, pp 295–298

24. Roy MS, Gunkel RD, Podgar MJ (1986) Color vision defects in early diabetic retinopathy. Arch Ophthalmol 104: 225–228
25. Zisman F, Adams AJ (1982) Spectral sensitivity of cone mechanisms in juvenile diabetics. Doc Ophthalmol 33: 127–131
26. Huie K, Adams AJ, Schefrin BE (1985) A simple clinical test of blue cone sensitivity. Invest Ophthalmol Vis Sci (Suppl) 26: 215
27. Witkin SR, Bresnick GH, Friedberg M, et al. (1986) Blue cone sensitivity and hue discrimination in diabetic retinopathy. Invest Ophthalmol Vis Sci (Suppl) 27: 308
28. Aspinall PA, Kinnear PR, Duncan LP, Clarke B (1983) Prediction of diabetic retinopathy from clinical variables and color vision data. Diabetes Care 6: 144–148
29. Thompson PG, Howarth F, Taylor H, Levy IS (1979) Defective color vision in diabetics: a hazard to management. Br Med J i: 859–860
30. Bresnick GH, Groo A, Palta M, et al. (1984) Urinary glucose testing inaccuracies among diabetic patients: effect of acquired color vision deficiency caused by diabetic retinopathy. Arch Ophthalmol 102: 1489–1496
31. Zisman F, Adams AJ, Linfoot J, et al. (1984) Diabetic blood glucose monitoring: influence of color deficiencies. Invest Ophthalmol Vis Sci 25 (Suppl): 178
32. Verriest G, Van Laethem J, Uvijls A (1982) A new assessment of the normal ranges of the Farnsworth–Munsell 100-hue test scores. Am J Ophthalmol 93: 635–642
33. Ferris FL, Kassoff A, Bresnick GH, et al. (1982) New visual acuity charts for clinical research. Am J Ophthalmol 94: 91–96
34. Sokol S, Moskowitz A, Skarf B, et al. (1985) Contrast sensitivity in diabetics with and without background retinopathy. Arch Ophthalmol 103: 51–54
35. Shafour M, Foulds WS, Allan D, et al. (1982) Contrast sensitivity in diabetic subjects with and without retinopathy. Br J Ophthalmol 66: 492–495
36. Hyvarinen L, Laurinen P, Rovamo J (1983) Contrast sensitivity in evaluation of visual impairment due to diabetes. Acta Ophthalmol 61: 94–101
37. Hirsch J, Puklin JE (1983) Reduced contrast sensitivity may precede clinically observable retinopathy in type 1 diabetes. In Henkind P (ed) Acta XXIV International Congress of Ophthalmology. Lippincott, San Francisco, New York, pp 719–724
38. Frost-Larsen K, Larsen HW (1983) Nyctometry: a new screening method for selection of patients with simple diabetic retinopathy who are at risk of developing proliferative retinopathy. Acta Ophthalmol 353–361
39. Frost-Larsen K, Larsen HW, Simonsen SE (1980) Oscillatory potential and nyctometry in insulin-dependent diabetics., Acta Ophthalmol 58: 879–888
40. Federman JL, Lloyd J (1984) Automated static perimetry to evaluate diabetic retinopathy. Trans Am Ophthalmol Soc 82: 358–370
41. Bell JA, Feldon SE (1984) Retinal microangiopathy. Correlation of OCTOPUS perimetry with fluorescein angiography. Arch Ophthalmol 102: 1294–1298
42. Sample PA, Weinreb RN, Boynton RM (1986) Blue-on yellow color perimetry and glaucoma assessment. Invest Ophthalmol Vis Sci (Suppl) 27: 159
43. Karpe G, Kornerup T, Wulfing B (1958) The clinical electroretinogram. VIII. The electroretinogram in diabetic retinopathy. Acta Ophthalmol 36: 281–291
44. Francois J, Derouck A (1954) L'electroretinographie dans la retinopathie diabetique et dans la retinopathie hypertensive. Acta Ophthalmol 32: 391–404
45. Speros P, Price J (1981) Oscillatory potentials. History, techniques and potential use in the evaluation of disturbances of retinal circulation. Survey Ophthalmol 25: 237–252
46. Simonsen SE (1975) Prognostic value of ERG (oscillatory potential) in juvenile diabetics. Acta Ophthalmol Suppl 123: 223–224
47. Simonsen SE (1981) The value of the oscillatory potential in selective juvenile diabetics at risk of developing proliferative retinopathy. Meta Pediatr Ophthalmol 5: 55–61

48. Bresnick GH, Korth K, Groo A, Palta M (1984) Electroretinographic oscillatory potentials predict progression of diabetic retinopathy. Arch Ophthalmol 102: 1307–1311
49. Bresnick GH, Palta M: Oscillatory potential amplitudes: relation to severity of diabetic retinopathy. Submitted for publication
50. Steno Study Group (1982) Effect of 6 months of strict metabolic control on eye and kidney function in insulin-dependent diabetics with background retinopathy. Lancet i: 121–124
51. Lauritzen T, et al., and the Steno Study Group (1983) Effect of 1 year of near-normal blood glucose. Lancet i: 200-204

Diabetic Complications: Early Diagnosis and Treatment
Edited by D. Andreani, G. Crepaldi, U. Di Mario and G. Pozza


CHAPTER 9

# *Diabetic Macular Edema: Diagnosis and Treatment*

J. G. Cunha-Vaz
*Clinica Oftalmologica, University Hospital, Coimbra, Portugal*

Diabetic macular edema is the largest cause of visual acuity reduction in diabetes (1). It affects central vision from the early stages of retinopathy and is extremely frequent, particularly in older Type 2 diabetic patients. Its role in the process of vision loss in diabetic patients and its occurrence in the evolution of retinopathy is being increasingly recognized.

In this chapter I will attempt to characterize and define diabetic macular edema, list and compare the available methods of assessment, discuss the possible pathophysiological mechanisms involved and, finally, outline its treatment.

## DEFINITION

Macular edema consists of an accumulation of fluid in the retinal layers around the fovea, causing a thickening of the retina (2).

The pathological picture of this condition is an accumulation of edema fluid in the outer plexiform (Henle's) and inner nuclear layers of the retina, centred around the fovea. There is, usually, evidence of leakage of fluorescein from the small paramacular capillaries with accumulation of fluorescein.

Macular edema is a non-specific sign of ocular disease, not a specific entity. It should be viewed as a special type of macular response to disease. It has been described in a variety of ocular situations such as uveitis, trauma, after intraocular surgery, vascular retinopathies, hereditary dystrophies such as retinitis pigmentosa, etc.

It is to be realized that diabetic macular edema is only one of the alterations that may occur in the macula and is not synonymous with diabetic maculopathy.

Diabetic maculopathy includes all the pathological alterations that may affect the macula in diabetes, such as vitreous traction with macular 'dragging' or detachment, macular ischemia due to non-perfusion of the perifoveal capillaries, intra- or preretinal hemorrhages in the macula and macular hole formation, aside from diabetic macular edema.

In this chapter, I will discuss only diabetic macular edema as an entity, occurring in its pure form more frequently in the earlier stages of diabetic retinopathy.

## DIAGNOSIS

The clinical evaluation of macular edema is difficult. Documentation of thickening of the retina and leakage of fluorescein or other tracer, the two major indicators of macular edema, is needed to establish a diagnosis. Unfortunately, the clinical methods available to assess the presence of abnormal fluid in the macula have limited sensitivity. Furthermore, they generally demonstrate only one component of the picture, either thickening or leakage.

Direct and indirect ophthalmoscopy may reveal nothing but an alteration of the foveal reflexes. Stereo slit-lamp microscopy may demonstrate changes in retinal volume in the macular area, namely, thickening and cystoid space formation. This thickening is well documented by stereo fundus photography and both slit-lamp examination and fundus photography play a fundamental role in the diagnosis of diabetic macular edema. The limitations of the photographic method are, however, well demonstrated by the grading, proposed by the Early Treatment Diabetic Retinopathy Study (ETDRS) to analyse retinal thickening (3).

Hard exudates are also detected by fundus photographs, and, although they are an indicator of previous leakage, the actual significance of their presence at a certain point of time in the fundus is not clear.

Fluorescein angiography permits a dynamic evaluation of local circulatory disturbances and the distribution of the edema fluid in the region. It can demonstrate the characteristic cystoid spaces and gives a gross estimation of blood–retina barrier permeability (leakage). It is, however, only semiquantitative and its reproducibility depends on the variable quality of the angiograms.

Finally, vitreous fluorophotometry appears to be the only available method that can quantify, in a reproducible manner, one of the major alterations occurring in diabetic macular edema: the alteration of the blood–retina barrier.

Several investigators have addressed the question of the appropriate definition of macular edema. The major problem has been associated with the methods available to document thickening. Situations of mild macular edema are excluded due to the difficulty of distinguishing a slightly thickened retina from a normal retina. Similarly, leakage detected with more sensitive methods is frequently observed in maculas that apparently are not thickened (1).

In the ETDRS (4) it was agreed that a set of characteristics, when present, would indicate 'clinically significant macular edema':

1. Retinal thickening (as seen either by slit-lamp biomicroscopy or by stereo fundus photography) at or within 500 $\mu$m of the centre of the macula;

2. Hard exudates at or within 500 $\mu$m of the centre of the macula, if associated with thickening of adjacent retina (no residual hard exudates remaining after the disappearance of retinal thickening); or
3. A zone, or zones, of retinal thickening one disc diameter or larger, any part of which is within one disc diameter of the centre of the macula.

This definition is useful because it gives a reference for comparison between studies, particularly in a subject that is difficult to characterize clinically.

Recently, I have performed a cross-sectional study of 34 diabetic patients with clinically significant macular edema, as defined by ETDRS criteria, in order to compare the different methods of clinical assessment (5).

Patients underwent visual acuity testing, stereo fundus photography (graded for retinal thickening and hard exudates), fluorescein angiography (evaluated for macular leakage and the outline of the foveal avascular zone (FAZ)) and vitreous fluorophotometry (whereby penetration ratios were calculated).

The vitreous fluorophotometry penetration ratio provided the highest single correlation with visual acuity (correlation coefficient $r = 0.69$, $p = 0.0001$). The next highest correlations with visual acuity were found with age ($r = 0.45$, $p = 0.008$) and FAZ grading ($r = 0.43$, $p = 0.014$). Multivariate regression confirmed that these three variables together gave the best model for prediction of visual acuity. Lesser correlations with visual acuity were obtained with angiographic leakage ($r = 0.37$, $p = 0.033$) and fundus photography grading (NS).

Table 1.

| | Visual acuity | Duration | VFPR | Thickening field (No. 2) | Leakage (FA) | FAZ (FA) |
|---|---|---|---|---|---|---|
| Visual acuity | *1.0 (0.0) | | | | | |
| Duration | NS | 1.0 (0.0) | | | | |
| VFPR | 0.69 (0.0001) | NS | 1.0 (0.0) | | | |
| Thickening field (No. 2) | NS | NS | 0.39 (0.023) | 1.0 (0.0) | | |
| Leakage (FA) | 0.37 (0.033) | NS | 0.44 (0.009) | 0.64 (0.0001) | 1.0 (0.0) | |
| FAZ (FA) | 0.43 (0.014) | NS | NS | NS | NS | 1.0 (0.0) |

* Values are $r$ ($P$): NS indicates not significant.
VFPR = vitreous fluorophotometry penetration ratio.
FAZ = foveal avascular zone.
FA = fluorescein angiography.

This study showed that retinal thickening (criteria for eligibility as documented by stereo fundus photography) correlates in a statistically significant manner with the alteration of the blood–retina barrier measured by vitreous fluorophotometry and leakage grading on fluorescein angiography.

All three of these variables appear clearly interrelated (Table 1). Vitreous fluorophotometry appears in this study to be the most sensitive and reliable method. In diabetic patients with macular edema the predictability of visual acuity increases to 69% when fluorophotometry replaces the grading of the angiographic leakage.

Regarding the different methods of examination available, fundus photography appears to have very limited value when applied to macular edema studies. Fluorescein angiography provides more useful information than fundus photography, but vitreous fluorophotometry appears to offer the only quantifiable, sensitive outcome variable of diabetic macular edema presently available. The fluorescein penetration ratio measures the alteration of the blood–retina barrier and our findings show that in diabetic macular edema this ratio correlates better with visual acuity than any other method or grading system.

## NATURAL COURSE

Diabetic macular edema is frequently a chronic process resulting from multiple leaking points. It may, however, spontaneously resolve, particularly in the early stages of retinopathy.

The typical picture presents one or more 'leakage' sites associated with thickening of the retina and deposition of intraretinal lipid exudates. Fluid accumulation appears to be particularly pronounced in the macula, around the fovea, apparently because of the larger potential extravascular spaces created by the obliquely running nerve fibres in the Henle layer.

Another characteristic appearance of localized leakage and edema is the circinate ring. Generalized diffuse leakage from the capillary bed with thickening of the macula is another common occurrence.

Visual acuity decreases in association with macular edema and this degeneration generally worsens as the process is repeated and becomes chronic. Loss of vision, however, appears to be relatively slow. It has been reported that 2 years are necessary for half of the patients with diabetic macular edema in a particular study to lose two or more lines of vision (6).

## PATHOPHYSIOLOGY

In the retina, fluid movement between the blood and the retina is restricted by the blood–retina barrier. This selective barrier is located fundamentally at two levels: chorioepithelial interface and retinal vessels.

The main structures involved are the retinal pigment epithelium and the endothelial membrane of the retinal vessels. These structures are involved in both the filtration and the removal of fluid from the retinal tissue. It is this equilibrium between filtration and removal that keeps the retina dry. With regard to filtration and following the reasoning expressed by Rapoport (7) concerning the blood–brain barrier, the 'force' $F$ driving fluid across the retinal vessels is the result of a hydrostatic pressure difference $\Delta P$ ($P$ plasma $-$ $P$ tissue) and an effective osmotic pressure difference $\sigma\Delta\pi$ ($\pi$ plasma $-$ $\pi$ tissue). This equation is, therefore $F = Lp\ (\Delta P = \sigma\Delta\pi)$ where $Lp$ is the 'membrane permeability' and an osmotic reflection coefficient.

In diabetic retinopathy an increased $F$ with $\sigma$ resulting in abnormal collection of fluid in the retina (edema) may be associated with:

1. Increased hydrostatic pressure difference, due to increased blood pressure, loss of autoregulation or decreased tissue compliance (2).
2. Decreased osmotic pressure difference most probably resulting from possible increase in tissue osmotic pressure.
3. Increased 'membrane permeability' due to an alteration of the blood–retina barrier.

There is, indeed, a wealth of evidence supporting the occurrence of these mechanisms in the retina in diabetes. An alteration of the blood–retina barrier has been repeatedly found to be one of the earliest changes known to occur in the diabetic retina (8, 9). Loss of autoregulation of the retinal vasculature, possibly associated with pericyte damage, has also frequently been invoked to explain the observation of early vasodilation (10).

Hypertension is a well-known associate of diabetes. Finally, an increase in tissue osmotic pressure, although never directly demonstrated, is a likely result of the disordered carbohydrate metabolism and may be due to sorbitol accumulation.

Regarding the removal of fluid from the retina, there is new evidence available from an experimental model recently developed to study permeability of individual retinal vessels in vitro using microperfusion techniques (11). An important finding of this study was the observation of a fluid flux across the normal retinal vessel wall from bath to lumen. This bath-to-lumen fluid flux was temperature-dependent and apparently coupled to the organic anion transport (Figure 1). When similar studies were repeated in diabetic retinal vessels, this fluid flux was 43% lower, suggesting that in the diabetic animal there is decreased fluid removal from the retina (12). The retinal vessels and possibly the retinal pigment epithelium may be functioning as selective membranes which facilitate the penetration of oxygen and glucose into the retina, but may have a very active fluid flux from the retina into the blood, thus keeping the retina relatively dry and maintaining the appropriate environment for optimal neural function. Alterations of fluid flux from retina and vitreous to blood may well be the principal cause of retinal edema.

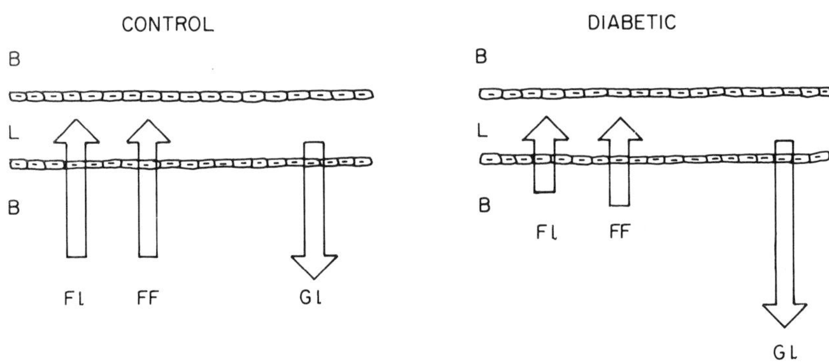


Figure 1. Retinal vessels. B = bath, L = lumen of the vessel, Fl = organic anion (fluorescein) transport from bath to lumen, FF = reabsorptive fluid flux, Gl = glucose transport from lumen to bath.

## TREATMENT

### Medical Therapy

The development of a therapeutic agent that, when given in the early stages of the disease, may prevent or stabilize retinopathy and other diabetic complications is a most desirable goal, but also one that has not yet been achieved. Resolving the complications of diabetes has been difficult because the treatment options have been limited to the alteration of symptoms rather than the reversal of the pathological process, and, therefore, there has been relatively little impetus to develop new techniques for the early detection of complications. In brief, there are no therapies available because few techniques for early detection have been developed, and there are not enough techniques for early detection because it did not seem worthwhile to detect early changes when a therapy was not available.

An important step towards a solution of this problem is the demonstration of a pathophysiological mechanism by which the complications of diabetes may develop, thus opening realistic perspectives for the development of a therapeutic agent. In the early 1970s, the polyol pathway and aldose-reductase activity were identified as one possible mechanism by which many of the complications of diabetes might be initiated. Since then experimental and clinical data have been accumulating to give strong support to this hypothesis.

Recently, two double-masked studies were reported examining the effect of two different aldose-reductase inhibitors on the early alteration of the blood-retina barrier occurring in human diabetes (13, 14). Both drugs tested showed a statistically significant beneficial effect on the breakdown of the blood–retina barrier, as shown by vitreous fluorophotometry. It is necessary now to confirm these results by long-term studies to determine if the progression and development of the full picture of vascular complications of diabetes can be prevented by the administration of aldose-reductase inhibitors. The major problems of such clinical trials reside in the definition of clinically significant outcome variables that are objective and quantitative, and in the characterization of the benefit to risk ratio.

Other therapeutic agents that should be considered are the inhibitors of prostaglandin synthesis and the oxygen radical 'scavengers'. Studies suggesting that arachidonic acid and ATPase may be involved in the chain of events leading to the development of diabetic complications indicate a possible role for these types of drugs (15).

In summary, although no medical therapy for diabetic retinopathy has been proven to be effective, work now in progress indicates that this situation may change in the very near future. In the meantime, focal photocoagulation remains the treatment of choice.

## Photocoagulation Therapy

For years, many reports have suggested a beneficial effect of photocoagulation on diabetic macular edema. Recently, the results published by the ETDRS show that focal photocoagulation of 'clinically significant' diabetic macular edema substantially reduces the risk of visual loss (4). In this randomized clinical trial, supported by the National Eye Institute, 754 eyes with macular edema and mild to moderate diabetic retinopathy were randomly assigned to focal argon laser photocoagulation, while 1490 such eyes were randomly assigned to deferral of photocoagulation. The beneficial effects of treatment demonstrated in this trial suggest that all eyes with clinically significant diabetic macular edema should be considered for focal photocoagulation.

The major points that have to be understood in this study are the definition of 'clinically significant' macular edema, the characterization of 'treatable' lesions and the understanding of the treatment strategies used.

The characteristics of clinically significant macular edema have already been listed above. The treatable lesions are identified by a pretreatment fluorescein angiogram and include: all focal leaks (most of these are microaneurysms); areas of diffuse leakage (associated with microaneurysms, intraretinal vascular abnormalities or diffuse capillary leakage); retinal avascular zones. Finally, the main treatment strategies are related to whether treatment is for focal leaks, or diffuse leaks and avascular zones. In the first case, direct impact, preferably using smaller spots to obtain darkening/whitening of the lesion, is used. In the second, moderate intensity burns in a grid-like pattern, one burn-width apart, are applied, avoiding treatment within 500 $\mu$m of the centre of the macula.

Two aspects of the treatment protocol used in the ETDRS seem particularly important. Firstly, great care must be taken to identify and photocoagulate treatable lesions. Secondly, follow-up visits are essential and additional treatment must be given for persistence or recrudescence of macular edema.

Another slightly different treatment strategy using grid photocoagulation of the posterior pole in a generalized and relatively uniform pattern has been advocated for diffuse macular edema (16, 17).

The presence of capillary closure and ischemia complicating diabetic macular edema appears to remain an obstacle for useful focal photocoagulation. When analysing their results with photocoagulation for treatment of diabetic ischemic maculopathy, Whitelocke et al. (16) suggest that only panretinal photocoagulation may be beneficial for these eyes. They found that 32% of eyes with ischemic maculopathy produced new vessels on the optic disc within the 2-year period of the study and suggest the use of preventive panretinal photocoagulation as a possible therapeutic alternative.

The ETDRS treatment protocol recommends the treatment of lesions up to 300 $\mu$m from the centre of the macula, unless there is perifoveal capillary drop-out, which might be worsened by this treatment. The generalized clinical impression is that photocoagulation for diabetic macular edema should be avoided, or only performed with great caution, whenever widening of the foveal avascular zone due to capillary closure dominates the picture.

## REFERENCES


1. Ferris FL III, Patz A (1984) Macular edema. A complication of diabetic retinopathy. Survey Ophthalmol 28: 452–461
2. Cunha-Vaz JG, Travassos A (1984) Breakdown of the blood–retina barriers and cystoid macular edema. Survey Ophthalmol 28: 485–492
3. Manual of Operations (1976) Diabetic Retinopathy Study. Baltimore, Maryland, DRS Coordinating Center
4. Early Treatment Diabetic Retinopathy Study Research Group (1985) Photocoagulation for diabetic macular edema. Early Treatment Diabetic Retinopathy Study Report Number 1. Arch Ophthalmol 103: 1796–1806
5. Smith RT, Lee CM, Charles HC, Farber M, Cunha-Vaz JG (1987) Quantification of diabetic macular edema. Arch Ophthalmol (in press)
6. Patz A, Bevrow JW (1967) Visual and systemic prognosis in diabetic retinopathy. Trans Am Acad Ophthalmol Otolaryngol 71: 253–258
7. Rapoport SI (1976) Blood–brain barrier in physiology and medicine. Raven Press, New York
8. Cunha-Vaz JG, Fairia de Abreu JR, Campos AJ, Figo GM (1975) Early breakdown of the blood–retina barrier in diabetes. Br J Ophthal 59: 649–656
9. Waltman SR (1984) Sequential vitreous fluorophotometry in diabetes mellitus: a five-year prospective study. Trans Am Ophthalmol Soc 82: 827–849
10. Kohner E (1974) Retinal blood flow in diabetes mellitus. In: Lynn JR, Snydder WB, Vaiser A (eds) Diabetic retinopathy. Grune & Stratton, New York
11. Murta JN, Cunha-Vaz JG, Sabo CA, Jones CW, Laski ME (1987) Microperfusion studies on the permeability of retinal vessels. I. A new model demonstrating organic anion transport and reabsorptive fluid flux. Invest Ophthalmol (in press)
12. Murta JN, Cunha-Vaz JG, Sabo CA, Laski ME (1987) Microperfusion studies of diabetic retinal vessels: organic anion transport and reabsorptive fluid flux. 1987 ARVO Meeting, Sarasota, USA
13. Cunha-Vaz JG, Mota MC, Leite EB, Faria de Abreu JR, Ruas MA (1986) Effect of

sulindac on the blood-retina barrier in the early diabetic retinopathy. Arch Ophthalmol 103: 1307–1311

14. Cunha-Vaz JG, Mota MC, Leite EB, Faria de Abreu JR, Ruas MA (1986) Effect of sorbinil on the blood–retina barrier in the early diabetic retinopathy. Diabetes 35: 575–578
15. Greene DA, Latimer SA (1984) Action of sorbinil in diabetic peripheral nerve. Relationship of polyol (sorbitol) pathway inhibitors to myo-inositol-mediated defect in sodium–potassium ATPase activity. Diabetes 33: 712–716
16. Whitelocke RAF, Kearns M, Black RK, Hamilton AM (1979) The diabetic maculopathies. Trans Ophthalmol Soc UK 99: 314–320
17. Olk RJ (1986) Modified grid argon (blue-green) laser photocoagulation for diffuse diabetic macular edema. Ophthalmology 93: (7): 938–950

Diabetic Complications: Early Diagnosis and Treatment
Edited by D. Andreani, G. Crepaldi, U. Di Mario and G. Pozza


CHAPTER 10

# *The Treatment of Diabetic Retinopathy*

R. Brancato and F. Bandello
*Clinica Oculistica dell'Università, Ospedale S. Raffaele, Milan, Italy*

Since the introduction of insulin treatment the mean duration of life for diabetic patients has been prolonged, but its benefits have been offset by an increased incidence of microvascular complications. Among these, particular attention should be paid to diabetic retinopathy on account of its severe effects on vision and the consequent economic and social involvement. The increased incidence of retinopathy indirectly suggests that current medical treatment is ineffective. Confusion on the matter is also generated by the failure to identify definite stages in the pathogenesis of the complication which seems to be a multifactorial disease in which connected but independent factors concur. The relation between metabolic control and microvascular complications is also rather unclear. The diffuse clinical impression of most ophthalmologists is that good metabolic control can delay the occurrence of diabetic retinopathy, but this cannot be assumed to be a scientific truth.

In the light of these considerations, it may be understood why a large number of drugs have been used time after time in the treatment of diabetic retinopathy: salicylates, dipiramidol, pentoxiphylline, vitamin $B_{12}$, testosterone, oestrogens, calcium dobesilate, chromocarbdiethylamine, and so forth. Although all of these drugs have a rational point of action in the pathophysiological sequence of diabetic retinopathy, none has definitely demonstrated its effectiveness so far (1). Since hypophysectomy has been progressively discontinued, photocoagulation remains the only treatment whose reliability and effectiveness have been convincingly demonstrated. This technique was first introduced into clinical practice in 1949 by Gerd Meyer-Schwickerath using xenon arc lamp photocoagulation. Technological progress and the advent of lasers have increased the number of clinical conditions in ophthalmology for which photocoagulation may be used, but diabetic retinopathy still represents the main clinical application. Photocoagulation is a disruptive treatment which exploits the conversion of light energy into thermal energy. The argon laser is the most commonly used light source currently available, followed, in recent years, by the krypton and dye lasers. The aim of photocoagulation is to stop or slow down the progress of diabetic retinopathy, preventing the more advanced stages of the disease and its complications, such as macular edema, vitreous hemorrhage, retinal detachment and neovascular glaucoma. The indications for and the technique of performing laser treatment are dependent on the type of diabetic retinopathy and its stage of evolution. It is worth reproducing here the most widely used classification of diabetic retinopathy which is also used in our clinic (Table 1). This classification was drawn up by the Diabetic Retinopathy Study Research Group in 1981 (2).

Table 1. Classification of diabetic retinopathy (Diabetic Retinopathy Study Research Group, 1981)

| |
|---|
| NON-PROLIFERATIVE (BACKGROUND) RETINOPATHY |
| *Simple background retinopathy* |
| Microaneurysms |
| Dot and blot hemorrhages |
| Hard exudates |
| (Macular edema) |
| *Preproliferative retinopathy* |
| Beaded veins |
| Soft exudates |
| Intraretinal microvascular abnormalities (IRMA) |
| (Extensive intraretinal hemorrhages) |
| PROLIFERATIVE DIABETIC RETINOPATHY |
| Neovascularization at the disk (NVD) |
| Neovascularization elsewhere in the retina (NVE) |
| Fibrovascular proliferation |
| Vitreous hemorrhage |

## PHOTOCOAGULATION OF PROLIFERATIVE DIABETIC RETINOPATHY

Following the first studies by Aiello et al. (3) and James and L'Esperance (4) in the early 1970s, two multicentre studies were undertaken to evaluate the effectiveness of photocoagulative treatment of proliferative diabetic retinopathy. The first trial, the Diabetic Retinopathy Study (DRS), began in 1971 and enrolled more than 1700 patients in 15 centres. One eye in each patient was randomly chosen as a control, while the other was assigned to either argon laser or xenon arc lamp therapy groups. The treatment consisted of panretinal photocoagulation, focal treatment of epiretinal neovascularizations and, in the argon laser group, treatment of papillary neovascularizations (5).

The second multicentre study was carried out in Great Britain by the British Multicentre Study (BMS) group. It included 99 subjects affected by proliferative diabetic retinopathy at the same stage of evolution. One eye was assigned to xenon-arc treatment, while the other served as a control (6).

Both trials demonstrated that photocoagulative treatment is effective in preventing the most serious visual complications caused by diabetic retinopathy.

Subsequent reports of the DRS revealed a reduction of blindness due to diabetic retinopathy ranging from 16.3% in the non-treated group to 6.4% in treated patients, with a difference of 61%. In other words, the rate of blindness in non-treated patients was three times as high as in the photocoagulated group. The DRS also identified as high risk factors, predictive of severe visual loss, neovascularizations that had already caused preretinal or intravitreal hemorrhages, and early neovascularizations with preretinal or peripapillary hemorrhages (7). The use of laser treatment on eyes showing these characteristics reduced blindness by more than 50% after 4 years of follow-up. Similar results were reported by the BMS.

A study undertaken at our clinic showed that laser photocoagulation of diabetic retinopathy with optic disk neovascularization led to a marked regression of the disease in 69.5% of cases; fluoroangiographic aspects remained unchanged in 19.5% of patients, and deteriorated in 11% (8). Follow-up was between 6 months and 3 years.

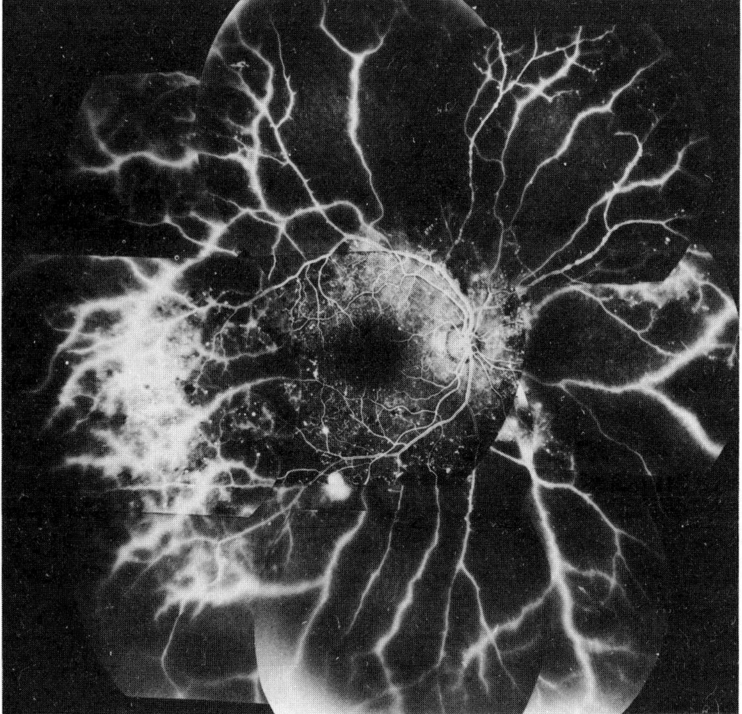

Figure 1. Panretinal fluoroangiography is able to demonstrate clearly the extension of retinal non-perfusion. Photocoagulation can thus be precisely directed on to retinal ischemic areas.

Fluorescein retinal angiography is of substantial value in identifying appropriate treatment. Panretinal fluoroangiography performed on the whole fundus is the only test able to highlight the extension of retinal non-perfusion, thus allowing a full picture of the lesions to be obtained (Figure 1). Photocoagulation, performed after panretinal angiography, must initially be directed on non-perfused retinal areas. 'Rational' photocoagulation can then gradually be started, first covering the ischemic areas. As for the various clinical pictures, the treatment is progressively extended during subsequent sessions, until the whole retina outside the temporal vascular arcades is included and the papilla is nasally licked (panretinal photocoagulation). This strategy is based on the conviction, shared by all authors, that the non-perfused retina is responsible for the production and release of a still unidentified angiogenic factor, which leads to the formation of new vessels. Photocoagulation of non-perfused areas thus represents an indirect treatment of retinal and papillary neovascularizations. Photocoagulation can be performed on one retinal quadrant at a time (inferior quadrants generally are treated first, since they may become unapproachable in the event of endovitreal hemorrhage). Spots are also applied concentrically from the periphery towards the posterior pole. Treatment sessions are preferably spaced over at least 24 hours. During each session 500–600 burns of at least 500 $\mu$m in diameter are placed contiguously at a power sufficient to produce a whitening of the retina. Moderately heavy (yellowish-grey to greyish-white) photocoagulation lesions are usually produced. Three to four sessions using this procedure are generally sufficient to complete a panphotocoagulation (Figure 2). In some cases, however, the panphotocoagulation is performed in a single session. Peripheral spots must be more confluent, while in more central areas it is preferable that a space should be kept between the burns to avoid the formation of wide visual field defects. When, despite the observation of the above-mentioned rules, neovascularization persists, direct photocoagulation of the new vessels may be considered. Laser wavelengths which show affinity with hemoglobin and oxyhemoglobin are particularly suitable. In this respect, the dye laser appears to be the most useful, since it provides a wavelength of 577 nm (yellow) with maximum absorption on neovascularizations (9). The monochromatic green argon laser has also been effectively employed in these cases. Following the advent of the red krypton laser in clinical practice, even advanced stages of proliferative diabetic retinopathy, previously unsuitable for treatment, have been photocoagulated (10). Among these borderline conditions may be listed proliferative diabetic retinopathy with vitreous hemorrhage, the presence of a well-developed fibrosis and marked opacities of the optical means. In the first case, the low affinity of the red light for hemoglobin and oxyhemoglobin allows an effective photocoagulation to take place even when the argon beam cannot reach the retina at sufficient power. When a marked fibrotic component is present, the use of the krypton laser allows the energy dispersion towards contiguous fibrosis to be reduced. The dangers of fibrotic retraction to the heat and the resulting secondary retinal detachment are diminished. In the event of opacity of the dioptric means, the limited scattering of the red light permits treatment that cannot be otherwise performed using the argon laser. With the exception of these extreme cases, the various wavelengths available yield results that are basically superimposable, as is demonstrated by the preliminary findings of a randomized study underway at our clinic on the use of different wavelengths of the dye laser.

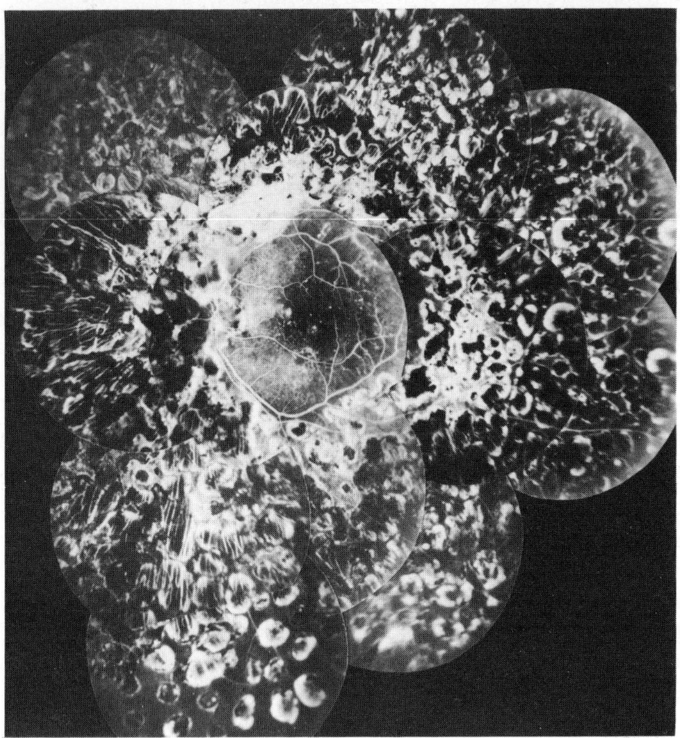

Figure 2. Panphotocoagulation performed up to the retinal vascular arcades determines the disappearance of the new vessels.

## PHOTOCOAGULATION OF PREPROLIFERATIVE DIABETIC RETINOPATHY

This is an evolutive phase of diabetic retinopathy characterized by the presence of cottonwool spots, IRMA, extended retinal hemorrhages and marked alterations of the vessels, mainly on the venous site. Retinal fluoroangiography reveals the presence of wide areas of capillary non-perfusion, whereas new vessels are still absent. Laser treatment at this stage of diabetic retinopathy should be subject to individual considerations, such as the level of patient compliance (frequency of examinations, distance of the ophthalmological centre from home, etc.) (11). Treatment may be delayed for patients who can follow a regular control schedule, while less compliant subjects should preferably be treated. The criteria and procedure for laser treatment have already been described.

## PHOTOCOAGULATION OF BACKGROUND DIABETIC RETINOPATHY

Maculopathy in non-proliferative diabetic retinopathy represents one of the main causes of visual reduction and legal blindness. Medical management of this problem has been largely ineffective. Although undoubtedly more effective, the use of laser treatment is still debated. Maculopathy in non-proliferative diabetic retinopathy is the clinical expression of a blood–retina barrier breakdown whose causes are still unclear. The results of the Early Treatment Diabetic Retinopathy Study (ETDRS) (1985) (12) demonstrated that laser photocoagulation effectively improves diabetic maculopathy. In this American multicentre prospective randomized trial, focal treatment was carried out on retinal areas responsible for the edema. Other authors had previously come to the same conclusions (13, 14). Encouraging results have been recently reported with a 'grid' treatment technique in which diffuse photocoagulation of the posterior pole is performed (15). A prospective randomized trial carried out at our clinic demonstrated a more favourable functional evolution in patients treated with scattered versus focal photocoagulation when examined 12 months after treatment (16). At present, the most rational approach is, in our opinion, the direct treatment of microvascular alterations, especially those located in the centre of hard exudates. Maculopathies with diffuse posterior edema of the macular area can be successfully treated with scattered photocoagulation. The two techniques can be associated in diffuse macular edema showing discrete areas of microvascular alterations. Green argon laser and yellow (577 nm) dye laser are the most suitable tools for focal photocoagulation, while lasers with longer wavelengths, such as red krypton, are appropriate for scattered treatment. The two procedures of treatment can be summarized as follows.

### Focal Photocoagulation

Microaneurysms and other distinct areas of fluorescein focal leakage are treated with spots 100–200 $\mu$m in diameter to obtain a whitening of the lesions. Treatment is always guided by previous identification on fluoroangiographic pictures of the leakage points responsible for the retinal edema (Figure 3).

### Scattered Photocoagulation

Spots 100-200 $\mu$m in diameter are applied to the whole posterior pole, one to two spots apart. The foveal avascular zone is untouched. In patients treated bilaterally, the spots are placed further apart in the temporal paramacular region of the right eye and the nasal paramacular region of the left eye to prevent, where possible, the development of deep scotomas which could hinder reading (Figure 4).

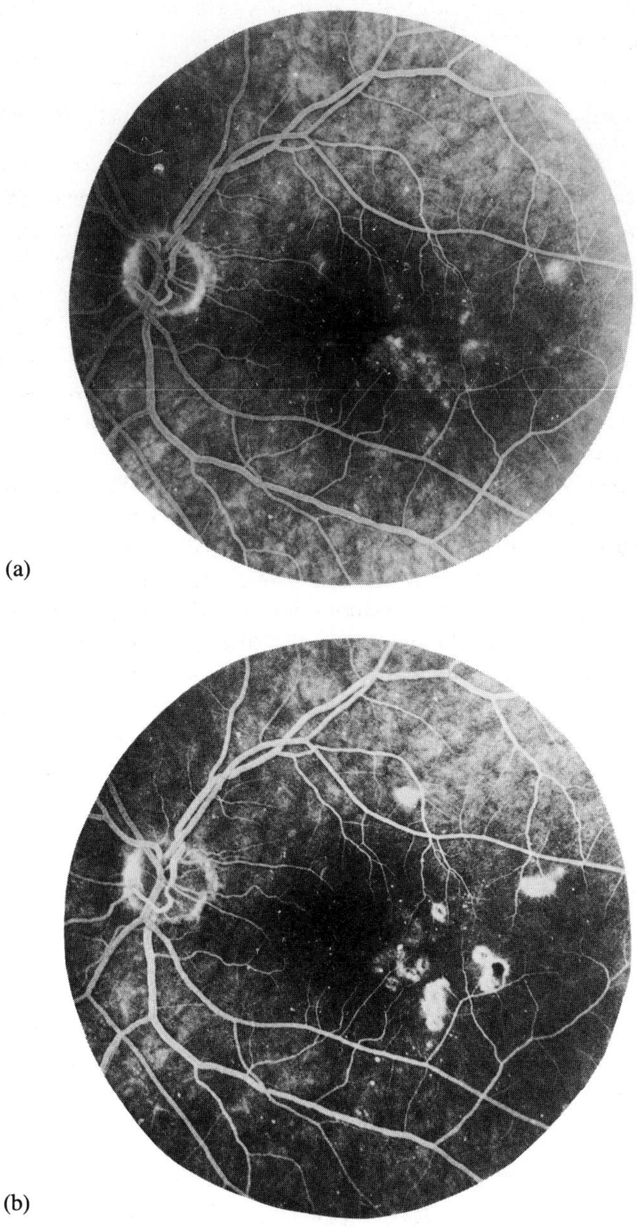


Figure 3. Fluoroangiographic pictures permit the identification of dye leakage points responsible for the retinal edema (a). Focal treatment performed on leakage sites leads to a decrease in the edema (b).

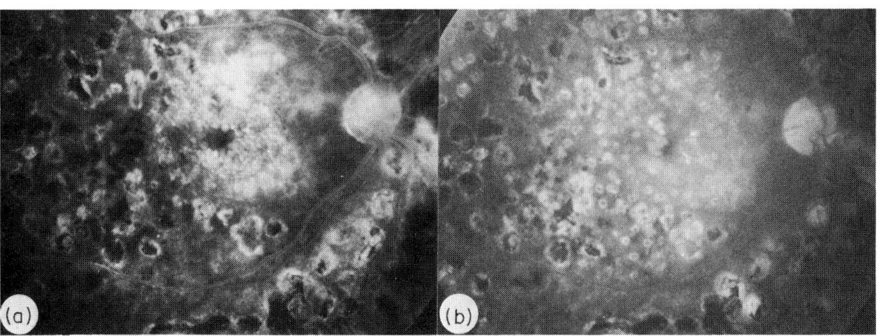


Figure 4. Retinal fluoroangiography performed before (a) and after (b) grid photocoagulation reveals a marked reduction in the cystoid macular edema.

A mechanism of direct obliteration of microvascular alterations is postulated for focal treatment to be effective. The mechanism yielding positive results with the scattered technique is more controversial. Among the most reliable hypotheses may be included: proliferation of pigment epithelial cells brought about by a mild photocoagulation, followed by an improved efficiency of the external blood–retina barrier (17); proliferation of capillary endothelial cells, followed by an improvement in the internal blood–retina barrier (18); improvement of the retinochoroidal metabolic exchanges through the passages opened between choroid and retina (19); and, finally, the release of coagulative necrosis of a factor able to improve the efficiency of the blood–retina barrier.

## VITRECTOMY

Vitrectomy must be considered in the presence of dense non-resorbing vitreous hemorrhages or taut vitreoretinal tractions. This surgical technique consists of the section and change of the vitreous using a cannula introduced via the pars plana. In this way, blood, membranes and fibrin can be carefully removed and replaced by Ringer solution. The results of vitrectomy via the pars plana are most satisfactory when visual loss is caused only by vitreal opacification by blood and fibrotic membranes. Of course, the results will be functionally much less dramatic if the retina has already been damaged by retinopathy, fibrosis, or other degenerative diseases. Echography and electroretinography prior to the intervention are useful for prognostic values. The Diabetic Retinopathy Vitrectomy Study (DRVS), which was started in the USA in 1976, pointed out the following positive prognostic indications for vitrectomy (20):

1. absence of new vitreal hemorrhages for at least 6 months;
2. no evidence of spontaneous reabsorption for at least 6 months;

3. presence of light perception with good projection in at least 2 quadrants;
4. no echographical evidence of detachment in eyes with uncertain light projections;
5. no fibrosis or detachments previously documented;
6. positive electroretinographical response;
7. understanding of the procedure by the patient and informed consent.

Vitrectomy can also be performed in the event of retinal detachment secondary to vitreoretinal fibrosis (this is a frequent complication of advanced proliferative diabetic retinopathy). On account of the risks involved, this surgical technique is not performed until tractions are revealed which threaten the macula. Until then, neodymium YAG (Nd : YAG) laser vitreolysis may be utilized, since it reduces intraoperative and postoperative risks and has all the advantages of an ambulatorial treatment (21). The most frequent complications of vitrectomy include rubeosis iridis, cataract, retinal breaks and recurrent hemorrhages (22). In view of the risks associated with this surgical technique, the possibility of using pulsed Nd : YAG laser vitreolysis to treat some vitreal complications has recently been considered. Laser treatment cannot of course replace surgical vitrectomy, but it should receive increasing attention since it is able to solve a number of clinical problems, obviating in special cases the risks of surgical intervention. Nd : YAG laser vitreolysis is a non-invasive technique, which is transpupillary and performed in non-hematic clear vitreous, to perforate and dissect membranes along the optical axis and to resect bands and strands that exert traction on the retina.

## REFERENCES

1. Murphy RP, Patz A (1983) The natural history and management of nonproliferative diabetic retinopathy. In: Little HL, Jack RL, Patz A, Forsham PH (eds) Diabetic retinopathy. Thieme-Stratton, New York, pp 225
2. Diabetic Retinopathy Study Research Group (1981) A modification of the Airlie House classification of diabetic retinopathy. Invest Ophthalmol Vis Sci 21: 2
3. Aiello LM, Beetham WP, Balodimos MC, *et al.* (1969) Ruby laser photocoagulation in treatment of diabetic proliferative retinopathy. In: Goldberg M, Fine S (eds) Treatment of diabetic retinopathy. Department of Public Health, Washington DC, pp 437
4. James WA, L'Esperance FE (1969) Treatment of diabetic optic nerve neovascularization by extensive retinal photocoagulation. Am J Ophthalmol 78: 939
5. Diabetic Retinopathy Study Research Group (1976) Preliminary report on the effect of photocoagulation therapy. Am J Ophthalmol 81: 380
6. British Multicentre Study Group (1977) Proliferative diabetic retinopathy treatment with xenon-arc photocoagulation. Br Med J 81: 739
7. Diabetic Retinopathy Study Research Group (1979) Four risk factors for severe visual loss in diabetic retinopathy. Arch Ophthalmol 97: 654
8. Brancato R, Mahnic F, Michelone C, Pigiona L (1979) La neovascolarizzazione papillare nella retinopatia diabetica. Proc Congr Società Oftalmologicá Italiana, pp 8
9. Brancato R, Menchini U, Pece A, Bandello F (1986) Clinical applications of the tunable dye laser. Laser Ophthalmol 1 (2): 115

10. L'Esperance FA (1972) Clinical photocoagulation with the krypton laser. Arch Ophthalmol 87: 693
11. Brancato R, Menchini U, Bandello F (1985) Le complicanze oculari del diabete mellito. In: Proc LXXXVI Congr Soc Italiana Medicina Interna, Rome
12. Early Treatment Diabetic Retinopathy Study (1985) Report number one—Photocoagulation for diabetic macular edema. Arch Ophthalmol 103: 1796
13. Spalter HF (1971) Photocoagulation of circinate maculopathy in diabetic retinopathy. Am J Ophthalmol 71: 242
14. Patz A, Schatz H, Berkow JW, Gittelsohn AM, Ticko U (1973) Macular edema—an overlooked complication of diabetic retinopathy. Trans Am Acad Ophthalmol Otol 77: 34
15. Olk J (1986) Modified grid argon (blue green) laser photocoagulation for diabetic macular edema. Ophthalmology 93: 938
16. Brancato R, Menchini U, Scialdone A, Bandello F (1986) Focal versus scattered green argon in diffuse diabetic macular edema. A prospective randomized trial. In: Gitter A, Schatz H, Yannuzzi L (eds) Laser photocoagulation of the macula (in press)
17. Bresnick GH (1983) Diabetic maculopathy: a critical review highlighting diffuse macular edema. Ophthalmology 90: 1301
18. Marshall J, Clover G, Rothery S (1984) Some new findings on retinal irradiation by krypton and argon lasers. Doc Ophthalmol Proc Ser 32: 21
19. Peyman GA, Bock D (1972) Peroxidase diffusion in the normal and laser coagulated primate retina. Invest Ophthalmol 11: 35
20. Kupfer C (1976) The diabetic retinopathy vitrectomy study. Am J Ophthalmol 81: 687
21. Brancato R, Menchini U, Bandello F, Alberti M (1986) Fotoresezione di briglie retinovitreali mediante Nd : YAG laser eseguita in pazienti affetti da retinopatia diabetica proliferante. Clin Ocul Patol Ocul 4: 251
22. Rice TA, Michels RG (1983) Complications of vitrectomy. In: Little H, Jack RL, Patz A, Forsham PH (eds) Diabetic retinopathy. Thieme-Stratton, New York, pp 315

# Neuropathy

Diabetic Complications: Early Diagnosis and Treatment
Edited by D. Andreani, G. Crepaldi, U. Di Mario and G. Pozza


CHAPTER 11

# *New Trends in the Etiopathogenesis of Diabetic Neuropathy*

R. S. CLEMENTS JR.
*University of Alabama at Birmingham School of Medicine, Birmingham, Alabama, USA*

In the three decades since Fagerberg first attributed diabetic neuropathy to a malfunction of the blood vessels supplying the peripheral nerves, a number of potentially pathogenetic mechanisms have been proposed to explain the development of this complication (1). In fact, the large number of mechanisms that have been invoked testifies to the fact that the actual cause of diabetic polyneuropathy is not known. It is likely that no single mechanism predominates, and that various mechanisms can interact in varying degrees to culminate in the expression of diabetic neuropathy.

The currently popular mechanisms to explain this complication are presented in Table 1. They are listed in the chronological order in which they appeared in the literature. These mechanisms will be discussed in sequence.

Table 1. Proposed mechanisms for the etiopathogenesis of diabetic neuropathy

1. The vascular hypothesis
2. The osmotic hypothesis
3. The inositol hypothesis
4. The glycosylation hypothesis
5. The hypoxia hypothesis
6. The hormonal hypothesis

## THE VASCULAR HYPOTHESIS

The possibility that structural and functional changes involving the vasa nervorum could underlie the development of diabetic polyneuropathy was initially proposed by Fagerberg (1). By light microscopic examination of sural nerve biopsies he observed a consistent thickening of the walls of neural arterioles which was accompanied by an increased staining with the periodic acid–Schiff reagent in patients with clinically obvious diabetic polyneuropathy. On the basis of these observations he proposed that the nerves of the patient with diabetic neuropathy may be deprived of nutrients and that this could lead to neural degeneration. Furthermore, he made the interesting speculation that fluctuations in the permeability of the intraneural vessels might be responsible for the reversible forms of diabetic neuropathy.

Over the intervening years, this vascular hypothesis was overshadowed by the various metabolic hypotheses that came into vogue. However, during the past year two groups of investigators have provided convincing electron microscopical evidence that ischemic microvascular events may play a major role in the genesis of diabetic neural degeneration (2–4).

Support for the notion that abnormalities in vascular permeability might also participate in the pathogenesis of diabetic neuropathy has been recently provided by the findings of Williamson and his colleagues (5–7). They observed that when new blood vessels develop in a diabetic milieu they are excessively leaky to radioiodinated albumin. Similarly, the retina, the choroid and the sciatic nerve of the diabetic rat display increased permeability to albumin. These functional changes are reversed by successful pancreatic islet transplantation and can be prevented with aldose reductase inhibitors, dietary myoinositol supplementation, or castration of the male rat (8). While such abnormalities in vascular function could be speculated to lead to nerve damage, the responsible mechanisms have yet to be identified.

In addition to the possibility that abnormalities in the blood vessel wall could participate in the pathogenesis of diabetic polyneuropathy, it is possible that phenomena both within the vascular lumen as well as extravascular factors could also contribute. Timperley and his colleagues have described aggregates of platelets within the vasa nervorum of patients with diabetic peripheral neuropathy, a finding that could be related to the focal ischemic damage described by Dyck and Johnson (2–4, 9). In addition, Powell and his colleagues have observed that increased polyol pathway activity in the rodent nerve results in a chronic increase in endoneurial fluid pressure which can be abrogated by the administration of aldose reductase inhibitors (10). Such an increase in endoneurial fluid pressure is thought to decrease nerve blood flow and thereby to contribute to nerve fiber damage (11).

It is gratifying that nearly a century after Charcot is reported to have proposed that diabetic polyneuropathy is secondary to vascular disease, increasing evidence is accumulating to substantiate his conclusion. Of further interest is the apparent intertwining of the vascular hypothesis with the other hypotheses listed in Table 1. Aldose reductase inhibitor and myoinositol feeding studies link the vascular hypothesis with both the osmotic and the inositol hypotheses. Obviously, abnormalities in vascular structure and function influence the hypoxia hypothesis. Finally, the fact that castration of the male diabetic rat prevents abnormal vascular permeability provides a connection between the vascular and the hormonal hypotheses. During the next decade it is anticipated that we will gain considerable understanding of the molecular mechanisms by which vascular abnormalities contribute to the pathogenesis of diabetic polyneuropathy.

## THE OSMOTIC HYPOTHESIS

Both the enzymes (aldose reductase and sorbitol dehydrogenase) and the intermediates (sorbitol and fructose) of the polyol pathway have been recognized as constituents of mammalian peripheral nerve for nearly 30 years. In addition, it is known that the induction of experimental diabetes in rodents will raise the neural concentrations of sorbitol and fructose (albeit to a lesser degree than is observed in the lens) (12). By analogy to the lens, Gabbay proposed that the accumulation of sorbitol within the Schwann cell would result in water accumulation on an osmotic basis and that this osmotic stress could contribute to Schwann cell damage with subsequent demyelination (12). More recent morphological studies have indicated that this scenario does not occur. Instead of edema of the Schwann cell, the cytoplasm of this cell is decreased in hyperglycemic states (13). The water which does accumulate under these conditions is localized to the endoneurial space. Since this accumulation of fluid can be prevented with aldose reductase inhibitors, it is undoubtedly a consequence of increased polyol pathway activity. The hypothesis proposed by Powell to explain the increase in endoneurial fluid sodium (and pressure) is that sodium may comigrate with glucose into the endoneurial space and that the established sodium gradient is maintained by neural metabolism of glucose (or galactose) via the polyol pathway (10). In addition, since increased polyol pathway activity results in a decrease in nerve sodium–potassium ATPase activity, it is possible that the nerve exposed to hyperglycemia is unable to pump out sodium at a normal rate (14).

While the 'osmotic hypothesis' as originally proposed has not been substantiated, it is clear that increased polyol pathway activity is associated with a number of functional abnormalities within the diabetic nerve. Treatment of the diabetic (or galactosemic) rodent with aldose reductase inhibitors will correct the abnormalities in motor nerve conduction velocities, axoplasmic transport, sodium–potassium ATPase activity, oxygen uptake, as well as the increased water content and increased endoneurial fluid pressure (14–16). Similarly, the use of aldose reductase inhibitors has been found slightly to improve nerve conduction velocities in humans with diabetic neuropathy (17, 18). Since virtually all of the functional abnormalities associated with increased polyol pathway activity can be prevented or reversed by dietary myoinositol supplementation, it is likely that the polyol pathway does its damage by interfering with the neural metabolism of myoinositol, phosphoinositides and inositol phosphates.

## INOSITOL HYPOTHESIS

For years it has been recognized that whenever there is an increase in neural polyol pathway activity there is a reciprocal decrease in the concentration of free myoinositol within the peripheral nerve. This was not thought to be of physiological significance until Greene and his colleagues demonstrated that the abnormally lowered sciatic motor nerve conduction velocity of the rat with experimental diabetes could be corrected by dietary myoinositol supplementation (19). Since the improvement in nerve function occurred in the face of a persistently increased activity of the polyol pathway, and since aldose reductase inhibitors prevented the decrease in nerve myoinositol content, it became clear that the abnormality in nerve myoinositol metabolism was (at least in part) secondary to increased polyol pathway activity (14, 15, 20). Currently it is thought that hyperglycemia lowers nerve myoinositol content via two mechanisms. First, glucose competitively inhibits the sodium- and energy-dependent active transport of myoinositol by the nerve (20). Second, increased polyol pathway activity within the neural cells may induce the loss of myoinositol from those cells.

One consequence of this decrease in cellular myoinositol content is that it may limit the ability of the neurons to synthesize membrane phosphoinositides. It is now recognized that the phosphoinositides serve as reservoirs of potential signal molecules that can transmit messages across the cell membrane (21). When hydrolysed by phosphoinositide-specific phospholipase C, the phosphoinositides give rise to diacylglycerol and inositol phosphates. Further hydrolysis of diacylglycerol yields arachidonic acid, which can be converted into prostaglandins, thromboxanes and leukotrienes. The breakdown of the phosphoinositides is regulated by membrane lipid constituents (e.g. diacylglycerol), by calcium, and by guanine nucleotide binding proteins. In response to electrical stimulation of the nerve there is a rapid hydrolysis of phosphoinositides with production of diacylglycerol and inositol 1,4,5-triphosphate. The former stimulates protein kinase C activity, while the latter mobilizes intracellular calcium stores. Both phenomena tend to reinforce the hydrolysis of phosphoinositides and are instrumental in the orchestration of numerous intracellular processes. Obviously, any abnormality in the amount or in the rate of turnover of membrane phosphoinositides could have adverse effects upon peripheral nerve function. That there is, in fact, a defective incorporation of myoinositol into nerve phospholipids has been demonstrated in rats with experimental diabetes (22).

Another function of the phosphoinositides is that they can serve as boundary or regulatory phospholipids for various membrane-associated enzymes. Following the induction of experimental diabetes, there is nearly a 50% decrease in the activity of sodium–potassium ATPase which accounts for a 30% decrease in oxygen uptake by the nerve (20). These abnormalities (plus the associated slowing of nerve conduction velocity) develop in parallel and are completely corrected by in vivo dietary myoinositol supplementation. This suggests (but does not prove) that all of these abnormalities are linked to a defect in membrane phosphoinositide metabolism.

That there is a decrease in the myoinositol and phosphatidyl inositol content of human diabetic nerves has been shown by Hawthorne and his colleagues (23). The effect of dietary myoinositol supplementation upon peripheral nerve function in patients with diabetic neuropathy has been considerably less impressive than it has been in the rat. Some pilot studies have observed an improvement in peripheral nerve function after inositol feeding (24, 25) while others have not (26). Additional long-term studies using larger groups of patients will be needed before it can be concluded whether or not inositol feeding is of benefit in diabetic polyneuropathy.

## THE GLYCOSYLATION HYPOTHESIS

It has been recognized for a decade that, when various proteins are exposed to elevated concentrations of glucose, covalent attachment of the glucose molecules to the proteins will occur in proportion to the averaged glucose concentration. Subsequently, the attached glucose molecules undergo rearrangements which can result in the formation of fluorescent cross-linked proteins (27). Recently it has been found that there is a more than five-fold increase in the amount of glycosylated myelin in the peripheral nerves of the diabetic rat when compared to control rats (28). Furthermore, it is known that myelin proteins that are glycosylated are recognized by specific receptors and are endocytosed by macrophages (29). Since macrophage invasion of the peripheral nerve has been demonstrated in diabetic rodents (30), it is reasonable to speculate that a macrophage attack upon peripheral nerve glycosylated myelin proteins could contribute to the segmental loss of myelin that is seen in human diabetic neuropathy.

Another aspect of protein glycosylation that is linked to the vascular hypothesis is that they attract and trap soluble proteins such as immunoglobulins G and M. Since diabetic endoneurial capillaries are excessively permeable to plasma proteins (31), it is not surprising to find fourteen-fold and four-fold increases respectively for trapped IgM and IgG on the peripheral nerve myelin of human diabetic subjects (32). Obviously such trapped immunoglobulins would render the peripheral nerve susceptible to classical immunological attack with resultant cell damage.

Another mechanism whereby protein glycosylation could alter peripheral nerve function could be its interference with the function of tubulin. It is known that glycosylation of rat brain tubulin profoundly inhibits its GTP-dependent polymerization and renders it insoluble (33). If peripheral nerve tubulin is glycosylated (as is suggested in ref. 28) it could explain the impaired axonal transport observed in experimental diabetes.

Therapeutic approaches to the prevention of glycosylation-induced protein cross-linking are being developed and may prove to be of use in the treatment of the diabetic person whose glycemic fluctuations cannot be normalized by conventional means.

## THE HYPOXIA HYPOTHESIS

The peripheral nerves of diabetic rodents have a significant decrease in blood flow which is thought to be due to a combination of hyperviscosity of blood and to the microangiopathy described under the vascular hypothesis (34). This was found to result in a 25% decrease in the endoneurial oxygen tension of the diabetic rat nerve. Such a decrease in oxygen tension appears to parallel the decreases in motor nerve conduction velocity, myoinositol content, axoplasmic transport, sodium–potassium ATPase activity and oxygen consumption that have been previously described in the sciatic nerves of diabetic rats. Since all of these processes are dependent upon oxidative metabolism, it is easy to understand how oxygen deprivation could lead to nerve damage.

Support for this hypothesis is provided by the observations that hypoxia (10%) causes a decrease in motor nerve conduction velocities in non-diabetic rats and that oxygen supplementation (40%) prevents the resistance to ischemic block that is characteristic of diabetic nerves (35). As yet, the oxygen tension of human diabetic nerves has not been reported nor have studies on the effect of oxygen supplementation of peripheral nerve function been carried out in neuropathic diabetic persons.

## THE HORMONAL HYPOTHESIS

At present, three hormones are known to influence peripheral nerve function in diabetic polyneuropathy: male sex steroids, thyroxine and insulin. Williamson and his colleagues observed that castration of male diabetic rats prevents the subsequent decrease in collagen solubility and increase in vascular permeability, but that it has no effect upon non-enzymatic glycosylation of proteins (36). We recently observed that thyroid hormone treatment normalized the motor nerve conduction velocities, sodium–potassium ATPase activities, as well as the nerve free and lipid-bound inositol concentrations of the streptozotocin-diabetic rat (37). Neither of these hormonal manipulations are viable therapeutic options in man. Thyroid hormone administration rendered our diabetic rats extremely feeble and most men would reject the opportunity to undergo castration.

Obviously the ideal hormonal manipulation would be the optimization of insulin therapy to normalize the fluctuations of serum glucose in the insulin-taking diabetic person. Now that home blood glucose monitoring techniques are readily available, such intensive insulin treatment schemes as multiple daily injections of insulin or continuous subcutaneous insulin infusion render the achievement of euglycemia feasible in certain patients. Since all of the proposed mechanisms for the etiopathogenesis of diabetic polyneuropathy require hyperglycemia to be operative, it is reasonable to speculate that the establishment of euglycemia will prevent the development of this complication. Unfortunately, the majority of patients who take insulin cannot maintain euglycemia. For those patients it is of value that we continue to explore the mechanisms responsible for the development of diabetic polyneuropathy in the hope that we can develop pharmacological approaches to the prevention or to the reversal of this complication.

## REFERENCES

1. Fagerberg SE (1959) Diabetic neuropathy: a clinical and histological study on the significance of vascular affections. Acta Med Scand 164 (Suppl 345): 1–80

2. Dyck PJ, Lais A, Karnes JL, O'Brien P, Rizza R (1986) Fiber loss is primary and multifocal in sural nerves in diabetic polyneuropathy. Ann Neurol 19: 425–439
3. Dyck PJ, Karnes JL, O'Brien P, Okazaki H, Lais A, Engelstad J (1986) The spatial distribution of fiber loss in diabetic polyneuropathy suggests ischemia. Ann Neurol 19: 440–449
4. Johnson PC, Doll SC, Cromey DW (1986) Pathogenesis of diabetic neuropathy. Ann Neurol 19: 450–457
5. Kilzer P, Chang K, Marvel J, Rowold E, Jaudes P, Ullensvang S, Kilo C, Williamson JR (1985) Albumin permeation of new vessels is increased in diabetic rats. Diabetes 34: 333–336
6. Williamson JR, Chang K, Rowold E, Marvel J, Tomlinson M, Sherman WR, Ackermann KE, Kilo C (1985) Sorbinil prevents diabetes-induced increases in vascular permeability but does not alter collagen cross-linking. Diabetes 34: 703–705
7. Williamson JR, Chang K, Rowold E, Kilo C, Lacy PE (1986) Islet transplant in diabetic Lewis rats prevent and reverse diabetes-induced increases in vascular permeability and prevent but do not reverse collagen solubility changes. Diabetologia 29: 392–396
8. Williamson JR, Chang K, Rowold E, Marvel J, Tomlinson M, Kilo C (1985) Diabetes-induced increases in vascular permeability are prevented by castration and by sorbinil. Diabetes 34: 108A
9. Williams E, Timperley WR, Ward JD, Duckworth T (180) Electron microscopical studies of vessels in diabetic peripheral neuropathy. J Clin Pathol 33: 462–470
10. Mizisin AP, Powell HC, Myers RR (1986) Edema and increased endoneurial sodium in galactose neuropathy: reversal with an aldose reductase inhibitor. J Neurol Sci 74: 35–43
11. Low PA, Dyck PJ, Schmelzer JD (1982) Chronic elevation of endoneurial pressure is associated with low-grade pathology. Muscle Nerve 5: 162–165
12. Gabbay KH (1973) The sorbitol pathway and the complications of diabetes. N Engl J Med 288: 831–836
13. Jakobsen J (1976) Axon dwindling in early experimental diabetes: a study of cross-sectioned nerves. Diabetologia 12: 539–546
14. Greene DA, Lattimer SA (1984) Action of sorbinil in diabetic peripheral nerve: relationship of polyol (sorbitol) pathway to a *myo*-inositol mediated defect in sodium–potassium ATPase activity. Diabetes 33: 712–716
15. Tomlinson DR, Holmes PR, Mayer JH (1982) Reversal by treatment with an aldose reductase inhibitor, of impaired axonal transport and motor nerve conduction velocity in experimental diabetes mellitus. Neurosci Lett 31: 189–193
16. Robison WG (1984) Aldose reductase and diabetic neuropathy. In: Cogan DG (mod) Aldose reductase and complications of diabetes. Ann Intern Med 101: 82–91
17. Young RD, Ewing DJ, Clarke BF (1983) A controlled trial of sorbinil, an aldose reductase inhibitor, in chronic painful diabetic neuropathy. Diabetes 32: 938–942
18. Fagius J, Jameson S (1981) Effects of aldose reductase inhibitor treatment in diabetic polyneuropathy: A clinical and neurophysiological study. J Neurol Neurosurg Psychiatry 44: 991–1001
19. Greene DA, DeJesus PV, Winegrad AI (1975) Effects of insulin and dietary *myo*-inositol on impaired peripheral motor nerve conduction velocity in acute streptozotocin diabetes. J Clin Invest 55: 1326–1336
20. Greene DA (1986) A sodium-pump defect in diabetic peripheral nerve corrected by sorbinil administration: relationship to *myo*-inositol and nerve conduction slowing. Metabolism 35 (Suppl 1): 60–65
21. Majerus PW, Connolly TM, Deckmyn H, Ross TS, Bross TE, Ishii H, Bansal VS, Wilson DB (1986) The metabolism of phosphonositide-derived messenger molecules.

Science 234: 1519–1526
22. Clements RS, Stockard CR (1980) Abnormal sciatic nerve *myo*-inositol metabolism in the streptozotocin-diabetic rat: effect of insulin treatment. Diabetes 29: 227–235
23. Mayhew JA, Gillon KRW, Hawthorne JN (1983). Free and lipid inositol, sorbitol and sugars in sciatic nerve obtained post-mortem from diabetic patients and control subjects. Diabetologia 24: 13–15
24. Salway JG, Finnegan JA, Barnett D, Whitehead L, Karunanayaka A, Payne RB (1978) Effect of *myo*-inositol on peripheral nerve function in diabetes. Lancet ii: 1282–1284
25. Clements RS, Vourganti B, Kuba T, Oh SJ, Darnell B (1979) Dietary *myo*-inositol intake and peripheral nerve function in diabetic neuropathy. Metabolism 28 (Suppl 1): 477–483
26. Gregersen G, Borsting H, Theil P (1978) *Myo*-inositol and function of peripheral nerves in human diabetics. Acta Neurol Scand 58: 242–248
27. Brownlee M, Vlassara H, Cerami A (1985) Nonenzymatic glycosylation and the pathogenesis of diabetic complications. Ann Intern Med 101: 527–537
28. Vlassara H, Brownlee M, Cerami A (1983) Excessive nonenzymatic glycosylation of peripheral and central nervous system components in diabetic rats. Diabetes 32: 670–674
29. Vlassara H, Brownlee M, Cerami A (1985) Recognition and uptake of human diabetic peripheral nerve myelin by macrophages. Diabetes 34: 553–557
30. Carson KA, Bossen EH, Hanker JS (1980) Peripheral neuropathy in mouse hereditary diabetes mellitus. Neuropathol Appl Neurobiol 6: 361–374
31. Takekazn O, Poduslo JF, Dyck PJ (1985) Increased endoneurial albumin in diabetic polyneuropathy. Neurology 35: 1790–1791
32. Brownlee M, Vlassara H, Cerami A (1986) Trapped immunoglobulins on peripheral nerve myelin from patients with diabetes mellitus. Diabetes 35: 999–1003
33. Williams SK, Howarth NL, Devenny JJ, Bitensky MW (1982) Structural and functional consequences of increased tubulin glycosylation in diabetes mellitus. Proc Natl Acad Sci USA 79: 6546–6550
34. Tuck RR, Schmelzer JD, Low PA (1984) Endoneurial blood flow and oxygen tension in the sciatic nerves of rats with experimental diabetic neuropathy. Brain 107: 935–950
35. Low PA, Tuck RR, Dyck PJ, Schmelzer JD, Yao JK (1984) Prevention of some electrophysiologic and biochemical abnormalities with oxygen supplementation in experimental diabetic neuropathy. Proc Natl Acad Sci USA 81: 6894–6898
36. Williamson JR, Rowald E, Chang K, Marvel J, Tomlinson M, Sherman WR, Ackerman KE, Berger RA, Kilo C (1986) Sex steroid-dependency of diabetes-induced changes in polyol metabolism, vascular permeability and collagen cross-linking. Diabetes 35: 20–27
37. Clements RS, Kassira W, Garcia AR, Husband ME, Patton MA, Stockard CR (1986) Thyroid status and nerve function in experimental diabetes. Diabetes 35: 105A

Diabetic Complications: Early Diagnosis and Treatment
Edited by D. Andreani, G. Crepaldi, U. Di Mario and G. Pozza


CHAPTER 12

# *The Role of Metabolic Control in the Onset and Development of Diabetic Neuropathy*

D. PORTE JR.
*Diabetes Research Center, Veterans Administration Medical Center, University of Washington, Seattle, USA*

Some abnormality of nerve function is present in almost every individual with the diagnosis of diabetes mellitus within 2 years of the onset of hyperglycemia. While the balance of evidence suggests that hyperglycemia per se is the proximate cause of the disorder, variability of clinical presentation and severity suggests there are a host of modifying factors which complicate this relationship. Evidence that hyperglycemia is itself involved revolves around three different pieces of information:

1. Epidemiological studies of the prevalence and incidence of diabetic neuropathy in populations. These are based on retrospective, cross-sectional and, in a few instances, prospective assessment of nerve function in groups of diabetic patients.
2. Short- and medium-term trials of insulin or other oral hypoglycemic treatment in patients with asymptomatic or symptomatic neuropathy.
3. Experimental animal studies of nerve function indicating rapid progression of nerve dysfunction after the induction of hyperglycemia and its prevention or reversal by insulin therapy treatment with aldose reductase inhibitors.

## EPIDEMIOLOGICAL STUDIES

Epidemiological studies of diabetic neuropathy support the metabolic hypothesis, but definitive conclusions have been hampered by a lack of consistency in defining diabetic neuropathy, by the frequent mixture of Type 1 and Type 2 diabetic subjects in the population of patients under study, or by the inclusion of patients with focal or multifocal polyneuropathy together with patients who have symmetric distal somatic or autonomic polyneuropathy. Since the underlying pathophysiology for the focal and diffuse forms of neuropathy is likely to be different, there has been confusion regarding this relationship, particularly if highly selected populations are studied where rather more rare neuropathic syndromes may have an unusually high incidence.

The temporal dissociation between the onset of hyperglycemia and the onset of the clinical neurological disorder also makes for some confusion, even if the hyperglycemia is the cause, since the pathologic process takes a variable time to develop. This conclusion is supported by the observation that clinically detected diabetic neuropathy is rarely reported within the first 5 years of diabetes in Type 1 diabetic patients (1), and that the prevalence of diabetic neuropathy is initially very low, but increases progressively with the duration of diabetes in both Type 1 and Type 2 subjects (2). While there are patients who present soon after diagnosis with neuropathic symptoms, this finding appears almost exclusively in Type 2 diabetic subjects in whom the onset of hyperglycemia is often difficult to determine. Severe polyneuropathy early in Type 1 diabetic subjects is exceedingly rare, and here the early presenting severe symptoms are usually related to diffuse multifocal disease occurring in late-onset Type 1 patients, rather than the presence of symptomatic symmetrical distal somatic polyneuropathy. The similarity of reported prevalence rates for clinically symptomatic neuropathy in Type 1 and Type 2 diabetic patients supports the role of hyperglycemia in the etiology of the syndrome (3). However, there is great variation in the reported prevalence rate due to the variability of diagnostic criteria from study to study.

Perhaps the best view is provided by the unique observations of Pirart who for over 25 years followed a large population of diabetic subjects in just one clinical program (4). Using a consistent definition of neuropathy as a loss of achilles or patella reflexes or both, combined with diminished vibratory sensation, approximately 12% of patients were affected at the time of diabetes diagnosis. This prevalence increased linearly with duration of diabetes to nearly 50% after 25 years. The prevalence and incidence of neuropathy corrected for duration of diabetes did not differ substantially as a function of age at diagnosis and supports the conclusion that neuropathy occurs with similar frequency in Type 1 and Type 2 diabetic patients. However, the number of very young patients was relatively small in this series and this question remains somewhat open. Since normal aging affects function tests administered to assess the severity of neuropathy, and because assessment of the degree of control of hyperglycemia has been difficult until very recently (5), there are older studies in the literature which fail to find an association between the degree of hyperglycemia and either the prevalence or incidence of diabetic neuropathy (6).

Similarly, the often cited paradoxical precipitation of neuropathy following the institution of good control has raised questions regarding the etiology of diabetic neuropathy and its relationship to hyperglycemia. However, the syndrome that develops after treatment is usually related to the onset of painful symptoms, rather than to progressive signs of nerve disease (2, 7). Thus, these symptoms of pain may reflect repair and regeneration of damaged nerve fibers just as well as disease progression.

Since neuropathy occurs in non-genetic types of diabetes, such as diabetes after pancreatectomy, hemochromatosis, or non-alcoholic pancreatitis, there is other evidence for a causal relationship between hyperglycemia and diabetic neuropathy (8). The variability found in the quantitative relationship to hyperglycemia suggests the presence of other independent variables. Other risk factors may be involved since peripheral neuropathy is common in the general population due to nutritional, toxic (e.g. alcohol), metabolic (e.g. uremia), and mechanical anatomical factors (2, 9).

Similar variability has been found in the association between hyperglycemia and autonomic neuropathy. Some studies found very little or no correlation between glycosylated hemoglobin and heart rate response to the Valsalva maneuver or deep breathing (10). But others, particularly a recent prospective study by Young *et al.* (11), found a clear relationship between neurological cardiovascular function tests and poor glycemic control. Evidence from a number of prevalence studies suggests that similar percentages of abnormal cardiovascular reflex tests are found in insulin-dependent and non-insulin-dependent diabetic patients, supporting the hypothesis that hyperglycemia is a major factor in the pathogenesis of diabetic autonomic diffuse neuropathy (12–14). While abnormal cardiovascular autonomic function can be detected within 2 years of diagnosis (14), in general there is a relationship between the severity of autonomic damage and duration of diabetes in most retrospective analyses (15, 16). However, there is a great deal of variation in individual patients in the severity of diabetic autonomic neuropathy in comparison with somatosensory dysfunction, and between the degree of autonomic dysfunction in the various organ systems evaluated, such as the bladder, pupil, heart, blood vessels, and gastrointestinal system, suggesting again that other risk factors make an important contribution to the onset and severity of autonomic abnormalities in diabetic patients.

## CLINICAL STUDIES

Electrophysiologic studies of nerve conduction velocity in motor and sensory perception thresholds have been used as subclinical measures of nerve function in both small-scale epidemiological studies and trials to assess the relationship between plasma glucose control and neuropathy. Studies have shown that nerve conduction velocity in Type 1 diabetic patients is reduced at the time of diagnosis and improves rapidly with treatment (17). If control is worsened experimentally, there is a concomitant impairment of nerve conduction which is reminiscent of what occurs in diabetic animals (18). Parallel measurements of vibratory perception threshold are associated with similar changes in response to changes in glycemic control (19).

Nerve conduction velocity and sensory perception decline with time in both Type 1 and Type 2 diabetes, but in a group of stable hyperglycemic Type 2 patients there was still a relationship between the degree of hyperglycemia and the rate of nerve conduction velocity in the peroneal, median, and tibial motor nerves (20). While sensory nerve conduction velocities were abnormal, there was no relationship to the degree of hyperglycemia. In patients conventionally treated over a period of a year, there was improvement in motor nerve conduction velocity in all of the motor nerves tested, with the degree of improvement proportional to the degree of glycemic lowering in motor, but not sensory, nerves (21). In Type 1 diabetic patients short periods of intensified insulin treatment are usually associated with an improvement of motor nerve condution velocity within a month of therapy (22–24). However, in randomly controlled clinical trials of intensified insulin treatment, statistically significant differences between intensively treated and conventionally treated patients were only found after 7 months' treatment in one study (25), although these persisted for over 2 years in another (26). Both vibratory thresholds and motor nerve conduction velocity were found to show these changes. A long-term, randomized, prospective intervention trial is underway at the present time to test the ability to prevent diabetic neuropathy. This is an important issue since most studies with electrophysiologic or perception threshold end-points tend to show improvement which is small and not continuously progressive over time.

The lack of improvement in sensory nerve conduction velocity and the ability always to show improvement in motor nerve conduction with glycemic treatment, no matter how severe the defect is at the time of the metabolic intervention, suggests that there is a small reversible component which leads to chronic progressive irreversible loss of nerve function and that these occur in sequence; reversibility can therefore be demonstrated to a minor degree throughout the course of neuropathy, but a substantial reversal of abnormal function is unlikely. Thus, there is a need for a long-term control trial to determine whether neuropathy can be prevented by hypoglycemic treatment. The importance of this trial is the recognition that intensified insulin treatment increases the susceptibility to iatrogenic hypoglycemia (27) and the possibility that hypoglycemia itself may be damaging to the nerves (28). One of the contributory mechanisms to diabetic neuropathy may thus be the variability of plasma glucose itself, leading to both hyperglycemic and hypoglycemic damage to nerves. Support for this concept is derived from studies of experimental diabetes in animals in which atrophy of nerves without fiber loss and decreased nerve function is seen in hyperglycemic animals, whereas nerve fiber is found only in animals made hypoglycemic during treatment (29, 30). Human nerve abnormalities seem to consist of both atrophy and fiber loss. This combination has yet to be induced in experimental animals who have not been treated with insulin, suggesting that the human disease may be variably dependent upon both the type of metabolic dysfunction and its response to treatment.

## STUDIES IN EXPERIMENTAL ANIMALS

Studies in experimental animals strongly support the metabolic hypothesis. Reduction of nerve conduction velocity is found in rats and mice who have either experimentally induced or spontaneous genetic hyperglycemia (31). Studies in these animals are complicated by the fact that they are usually young and still growing at the time the lesion is induced and, as a result, nerve conduction velocity actually increases with age due to the effects of growth on nerve function, which even in the diabetic animal leads to larger, more rapidly conducting nerves. Nevertheless, there is always a large difference in conduction velocity between the control and the experimental diabetic animal. These changes can be prevented by insulin treatment given at the time of the induction of hyperglycemia or can be reversed by insulin treatment if glycemic control is instituted within 6 months of the development of hyperglycemia (32, 33). After this time, there is some reversibility, but not restoration to normal. In conjunction with this abnormality of function, there is an impairment of axonal anterograde and retrograde transport (34–36), as well as a shrinkage and diminution of axonal size (37). The longer after the development of hyperglycemia an examination is made, the more likely one is to find pathologic changes that include axonal degeneration and demyelination. Alterations in nerve conduction velocity are always found before pathologic changes are observed, indicating that these conduction velocity changes are likely to be due to functional, rather than structural, abnormalities. Nerve swelling has been observed and intracellular edema has been demonstrated morphologically, but the predominant area of swelling appears to be in the endoneurial space, examined by electron microscopy (38). This location has been of some concern as aldose reductase is found in Schwann cells rather than in the axon by immunohistochemical methods.

Similar findings of reduced induction velocity with early pathologic changes and a progressive abnormal nerve function have been reported in diabetic monkeys, chinese hamsters, mouse, and dog (31). The most extensive neuropathy has been described in the bb rat, which develops severe hyperglycemia of the Type 1 form at approximately 100 days of age. In these animals treatment with small doses of insulin, sufficient to prevent ketoacidosis but not to normalize glucose levels, is associated with reduced nerve conduction followed by axonal atrophy, shrinkage and wrinkling. Autonomic nervous system dysfunction is also seen in this animal model and it is associated with a variety of dystrophic autonomic axonal changes (39). Axonal transport is also abnormal and treatment with insulin prevents all of the changes observed, indicating the metabolic abnormality as a likely underlying factor.

Increased glucose metabolism via the sorbitol pathway has been suggested as a major mechanism for the etiology of these functional abnormalities ocurring after experimental or genetic hyperglycemia (40). Activation of this pathway leads by unknown mechanisms to myoinositol depletion. This depletion is associated with a reduction in protein kinase C and sodium–potassium ATPase activity. The reduction in sodium–potassium ATPase activity is associated with a reduced overall nerve oxygen consumption, an increase in intracellular sodium, and an impairment in nerve conduction velocity (41). It is postulated that this metabolic sequence then leads to the morphological changes seen in long-standing neuropathy.

Since the mouse appears to lack the enzyme aldose reductase, but still develops abnormal nerve conduction velocity and axonal dwindling, at least in some experimental models this mechanism cannot be invoked. Glycosylation of proteins also occurs as in experimental hyperglycemia (42) and glycosylation of nerve proteins is known to take place (43, 44). Therefore, there is at least a possibility that the metabolic consequences of hyperglycemia are complex and may vary from time to time and in different species. Support for the role of aldose reductase as a mechanism for the effects of hyperglycemia in diabetic neuropathy has been given by the use of aldose reductase inhibitors in rats (45, 46). Several different chemical classes of aldose reductase inhibitor have been used. All have been shown to reduce sciatic nerve sorbitol concentration and improve motor nerve conduction velocity. Most have also been shown to restore nerve myoinositol concentrations and prevent defects in axonal transport. These same compounds have also been found to prevent galactosemic retinal capillary basement thickening, partially to reverse diabetic proteinuria in experimental diabetic rats, and to reduce the concentration of sorbitol in isolated glomeruli (47). Studies in man have been much less extensive, but clear-cut, short-term improvement in nerve function has also been found (48, 49).

## SUMMARY AND CONCLUSION

Clinical, epidemiological and experimental studies in animals and man suggest that hyperglycemia, per se, plays an important role in the etiology and pathogenesis of diabetic neuropathy. Experimental studies suggest that aldose reductase is important at least initially, but further studies concerning alternative mechanisms, including protein glycosylation, need further experimental evaluation. Long-term prospective randomized trials will be necessary to assess the ability to prevent or reverse diabetic neuropathy in man, using either intensified insulin treatment regimens or compounds designed to interfere with one or more of the proposed pathogenic mechanisms. At this time, however, diabetic neuropathy probably represents the best example of a diabetic complication in which the role of metabolic control has been demonstrated. Since the syndrome remains heterogeneous within the diabetic population, the important modifying factors that must participate in this complication need to be further elucidated and the mechanism of their interaction with hyperglycemia determined.

## REFERENCES


1. Eng GD, Hung W, August GP, Smokvina MD (1976) Nerve conduction velocity determinations in juvenile diabetes: continuing study of 190 patients. Arch Phys Med Rehabil 51: 1
2. Brown MJ, Asbury AK (1984) Diabetic neuropathy. Ann Neurol 15: 2
3. Thomas PK, Ward JD, Watkins PJ (1982) Diabetic neuropathy. In: Keen H, Jarrett J (eds) Complications of Diabetes. Edward Arnold, London, pp 109–136
4. Pirart J (1978) Diabetes mellitus and its degenerative complications: a prospective study of 4400 patients observed between 1947 and 1973. Diabetes Care 1: 68 and 252
5. National Diabetes Data Group (1984) Report of the expert committee on glycosylated hemoglobin. Diabetes Care 7: 602–606
6. Gregersen G (1967) Diabetic neuropathy: Influence of age, sex, metabolic control and

duration of diabetes on motor conduction velocity. Neurology 17: 972
7. Thomas PK, Eliasson SG (1984) Diabetic neuropathy. In: Dyck PJ et al. (eds) Peripheral neuropathy, second edition WB Saunders, Philadelphia, pp 1773–1810
8. Thomas PK, Ward JD, Watkins PJ (1982) Diabetic neuropathy. In: Keen H, Jarrett J (eds) Complications of diabetes. Edward Arnold, London, pp 109–136
9. McCulloch DK, Campbell IW, Prescott RJ, Clarke BP (1980) Effect of alcohol intake on symptomatic peripheral neuropathy in diabetic men. Diabetes Care 3: 245
10. Smith SE, Smith SA, Brown PM (1981) Cardiac autonomic dysfunction in patients with diabetic retinopathy. Diabetologia 21: 525
11. Young RJ, MacIntyre CA, Martyn CN, et al. (1986) Progression of subclinical polyneuropathy in young patients with Type 1 (insulin-dependent) diabetes: associated with glycaemic control and microangiopathy (microvascular complications). Diabetologia 29: 156
12. Fernandez-Castaner M, Mendola G, Levy I, Gromis R, Figuerola D (1985) The prevalence and clinical aspects of the cardiovascular autonomous neuropathy in diabetic patients. Med Clin 84: 215
13. Masaoka S, Lev-Ran A, Hill LR, Vakil G, Hon EHG (1985) Heart rate variability in diabetes: relationship to age and duration of the disease. Diabetes Care 8: 64
14. Pfeifer MA, Weinberg CR, Cook DL, et al. (1984) Autonomic neural dysfunction in recently diagnosed diabetic subjects. Diabetes Care 7: 447
15. Masaoka S, Lev-Ran A, Hill LR, Vakil G, Hon EHG (1985) Heart rate variability in diabetes: relationship to age and duration of the disease. Diabetes Care 8: 64
16. Sundvist G (1981) Autonomic nervous dysfunction in asymptomatic diabetic patients with signs of peripheral neuropathy. Diabetes Care 4: 529
17. Ward JD, Fisher DJ, Barnes CG, Jessop JD (1971) Improvement in nerve conduction following treatment in newly diagnosed diabetics. Lancet i: 428
18. Gregersen G (1968) Variations in motor conduction velocity produced by acute changes of the metabolic state in diabetic patients. Diabetologia 4: 273
19. Terkildsen AB, Christensen NJ (1971) Reversible nervous abnormalities in juvenile diabetics with recently diagnosed diabetes. Diabetologia 7: 113
20. Graf RJ, Halter JB, Halar E, Porte D Jr (1979) Nerve conduction abnormalities in untreated maturity-onset diabetes: relation to levels of fasting plasma glucose and glycosylated hemoglobin. Ann Intern Med 90: 298
21. Graf RJ, Halter JB, Pfeifer MD, Halar E, Brozovich F, Porte D Jr (1981) Glycemic control and nerve conduction abnormalities in non insulin-dependent diabetic subjects. Ann Intern Med 94: 307
22. Gallai V, Agostini L, Rossi A, et al. (1978) Evaluation of the motor and sensory conduction velocity (MCV, SCV) in diabetic patients before and after a three-day treatment with the artificial beta cell (Biostator). In: Canal N, Pozza G (eds) Peripheral neuropathies. Elsevier/North-Holland Biomedical Press, Amsterdam, pp 287–289
23. Golden M, Nudleman K, Myers G, Charles A (1980) Improvement in peripheral nerve function in diabetes after short-term treatment with an artificial pancreas. Diabetes 29: 58
24. Pietri A, Ehle A, Raskin P (1980) Changes in nerve conduction velocity after six weeks of glycoregulation with portable insulin infusion pumps. Diabetes 29: 668
25. Service FJ, Rizza RA, Daube JR, et al. (1985) Near normoglycaemia improved nerve conduction and vibration sensation in diabetic neuropathy. Diabetologia 28: 722
26. Holman RR, White VM, Orde-Pecker C, et al. (1983) Prevention of deterioration of renal and sensory-nerve function by more intensive management of insulin-dependent diabetic patients. A two-year randomized prospective study. Lancet i: 204
27. The DCCT Research Group (1986) Results of feasibility phase of the diabetes control

and complications trial (DCCT): glycemic control, follow-up and complications of therapy. Diabetes (Suppl 1): 3A

28. Jakobsen J, Sidenius P (1987) Hypoglycemic neuropathy. In: Dyck PJ, Thomas PK, Asbury AK, Weinegrad AI, Porte D Jr (eds) Diabetic neuropathy. WB Saunders, Philadelphia, pp 94–99
29. Sidenius P, Jakobsen J (1983) Peripheral neuropathy in rats induced by insulin treatment. Diabetes 32: 383
30. Jakobsen J (1979) Early and preventable changes of peripheral nerve structure and function in insulin-deficient diabetic rats. J Neurol Neurosurg Psychiatry 42: 509
31. Sharma AK, Thomas PK (1987) Animal models: pathology and pathophysiology. In: Dyck JP, Thomas PK, Asbury AK, Winegrad AI, Porte D Jr (eds) Diabetic neuropathy. WB Saunders, Philadelphia, pp 237–252
32. Greene DA, DeJesus PV, Winegrad AI (1975) Effects of insulin and dietary myoinositol on impaired peripheral motor nerve conduction velocity in acute streptozotocin diabetes. J Clin Invest 55: 1326
33. Jakobsen J (1979) Early and preventable changes of peripheral nerve structure and function in insulin-deficient diabetic rats. J Neurol Neurosurg Psychiatry 42: 509
34. Jakobsen J, Sidenius P (1980) Decreased axonal transport of structural proteins in streptozotocin diabetic rats. J Clin Invest 66: 292
35. Jakobsen J, Sidenius P (1979) Decreased axonal flux of retrogradely transported glycoproteins in early experimental diabetes. J Neurochem 33: 1055
36. Tomlinson DR, Mayer JH (1984) Defects of axonal transport in diabetes mellitus—a possible contribution to the etiology of diabetic neuropathy. J Auton Pharmacol 4: 59
37. Jakobsen J (1976) Axonal dwindling in early experimental diabetes. 1. A study of cross sectioned nerves. Diabetologia 12: 539
38. Jakobsen J (1978) Peripheral nerves in early experimental diabetes. Expansion of the endoneurial space as a cause of increased water content. Diabetologia 14: 113
39. Sima Anders AF, Brismar T, Yagihashi S (1987) Neuropathies encountered in the spontaneously diabetic BB wistar rat. In: Dyck PJ, Thomas PK, Asbury AK, Winegrad AI, Porte D Jr (eds) Diabetic neuropathy. WB Saunders, Philadelphia, pp 253–259
40. Clements RS (1979) Diabetic neuropathy: new concepts of its etiology. Diabetes 28: 604
41. Greene DA, Lattimer S, Ulbrecht J, Carroll P (1985) Glucose-induced alterations in nerve metabolism: Current perspective on the pathogenesis of diabetic neuropathy, and future directions for research and therapy. Diabetes Care 8: 290
42. Proceedings of a conference on nonenzymatic glycosylation and browning reactions: their relevance to diabetes mellitus (1982) Diabetes 31 (Suppl 3): V–VI
43. Williams SK, Howarth NL, Devenny JJ, Bitensky MW (1982) Structural and functional consequences of increased tubulin glycosylation in diabetes mellitus. Proc Natl Acad Sci USA 79: 6546
44. Vlassara H, Brownlee M, Cerami A (1983) Excessive nonenzymatic glycosylation of peripheral and central nervous system myelin components in diabetic rats. Diabetes 32: 670–674
45. Service FJ, Daube JR, O'Brien PC, Dyck PJ (1981) Effect of artificial pancreas treatment on peripheral nerve function in diabetes. Neurology 31: 1375
46. Troni W, Carta Q, Cantello R, Caselle MT, Rainero I (1984) Peripheral nerve function and metabolic control in diabetes mellitus. Ann Neurol 16: 178
47. Zimmerman BR (1987) Aldose reductase inhibitors. In: Dyck PJ, Thomas PK, Asbury AK, Winegrad AI, Porte D Jr (eds) Diabetic neuropathy WB Saunders, Philadelphia, pp 190–193
48. Judzewitsch RG, Jaspan JB, Polonsky KS, et al. (1983) Aldose reductase inhibition improves nerve conduction velocity in diabetic patients. N Engl J Med 308: 119

49. Fagius J, Brattburg A, Jameson S, Berne C (1985) Limited benefit of treatment of diabetic polyneuropathy with an aldose reductase inhibitor: a 24-week controlled trial. Diabetologia 28: 323

Diabetic Complications: Early Diagnosis and Treatment
Edited by D. Andreani, G. Crepaldi, U. Di Mario and G. Pozza


CHAPTER 13

# *New Methodological Approaches in the Diagnosis of Autonomic Neuropathy*

D. J. Ewing
*Wellcome Trust, University of Edinburgh, UK*

There is increasing realization that damaged autonomic nerves play an important role in the development of diabetic complications. The clinical picture of diabetic autonomic neuropathy is well recognized, but more subtle abnormalities of autonomic function are now being found in, for example, the lungs and the kidneys. Cardiovascular reflex evidence of deranged autonomic function is present in 20–40% of all diabetic subjects. The question has to be asked, however, as to how reliable current methods of detection are, and what new approaches are being developed for the objective diagnosis of diabetic autonomic neuropathy.

This brief review will examine some of the current problems inherent in non-invasive cardiovascular reflex testing, describe several new methods for detecting early cardiovascular reflex damage, and discuss the development of some other new approaches to the diagnosis of autonomic abnormalities elsewhere.

## CARDIOVASCULAR REFLEX TESTING

There is widespread agreement that non-invasive cardiovascular reflex tests can give objective evidence of autonomic involvement. Over the past 10 years or so the possible test options have been considerably refined. Some tests have been discarded as unsuitable for a variety of reasons, while others have been added to the existing battery of available tests. Five tests are emerging as the most popular and reliable. These are the heart rate responses to the Valsalva manoeuvre, deep breathing and standing up, and the blood pressure responses to standing up and sustained handgrip. A number of other cardiovascular tests have been proposed and used, but all have certain disadvantages. For example, although the normal response to the cold pressor test, mental stress, or a loud noise is a rise in blood pressure, this is usually small and does not invariably occur. This, of course, makes interpretation of an 'abnormal' response very difficult. Neck suction and lower body negative pressure are useful physiological manoeuvres, but need special apparatus and are not appropriate for more general use. Apneic face immersion requires the subject to dip his or her face in a bowl of water. Atropine and propranolol need intravenous injections and careful heart rate monitoring. Atropine also has a number of other physiological effects which are not always pleasant.

What then are some of the pitfalls associated with the five tests mentioned above? They are all non-invasive, easy to perform, have good repeatability, and the results clearly differentiate normal responses from abnormal. Problems arise more with the operators than with the tests themselves. Firstly, there is the danger of relying on a single test to diagnose autonomic neuropathy. It is better to use a battery of tests to avoid overinterpretation of a doubtful or borderline single result. Using several tests also enables the severity of the autonomic neuropathy to be established more easily. Secondly, there is an assumption that is sometimes forgotten that is implicit in the use of these tests. They measure cardiovascular reflexes and damage elsewhere is only inferred. The evidence for this is good, as autonomic neuropathy in diabetes appears to affect all parts of the body, but it does not always follow.

Thirdly, although the five tests are widely applied, there is considerable controversy surrounding the precise techniques used, how the results are calculated and the normal reference ranges. For example, heart rate variation during breathing can be measured with the subject sitting or lying, breathing quietly or deeply, and taking a single or repeated deep breaths. Results have been expressed as the maximum minus minimum heart rate, the expiration inspiration (EI) ratio, the coefficient of variation, and the standard deviation of the heart rate. Some groups have taken age into account when calculating normal ranges, whereas others have not. Similar problems occur with each of the other tests. There is clearly a need for standardization so that the tests can be readily applied and results compared in different centres. From a practical point of view, while there is no absolute right or wrong method for performing the tests or calculating the results, the techniques we have used in Edinburgh and our criteria for normal ranges (1) are being increasingly adopted. We now use an on-line microcomputer system for performing the tests and measuring the results.

The categorization of autonomic damage presents a further difficulty. Although previously we classified autonomic neuropathy into 'parasympathetic' and 'parasympathetic plus sympathetic', it is clear that the pathways subserving the cardiovascular reflexes are extremely complex and it is not physiologically precise to categorize the damage in these terms. We now classify subjects as 'normal', 'early', 'definite', 'severe', or 'atypical', depending on their responses to the five tests (1).

## SOME NEWER METHODS TO DETECT CARDIOVASCULAR REFLEX DAMAGE

### Analysis of 24-Hour ECG Recordings

Heart rates have been recorded over 24-hour periods in a number of diabetic subjects. In one study (2), 64 diabetic subjects with different degrees of autonomic damage, ranging from none to very severe, underwent 24-hour ambulatory electrocardiogram (ECG) monitoring. The diabetic patients had higher mean hourly heart rates, and reduced diurnal variations with increasing severity of autonomic damage. In particular, the normal fall in heart rate at night was much less obvious, so that the mean sleeping heart rates were considerably increased when compared with an age-matched control group. Two other groups have now confirmed these findings (3, 4).

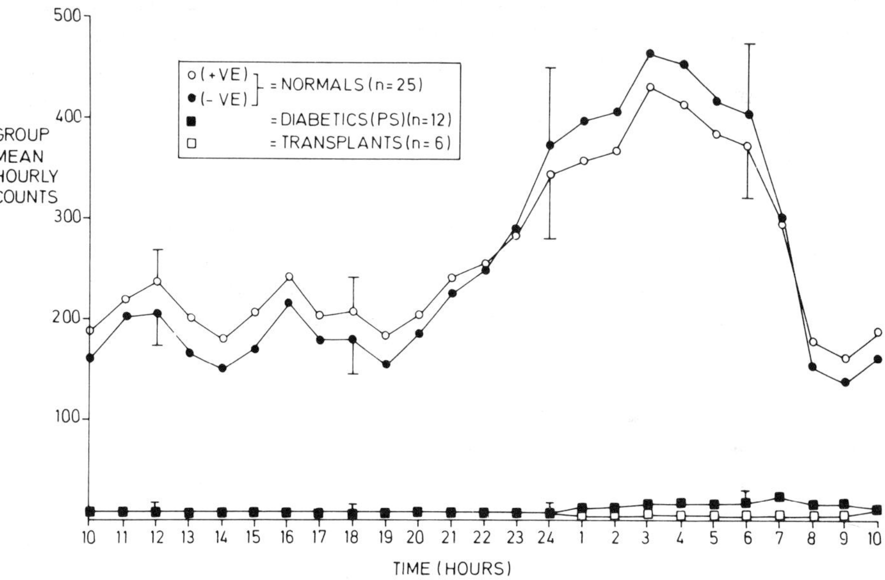


Figure 1. Group mean hourly R-R interval step counts in normal subjects, diabetic subjects with cardiac parasympathetic damage, and cardiac transplant patients. Bars represent SEM. Reproduced from Ewing et al. (5) with permission.

A different approach to the analysis of the 24-hour heart rate signal has also been undertaken by us (5). Examination of heart rate records reveals that in normal subjects, in addition to the well-known small cyclical variations of sinus arrhythmia, there are a large number of irregular abrupt changes in R-R interval cycle length. If these are counted, then changes in successive R-R intervals of more than 50 msec occur on average about 200 times per hour during the day and 400 times per hour at night. Diabetic subjects with cardiac parasympathetic damage, and cardiac transplant subjects, both had extremely low counts (Figure 1). This and other evidence suggests that this method of 'counts' provides a very sensitive and reliable index of cardiac parasympathetic activity, which can be applied over prolonged periods. Instead, therefore, of an indication of parasympathetic activity for just over a few seconds, as with conventional cardiovascular reflex tests, this method has the potential for monitoring cardiac parasympathetic activity continuously over long periods. As the autonomic nervous system is in a dynamic state of flux, such an approach could be used to examine the autonomic responses to a successive variety of everyday stimuli.

### Computer Analysis of Heart Rate Variation

As heart rate variation is extremely complex, a number of workers have developed complex computer analyses of the heart rate rhythm and its relation to the respiratory cycle. The principle behind this approach has been that, by use of spectral analysis and cross-correlation techniques, the heart rate pattern can be broken down into a series of rhythms of different frequencies, and related to other factors such as respiration, blood pressure changes and temperature. Inevitably, diabetic subjects with autonomic neuropathy have provided a most useful group to study in comparison with normal subjects. As might be expected, such diabetic subjects have lower heart rate variations and fewer cross-correlations with respiration (6). While such a complex approach may be mathematically sound, it has yet to be established that this type of analysis will produce physiologically interpretable results or more accurate bedside methods for diagnosing autonomic neuropathy.

### Heart Rate Response to Coughing

Coughing produces rapid intrathoracic pressure fluctuations with consequent hemodynamic and cardiovascular reflex effects. Normally a brief cough produces an immediate shortening of the R-R interval (or an increase in heart rate) reaching a peak in 2–3 sec, and followed by the R-R interval lengthening back to the resting value over the next 18–20 sec. The cardiac acceleration is abolished by atropine, but not propranolol, showing that it is dependent on cardiac parasympathetic pathways (7). Diabetic subjects with autonomic neuropathy have a response similar to normal subjects after autonomic blockade, unlike diabetic subjects with intact cardiovascular reflexes. It is possible that this manoeuvre could be adopted as a further simple test of cardiac parasympathetic function.

### Immediate Heart Rate Response to Lying Down

When a normal subject lies down, there is a small but consistent immediate rise in heart rate over 3 or 4 beats, followed by a fall in heart rate to below the standing level over the next 25–30 beats. The first part of the response appears to be under cardiac parasympathetic control, while the latter is more under sympathetic control (8). This has been adapted as a further possible simple cardiovascular reflex test in diabetic subjects (9). In a recent study it has been suggested that the first part of the response, over the first five beats after starting to lie down ($S-L_1$), could be used as a test of parasympathetic integrity, while the later fall in heart rate ($S-L_2$) could be used as a mixed, but predominantly sympathetic, test (10). Further investigations are awaited to see whether or not this test will prove useful clinically.

### Baroreflex Abnormalities

There has been renewed interest in baroreflex function in diabetic subjects, using amyl nitrite inhalation and phenylephrine infusions (11, 12). These studies have shown abnormalities of baroreflex control in diabetic patients both with and without autonomic symptoms, signifying extensive defects of both parasympathetic and sympathetic innervation.

## SOME NEW APPROACHES TO THE DETECTION OF AUTONOMIC DAMAGE ELSEWHERE

### Pupillary Function

Two new and relatively simple techniques have recently been described. The first measures the diameter of the dark-adapted pupil, using a polaroid photograph of the eye taken by electronic flash. When standardized against the outer diameter of the iris, the diameter of the dark-adapted pupil provides a quantitative estimate of sympathetic innervation (13). The second technique, measurement of pupil cycle time (PCT), depends on the observation that regular oscillations of the pupil can be induced with a slit-lamp beam in normal subjects and timed with a stopwatch (14). Pharmacological testing confirms that PCT is a sensitive measure of parasympathetic dysfunction, and in diabetic patients with autonomic neuropathy it is considerably prolonged (Figure 2). These techniques provide two additional simple methods of testing autonomic reflexes independent of cardiovascular pathways.

### Sudomotor and Skin Tests

Local sweat output can now be measured by two techniques. The first is that of a quantitative sudomotor axon reflex test (QSART) in which local sweating is stimulated by acetylcholine iontophoresis (15). This method has recently been used to compare distal sympathetic function with cardiovascular reflex tests of vagal function in a large group of diabetic subjects. Abnormal QSART tests in the foot and abnormal heart rate variation were found in roughly equal proportions, and much more frequently than either orthostatic hypotension or sweating abnormalities in the

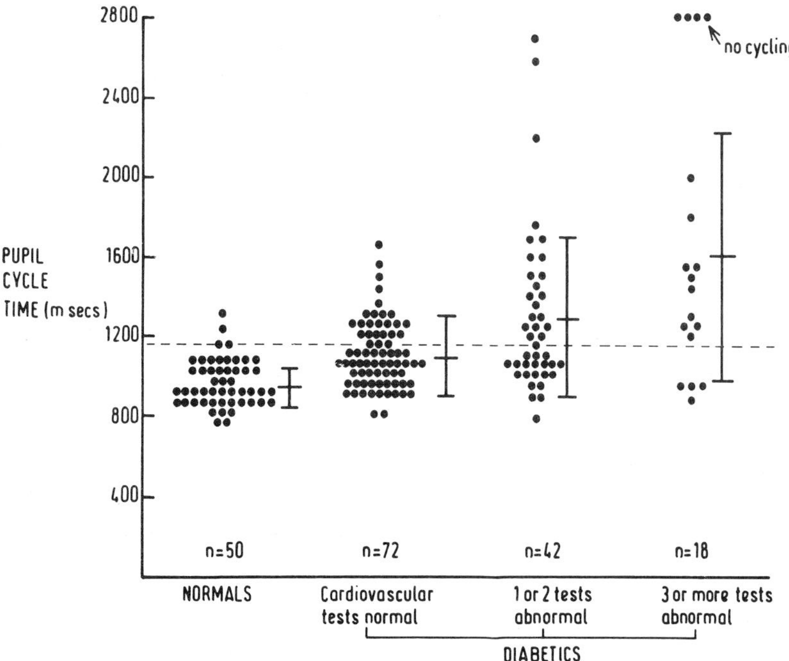


Figure 2. Pupil cycle times in normal and diabetic subjects. The diabetic subjects are grouped according to the number of abnormal cardiovascular reflex tests. The solid lines represent mean ± SD, and the dotted line indicates the upper limit of normal. Reproduced from Martyn and Ewing (14) with permission.

arm (16), thus supporting earlier suggestions that distal sympathetic function becomes abnormal early in the natural progression of diabetic autonomic neuropathy. The second sweat test technique is to count the number of imprints that sweat drops make in a soft silastic impression material after stimulation of local sweating with pilocarpine iontophoresis (17).

Other new approaches to testing skin reflexes have included the measurement of the skin flare responses to intradermal histamine before and after the addition of noradrenaline or terbutaline (adrenoceptor agonists). Diabetic patients with autonomic neuropathy showed no change in the size of the skin flare after noradrenaline, in contrast to normal subjects and diabetic subjects without neuropathy, thus suggesting a defect in these patients at the adrenoceptor level (18). This might provide a further simple test for distal autonomic neuropathy, but confirmatory studies are required.

Further tests of skin temperature responsiveness and blood flow have recently been proposed for the diagnosis of autonomic neuropathy. One group has described thermography of the leg after indirect heating of the other leg in a warm waterbath.

Normal subjects produced a rise in temperature, whereas some diabetic subjects had a flat response, and the authors felt that this provided a further measure of distal sympathetic function (19). Another group of workers found that temperature sensitivity thresholds in the lower limbs were impaired in diabetic subjects with clinical evidence of autonomic neuropathy, again indicating defects of distal sympathetic function (20). Patterns of fingertip blood flow, measured by a doppler technique, have been suggested as another possible way to detect autonomic neuropathy (21).

### Neuroendocrine Defects

With the realization that a variety of neuroendocrine abnormalities may be present in diabetic patients with autonomic neuropathy, considerable attention is now being paid to elucidating the pathophysiological mechanisms involved, although at this stage some of the results appear somewhat discrepant (22). One gastrointestinal hormone that may be useful as a marker of vagal function is pancreatic polypeptide (PP). In diabetic patients with autonomic neuropathy, reduced PP responses have been demonstrated during the early phase after a meal (Figure 3) (23, 24) and following sham feeding (25) and insulin-induced hypoglycemia (26).

Although plasma noradrenaline is widely used as an index of sympathetic activity, there are a number of assumptions implicit in the interpretation of results. Plasma levels represent only a small proportion of the catecholamine pool and are themselves the net result of the balance between noradrenaline production and utilization. Widely varying basal levels of noradrenaline have been reported in diabetic subjects, making interpretation extremely difficult. Noradrenaline turnover studies have been developed to try to obviate this difficulty. Two groups have found that in diabetic patients with autonomic neuropathy, while metabolic clearance was similar to those without autonomic neuropathy, noradrenaline production measured as plasma appearance rate was reduced (27, 28).

Recent interest has also focused on arginine vasopressins (AVP). Reduced AVP response to volume depletion (29) and upright posture (30) has been demonstrated in diabetic autonomic neuropathy. The pathways controlling AVP release are beginning to be understood and it is likely that other studies in diabetic autonomic neuropathy will uncover further abnormalities in this complex area.

### Gastrointestinal Function

Within the gastrointestinal tract a number of new approaches have been utilized and applied to diabetic patients with autonomic neuropathy. Esophageal motility disturbances, which are usually asymptomatic, are well recognized and have been studied by radiographic barium swallows and esophageal manometry. Manometric abnormalities include multipeaked esophageal peristaltic pressure waves which are much more prominent in diabetic subjects with autonomic abnormalities elsewhere (31).

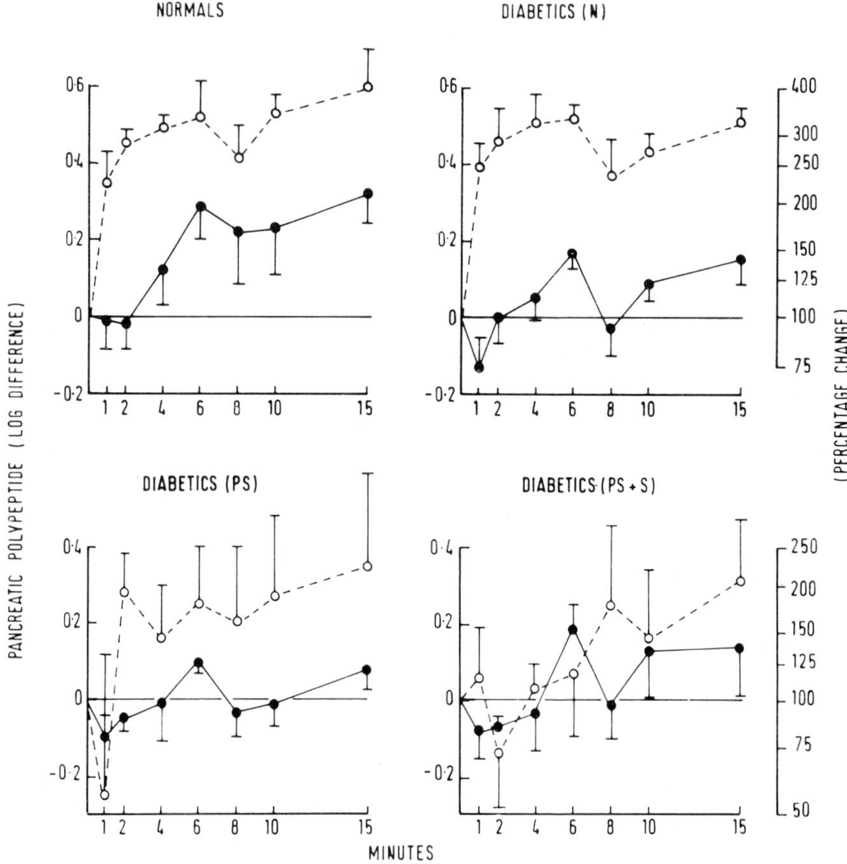


Figure 3. Group mean (± SEM) pancreatic polypeptide concentrations following a mixed meal (o- - -o) or intravenous edrophonium (●—●) in six normal subjects, five diabetic patients with normal cardiovascular reflexes, three with parasympathetic cardiac damage, and four with combined cardiac parasympathetic and sympathetic damage. Reproduced from Ewing et al. (23) with permission.

Esophageal emptying times have been measured using scintigraphic techniques. Diabetic patients with autonomic neuropathy had delayed emptying whether assessed by numbers of swallows, length of time to clear a solid bolus through the esophagus (32, 33), or water transit times (34).

Gastric function is also abnormal. Most observers have found that isotope clearance studies show normal liquid emptying, but slow emptying of solids (35, 36), although a recent study found abnormal liquid emptying as well in diabetic subjects and this correlated with cardiovascular evidence of autonomic neuropathy (33). Another report, however, suggested that gastric accommodation to distension was abnormal, and that this consequently gave rise to rapid early liquid emptying in these diabetic subjects (37). While, therefore, there is agreement about gastric emptying of solids being delayed, there is some disagreement about the patterns of liquid emptying from the stomach. Other new observations are pyloric sphincter dysfunction (38) and abnormal interdigestive migrating motor complexes (39) in diabetic patients with autonomic neuropathy.

## CONCLUSIONS

As will be seen from this brief review, a large number of different areas are being explored to try to understand further the pathophysiological abnormalities underlying diabetic autonomic neuropathy. While cardiovascular reflexes provide a simple and objective measure of autonomic damage, there are certain limitations that need to be understood. Further standardization of tests is required so that diagnosis can be made more easily. Several new cardiovascular approaches are being developed to provide more sensitive tests that will detect autonomic damage at a very early stage. Outside the cardiovascular system new approaches are also being explored, both to provide simple bedside diagnostic tests and to give further pathophysiological insights. With all these new ways of looking at diabetic autonomic neuropathy it is to be hoped that further progress will be made in reducing the morbidity and mortality of this particular complication of diabetes.

## REFERENCES

1. Ewing DJ, Martyn CN, Young RJ, Clarke BF (1985) The value of cardiovascular autonomic function tests: 10 years experience in diabetes. Diabetes Care 8: 491–498
2. Ewing DJ, Borsey DQ, Travis P, et al. (1982) Abnormalities of ambulatory 24 hour heart rate in diabetes mellitus. Diabetes 32: 101–105
3. Rubler S, Chu DA, Bruzzone CL (1985) Blood pressure and heart rate responses during 24-hour ambulatory monitoring and exercise in men with diabetes mellitus. Am J Cardiol 55: 801–806
4. Valensi P, Attali JR, Sachs R-N, et al. (1985) Abnormalities of 24-hour continuous electrocardiographic monitoring in diabetes mellitus: involvement of cardiac neuropathy and/or insulin treatment. Diabete Metab 11: 337–342
5. Ewing DJ, Neilson JMM, Travis P (1984) New method for assessing cardiac parasympathetic activity using 24 hour electrocardiograms. Br Heart J 52: 396–402
6. Bernardi L, Calciati A, Marti G, et al. (1986) Bedside diagnosis of cardiac autonomic damage by computerized analysis of heart rate–respiration relationship. Acta Diabetol Lat 23: 141–154
7. Cardone C, Bellavere F, Ferri M, Fedele D (1987) Autonomic mechanisms in the heart rate response to coughing. Clin Sci 72: 55–60
8. Bellavere F, Ewing DJ (1982) Autonomic control of the immediate heart rate response to lying down. Clin Sci 62: 57–64
9. Rodrigues EA, Ewing DJ (1983) Immediate heart rate response to lying down: simple test for parasympathetic damage in diabetes. Br Med J 287: 800
10. Bellavere F, Cardone C, Ferri M, et al. (1987) Standing to lying heart rate variations. A

new simple test in the diagnosis of diabetic autonomic neuropathy. Diabetic Med 4: 41–43
11. Olshan AR, O'Connor DT, Cohen IM, Mitas JA, Stone RA (1983) Baroreflex dysfunction in patients with adult-onset diabetes and hypertension. Am J Med 74: 233–242
12. Eckberg DL, Harkins SW, Fritsch JM, Musgrave GE, Gardner DF (1986) Baroreflex control of plasma norepinephrine and heart period in healthy subjects and diabetic patients. J Clin Invest 78: 366–374
13. Smith SA, Dewhirst RR (1986) A simple diagnostic test for pupillary abnormality in diabetic autonomic neuropathy. Diabetic Med 3: 38–41
14. Martyn CN, Ewing DJ (1986) Pupil cycle time: a simple way of measuring an autonomic reflex. J Neurol Neurosurg Psychiatry 49: 771–774
15. Low PA, Caskey PE, Tuck RR, Fealey RD, Dyck PJ (1983) Quantitative sudomotor axon reflex test in normal and neuropathic subjects. Ann Neurol 14: 573–580
16. Low PA, Zimmerman BR, Dyck PJ (1986) Comparison of distal sympathetic with vagal function in diabetic neuropathy. Muscle Nerve 9: 592–596
17. Kennedy WR, Sakuda M, Sutherland D, Goetz FC (1984) The sweating deficiency in diabetes mellitus: methods of quantitation and clinical correlation. Neurology (Cleveland) 34: 758–763
18. Hoffman A, Conen D, Leibundgut U, Berger W (1982) A skin test for autonomic neuropathy. Eur Neurol 21: 29–33
19. Fushimi H, Inoue T, Nishikawa M, Matsuyama Y, Kitagawa J (1985) A new index of autonomic neuropathy in diabetes mellitus: heat stimulated thermographic patterns. Diabetes Res Clin Pract 1: 103–107
20. Lehmann WP, Halsbeck M, Muller J, Mehnert H, Strian F (1985) Early diagnosis of autonomic diabetic neuropathy with the temperature sensitivity test. Deutsch Med Wochenschr 110: 639–642
21. Oimomi M, Nishimoto S, Mastsumoto S, et al. (1985) Evaluation of periflux blood flow measurements in diabetic patients with autonomic neuropathy. Diabetes Res Clin Pract 1: 81–85
22. Ewing DJ, Clarke BF (1986) Diabetic autonomic neuropathy: present insights and future prospects. Diabetes Care 9: 648–665
23. Ewing DJ, Bellavere F, Espi F, et al. (1986) Correlation of cardiovascular and neuroendocrine tests of autonomic function in diabetes. Metabolism 35: 349–353
24. Gambardella G, Felici MG, Annibale B, et al. (1986) Pancreatic polypeptide response to a protein-rich meal in diabetic patients with and without neuropathy. J Endocrinol Invest 9: 1–4
25. Buysschaert M, Donckier J, Dive A, Ketelslegers J-M, Lambert AE (1985) Gastric acid and pancreatic polypeptide responses to sham feeding are impaired in diabetic subjects with autonomic neuropathy. Diabetes 34: 1181–1185
26. Krarup T, Schwartz TW, Hilsted J, et al. (1979) Impaired response of pancreatic polypeptide to hypoglycaemia: an early sign of autonomic neuropathy in diabetics. Br Med J ii: 1544–1546
27. Hoeldtke RD, Cilmi KM (1984) Norepinephrine secretion and production in diabetic autonomic neuropathy. J Clin Endocrinol Metab 59: 246–252
28. Dejgaard A, Hilsted J, Christensen NJ (1986) Noradrenaline and isoproterenol kinetics in diabetic patients with and without autonomic neuropathy. Diabetologia 29: 773–777
29. Grimaldi A, Pruszczynski W, Thervet R, Ardaillou R (1985) Antidiuretic hormone response to volume depletion in diabetic patients with cardiac autonomic dysfunction. Clin Sci 68: 545–552
30. Cignarelli M, De Pergola G, Paternostro A, et al. (1986) Arginine-vasopressin response to supine–erect positive change: an index for evaluation of the integrity of the afferent

component of baroregulatory system in diabetic neuropathy. Diabete Metab 12: 28–33
31. Loo FD, Dodds WJ, Soergel KH, et al. (1985) Multipeaked esophageal peristaltic pressure waves in patients with diabetic neuropathy. Gastroenterology 88: 485–491
32. Maddern GJ, Horowitz M, Jamieson GG (1985) The effect of domperidone on oesophageal emptying in diabetic autonomic neuropathy. Br J Clin Pharmacol 19: 441-444
33. Horowitz M, Harding PE, Maddox A, et al. (1986) Gastric and oesophageal emptying in insulin-dependent diabetes mellitus. J Gastroenterol Hepatol 1: 97–113
34. Channer KS, Jackson PC, O'Brien I, et al. (1985) Oesophageal function in diabetes mellitus and its association with autonomic neuropathy. Diabetic Med 2: 378–382
35. Loo FD, Palmer DW, Soergel KH, Kalbfleisch JH, Wood CM (1984) Gastric emptying in patients with diabetes mellitus. Gastroenterology 86: 485–494
36. Wright RA, Clemente R, Wathen R (1985) Diabetic gastroparesis: an abnormality of gastric emptying of solids. Am J Med Sci 289: 240–242
37. Oliveira RB, Troncon LEA, Meneghelli UG, Dantas RO, Godoy RA (1984) Gastric accommodation to distension and early gastric emptying in diabetics with neuropathy. Brazilian J Med Biol Res 17: 49–53
38. Mearin F, Camilleri M, Malagelada JR (1986) Pyloric dysfunction in diabetics with recurrent nausea and vomiting. Gastroenterology 90: 1919–1925
39. Achem-Karam SR, Funakoshi A, Vinik AI, Owyang C (1985) Plasma motilin concentration and interdigestive migrating motor complex in diabetic gastroparesis: effect of metaclopramide. Gastroenterology 88: 492–499

Diabetic Complications: Early Diagnosis and Treatment
Edited by D. Andreani, G. Crepaldi, U. Di Mario and G. Pozza


# CHAPTER 14

# *Central Nervous Involvement in Diabetic Patients*

G. Comi and A. Martini*
*Istituto Scientifico S. Raffaele, Department of Neurology, University of Milan; *ENT Department, University of Padua, Italy*

Approximately two-thirds of patients with diabetes mellitus have clinical or subclinical peripheral neuropathy. Whether there is also a specific involvement of the central nervous system (CNS) has not yet been clarified. In 1950 De Jong (1) published a pathological study of a 28-year-old diabetic patient with severe histological CNS abnormalities and coined the term 'diabetic encephalopathy'. In 1965 Reske-Nielson et al. (2) described the neuropathological findings in the brains of 16 juvenile diabetic patients. A characteristic histological pattern was observed in all the cases consisting of diffuse degenerative abnormalities of the brain tissue. The authors concluded that the degenerative changes were probably due to a primary diabetic abnormality of the brain tissue variably associated to angiopathy. All the patients had severe and widespread vascular complications and retinopathy, while 11 out of 16 had nephropathy and 10 suffered from hypertension. A variable combination of these conditions can at least partially explain the pathological changes observed.

Hypoglycemic episodes can also induce severe changes in the CNS. Multifocal or diffuse necrosis of the cerebral cortex and chromatolysis of the ganglion cells have been described in patients dying of hypoglycemia (3, 4).

Some psychological tests seem to be altered in a significant number of diabetic patients. Using the Walton–Black test for auditory learning, Bale (5) found an abnormal score in 17% of adult insulin-dependent diabetic (IDDM) patients. However, these patients showed normal levels of intelligence in the WAIS (Wechsler Adult Intelligence Score). In another study in a group of IDD patients, Franceschi et al. (6) reported a significantly worse performance in global memory, abstract reasoning and eye–hand coordination tests in comparison with the control group. Similar results have been obtained by De Jong (7). In diabetic children cognitive processes seem to be normal (8, 9); mild deficits have been observed only in children with a very early onset of the disease.

In the light of all these neuropsychological studies, some subtle and selective deficit of cognitive function seems to occur in diabetic patients. Whether these deficits are caused by CNS dysfunction, or by the emotional influence of chronic illness on intellectual and educational development, is still unclear. Neurophysiological techniques are an important tool in investigating CNS function. The frequency of electroencephalogram (EEG) abnormalities varies between 19% and 76% (10, 11). The relationship between the EEG features and the clinical data of diabetic patients is often incomplete and divergent, especially with regard to the role of hypoglycemia, diabetic control and vascular complications. There is general agreement that the incidence of EEG changes is related to the frequency and severity of hypoglycemic states (12, 13). Haumont et al. (1979) found a significant positive correlation between EEG abnormalities and the degree of diabetic control: an abnormal EEG was observed in 7% of patients with good diabetic control and in 60% of patients with poor control. The use of evoked potentials is a recently developed technique that allows the nervous conduction along the auditory, visual and somatosensory pathways to be evaluated. All the modalities of evoked potentials have been employed to study CNS dysfunction in diabetes. It is the aim of this chapter to consider the results of these studies.

## VISUAL EVOKED POTENTIALS

Retinal microangiopathy is a frequent complication of diabetes mellitus. The severity of retinal dysfunction can be determined by fluorescein angiography and by flash electoretinography. The oscillatory potentials disappear early, sometimes before ophthalmoscopic signs of retinopathy can be demonstrated (14). The alterations of these potentials can be partially reversed by improving metabolic control (15). Later in the disease, an increase in the latency and a decrease in the amplitude of B and A waves can be observed.

It has been recently shown that contrast sensitivity (CS) is impaired in diabetic patients (16, 17) both with and without ophthalmoscopic signs of retinopathy. Some investigators (18) think that CS tests can be used to detect preclinical stages of retinopathy; however, no relationship between CS test abnormalities and fluorescein angiographic signs of retinopathy has yet been found. We studied CS in 92 diabetic children by using the Cambridge low-contrast gratings, a test which is very easy to perform, as described by Della Sala et al. (18). The mean score of the CS test was significantly lower in diabetic patients compared with normal controls (17.8 $\pm$ 3 vs 20.4); 20% of diabetic patients had abnormal scores. Analysis of correlations between the CS test scores and age, $HbA_{1c}$, and daily insulin doses showed them to be not significant. The correlation between duration of the disease and CS test scores was positive, but not significant. Also in our study there was no significant difference in the contrast sensitivity impairment between diabetic patients with and without retinopathy.

The problem of the involvement of the visual system in diabetes is made more complex by two other recent observations: both the pattern reversal visual evoked potential (PRVEP) and the pattern reversal electroretinogram (PERG) can be altered in diabetic patients.

PRVEP is a response recorded from the occipital cortex following the stimulation of the centre of the retina. The stimulus is the reversal of a black-and-white checkerboard generated by a television display. The presence of the major positive wave (P 100) of this potential indicates optic nerve pathology, provided that local ocular abnormalities, such as glaucoma and lesions of the vitreous lens, anterior chamber or cornea, are excluded. We evaluated PRVEP in 145 patients. P 100 mean latency was significantly prolonged in diabetic patients (Table 1). The response was abnormal in 22% of cases. The mean P 100 latency significantly increased with the duration of diabetes. We did not find any significant correlation between age, glycosylated hemoglobin, insulin requirements and PRVEP latency. There was a negative correlation between P 100 latency and motor and sensory nerve conduction velocities. The distribution of fluorangiographic alterations in patients with and without delayed PRVEP were not significantly different.

Table 1. Pattern reversal visual evoked potential (PRVEP) in 145 patients

| | P 100 Latency (msec) | | |
|---|---|---|---|
| | Diabetics | Controls | $p$ |
| 30′ check size | 112.8 ± 7.7 | 109.1 ± 4.8 | <0.001 |
| 15′ check size | 119.1 ± 10.5 | 112.8 ± 5.2 | <0.001 |

PERG is an evoked retinal response to pattern stimuli that probably originates in the ganglion cells (19). PERG has been studied by our group in 40 diabetic children and in 20 normal subjects, using stimuli of 60′ and 30′ checks and contrast of 100% and 50%. The mean PERG amplitude was significantly reduced in diabetic patients after all forms of stimulation (Tables 2 and 3). The frequency of abnormal PERG amplitude increased with a decrease in check size and contrast: with 15′ check size and 50% contrast, PERG was not detectable in 30 eyes. Simultaneous recording of PRVEP and PERG was performed in 35 patients.

There was a statistically significant correlation ($p < 0.01$) between reduced PERG amplitude and increased P 100 latency (Figure 1). PERG abnormalities were not related to retinal microangiopathy.

Abnormalities of PERG, PRVEP and CS have been considered to be a consequence of retinal microangiopathy (18, 20, 21). Retinopathy was rare in our patients and, when present, it was mostly mild and unrelated to the alterations observed in the diagnostic tests. For these reasons it seems unlikely that retinal microangiopathy can produce the alterations that we have observed, and other mechanisms must be taken into consideration. The correlations between PRVEP and PERG abnormalities and between PRVEP and peripheral nerve conduction, and the same influence of the duration of the disease on PRVEP and peripheral neuropathy, suggest common causal factors.

Table 2. PERG check size 60′ in diabetics (D) and normal controls (N)

| | | Contrast | | | |
|---|---|---|---|---|---|
| | | 100% | | 100% | |
| | | D | N | D | N |
| Latency | $\bar{m}$ | 54.4 | 53.8 | 52.9* | 51.6 |
| | SD | ±2.6 | ±2.3 | ±3.2 | ±2.3 |
| Amplitude | $\bar{m}$ | 1.55** | 1.93 | 0.87** | 1.40 |
| | SD | ±0.55 | ±0.54 | ±0.45 | ±0.62 |

*$p<0.05$.
**$p<0.001$.

Table 3. PERG check size 30′ in diabetics (D) and normal controls (N)

| | | Contrast | | | |
|---|---|---|---|---|---|
| | | 100% | | 100% | |
| | | D | N | D** | N |
| Latency | $\bar{m}$ | 55.1 | 54.9 | 54.1 | 53.2 |
| | SD | ±3.1 | ±3.1 | ±2.6 | ±2.4 |
| Amplitude | $\bar{m}$ | 1.23* | 1.59 | 0.88 | 0.97 |
| | SD | ±0.58 | ±0.48 | ±0.47 | ±0.33 |

*$p<0.005$.
**absent in 16 eyes.

In conclusion, the results of these studies suggest a primary involvement of ganglion cells, while damage to the subclinical optic nerve may be only a secondary phenomenon.

## AUDITORY EVOKED POTENTIALS

The acoustic stimulus-induced electrical activity of peripheral and central auditory pathways can be recorded in man. These electrical responses are classified on the basis of latency after stimulus.

Auditory brain responses (ABR) have the most diffuse clinical application at the present time. ABR are measures of electrical events generated along the auditory pathway, recorded from the scalp by far-field averaging methods. The response to

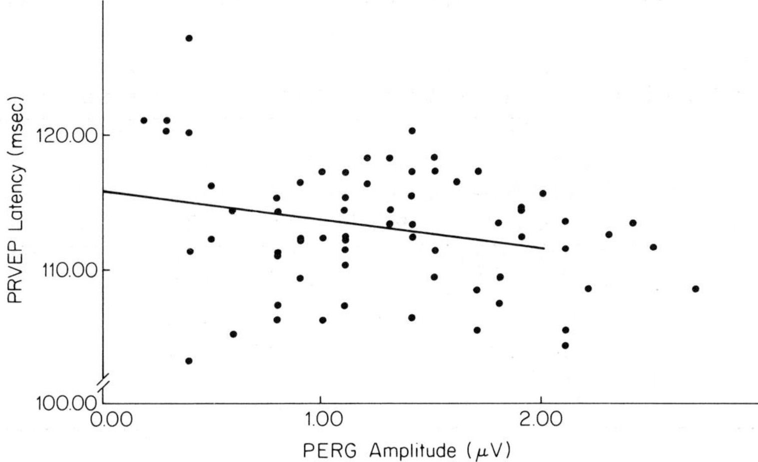


Figure 1. Relationship between P 100 latency and PERG amplitude in diabetic children. Each point represents the relationship in one eye.

a click (a particular acoustic stimulus which presents a large frequency spectrum and a short duration, usually 100 μsec) consists of 6 or 7 small vertex-positive waves recorded in the first 10 msec after the stimulus. These potentials may reflect sequential activation of relay nuclei in the auditory afferent pathways. The possible origins of the early auditory evoked potentials have given rise to much controversy.

Therefore, the I-V interval can be considered as the central transmission time (CTT).

In spite of the controversy over the origins of the waves, this test has been proved to provide an objective, clinically useful measure of auditory nerve and brainstem dysfunction, even in the absence of associated clinical symptoms or signs.

A preliminary functional study of the CNS in diabetic patients was reported by Donald et al. (22). Analysing the slow vertex evoked responses in a group of 10 diabetic patients, the authors noted that these subjects had greater suppression of high rates of stimulation response causing a slowing down of the recovery process in the CNS. It was also found, in a further study regarding ABR, that diabetic patients have longer interpeak latencies than normal subjects (23). Similar data have been reported in previous papers by our group (24, 25).

Recently, we recorded ABR in 60 normally hearing insulin-dependent diabetic patients (31 males and 29 females, aged 17–55 years), evaluating metabolic parameters together with some long-term diabetic complications (26). Glycemic control was monitored by glycosylated hemoglobin and mean daily plasma glucose, while of the late complications, somatic and autonomic neuropathy, nephropathy and retinopathy were evaluated. Pathological ABR was diagnosed when the I-V interval latency shift was more than 2 SD of the mean latency of a sex- and age-matched control group. We reported ABR abnormalities in 28.2% of the cases. This impairment affects the I-V interval, or CTT which is considered the most reliable index of brainstem function. In diabetic patients, we observed a significant correlation ($p<0.05$) between the I-V interval shift and an EMG proven reduction in motor conduction velocity (MCV) of the peroneal nerve (Figure 2). We also found a high incidence of ABR impairment (53%) in diabetic patients with cardiovascular autonomic failure. A 6-month follow-up study was performed on 20 patients in this group. ABR at the first check-up was pathological in 9 cases and normal in 11 patients. No significant mean variations of ABR latencies were noted in the impaired group (CTT analysed by *t* test for repeated measures).

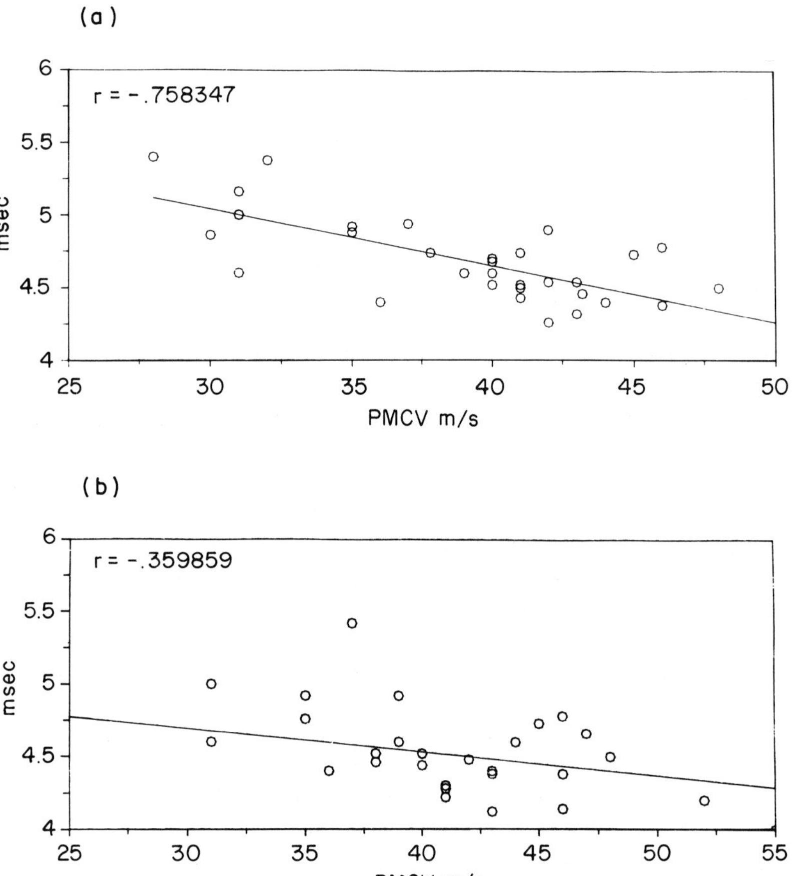


Figure 2. Relationship between I-V interpeak latency and motor conduction velocity of peroneal nerve PMCV in (a) diabetic males and (b) diabetic females.

## SOMATOSENSORY EVOKED POTENTIALS

Spinal cord disease in diabetes has been described as 'diabetic myelopathy' (27, 28) and 'pseudotabes diabetica' (29). The neuropathological findings include demyelination and axon cylinder loss, particularly in the posterior columns, and degeneration of the ganglion cells of the anterior and posterior horns (2, 30). These changes are prominent in proximity to the cervical and lumbar enlargements.

Somatosensory evoked potentials (SEP) following the stimulation of upper or lower limbs can provide information about conduction in both peripheral and central afferent pathways. The determination of central somatosensory conduction time (CCT) by the simultaneous recording of spinal and cortical SEP has become important in clinical diagnosis (31–33). We recorded cortical and spinal SEP after both median and tibial nerve stimulation in 30 insulin-dependent diabetic patients. Conduction along central somatosensory pathways was slow in 31.2% of patients after tibial nerve stimulation (increased $N_{24}-P_{40}$ interpeak) and in 20% of cases after median nerve stimulation (increased $N_{11}-N_{20}$ interpeak) (Table 4). Of 6 patients with abnormal conduction along central pathways of the median nerve, 4 also had prolonged peripheral conduction time. Gupta and Dorfman, using indirect estimates of conduction rates within spinal afferent pathways, found spinal conduction to be slow in about 40% of diabetic patients (34). Cracco et al. (35) found abnormal spinal conduction in 22% of patients with juvenile diabetes without clinical signs of peripheral or spinal involvement. Our study has shown that central conduction in diabetic patients may be affected as frequently as peripheral conduction along the somatosensory pathways.

The two abnormalities are frequently, but not always, associated, as has been pointed out in other studies (34, 35). In most cases, posterior column dysfunction seems to be secondary to ganglion cell involvement (36), which explains the good correlation between the abnormal $N_9$ latency and the abnormal $N_9-N_{13}$ interpeak latency that we found in the present study. Slowed spinal conduction could be a consequence of the loss from the peripheral nerve of the most rapidly conducting fibres, or it could be a result of axonopathy and/or demyelination of both the afferent branches of the ganglion cell, perhaps at different times. This latter hypothesis could explain our two patients with abnormal $N_{11}-N_{13}$ interpeak latency, but with normal peripheral conduction.

There might be selective involvement of the second and the third neurons of the somatosensory pathways in cases with only an abnormal $N_{13}-N_{20}$ interval. Another hypothesis is that these cases have a vascular pathology. In our two cases with both $N_{11}-N_{13}$ and $N_{13}-N_{20}$ abnormal conduction times, there must have been chance damage to the first, second and third neurons, in addition to transsynaptic degeneration.

Our study, like earlier ones, revealed no correlation between decreased spinal cord conduction velocity and the duration of diabetes, the levels of $HbA_{1c}$ or fasting blood glucose. However, correlations have been repeatedly demonstrated between

Table 4. Frequencies of abnormal median and tibial SEPs

| | SEP | Number of abnormalities | Total number | Percentage abnormalities |
|---|---|---|---|---|
| *Median* | | | | |
| | Erb | 9 | 30 | 30 |
| | $N_9$ | 9 | 30 | 30 |
| | $N_{11}$ | 9 | 30 | 30 |
| | $N_{13}$ | 10 | 30 | 33 |
| | $N_{20}$ | 11 | 30 | 37 |
| | $N_9-N_{11}$ | 7 | 30 | 23 |
| | $N_{11}-N_{13}$ | 5 | 30 | 17 |
| | Erb$-N_{11}$ | 7 | 30 | 23 |
| | $N_{13}-N_{20}$ | 3 | 30 | 10 |
| | $N_{11}-N_{20}$ | 6 | 30 | 20 |
| *Tibial* | | | | |
| | $N_{24}$ | 7 | 16 | 44 |
| | $P_{40}$ | 17 | 30 | 56 |
| | $N_{24}-P_{40}$ | 5 | 16 | 31 |
| | CCI | 7 | 16 | 44 |
| | PCI | 7 | 16 | 44 |

peripheral neuropathy and these factors (37). Dorsal column damage in diabetes could explain why some patients have sensory disturbances without electroneurographic abnormalities and why some are refractory both to drugs (38) and to the improvement of metabolic control (39), indeed both remyelination and axonal regeneration are slower in the spinal cord than in peripheral nerves.

## REFERENCES

1. De Jong RN (1950) The nervous system complications in diabetes mellitus with special reference to cerebrovascular changes. J Nerv Ment Dis 111: 181–206
2. Reske-Nielsen E, Lundbaek K, Rafaelsen OJ (1965) Pathological changes in the central and peripheral nervous system of young long-term diabetics. I. Diabetic encephalopathy. Diabetologia 1: 233–241
3. Lawrence RD, Meyer A, Nervin S (1942) The pathological changes in the brain in the fatal hypoglycaemia. J Med 35: 181–201
4. Greenfield JG (1960) Neuropathology. Edward Arnold, London, pp 245–247
5. Bale RN (1973) Brain damage in diabetes mellitus. Br J Psychiatry 122: 337–341
6. Franceschi M, Cecchetto R, Minicucci F, Smirne S, Baio G, Canal N (1984) Cognitive processes in insulin-dependent diabetes. Diabetes Care 7: 228–231
7. De Jong RN (1977) CNS manifestations of diabetes mellitus. Postgrad Med 61 (1): 101–107
8. Kubany A, Danowsky TS, Moses C (1956) The personality and intelligence of diabetics. Diabetes 5: 126–130

9. Ack M, Miller I, Weil WM (1961) Intelligence of children with diabetes mellitus. Pediatrics 28 (Suppl): 764–770
10. Laron Z, Karp M, Freinkel JJ (1972) Electroencephalographic examination—A study of rehabilitation of juvenile and adolescent diabetics in the central region of Israel. Kupat Holin Press, Petah Tikva, pp 35–37
11. Meik M, Schadlich M, Warnle M (1962) Das Elektroenzephalogramm des diabetischen Kindet. Z Inn Med 17: 616
12. Schlack H, Palm D, Jochmus I (1969) Der Einfluss rezidivierender Hypoglykemien auf das EEG des diabetischen Kindet. Mschr Monatssch Kinderheilk: 117–251
13. Abramowicz I, Margolis A, Wawrzynkiewicz T (1969) Zmiany elektroencefalograficzne u dzieci chorych na cukrzyce. Pediatr Pol 44: 693
14. Babel J, Stangos N, Korol S, Spiritus M (1977) Electrophysiology: a clinical and experimental study of electroretinogram, electrooculogram and visual evoked response. Thieme, Stuttgart, pp 1–172
15. Frost-Larsen K, Christiansen JS, Parving MM (1983) The effect of short term metabolic control on retinal nervous system abnormalities in newly diagnosed type 1 diabetic patients. Diabetologia 24: 207–209
16. Ghafour M, Foulds WS, Allan D, McClure F (1982) Contrast sensitivity in diabetic subjects with and without retinopathy. Br J Ophthalmol 66: 492–495
17. Hyvarinen L, Laurinen P, Rovamo J (1983) Contrast in evaluation of visual impairment due to diabetes. Acta Ophthalmol 61: 94–101
18. Della Sala S, Bertoni G, Somazzi L, Stubbe F, Wilkins AJ (1985) Impaired contrast sensitivity in diabetic patients with and without retinopathy: a new technique for rapid assessment. Br J Ophthalmol 69: 136–142
19. Maffei L, Fiorentini A (1981) Electroretinographic responses to alternating gratings before and after section of the optic nerve. Science 211: 953–955
20. Cirillo D, Gonfiantini E, De Grandis D, Bongiovanni L, Robert JJ, Pinelli L (1984) Visual evoked potentials in diabetic children and adolescents. Diabetes Care 7: 273–275
21. Collier A, Mitchell JD, Clarke BF (1985) Visual evoked potential and contrast sensitivity function in diabetic retinopathy. Br Med J 291–248
22. Donald MW, Bird CE, El-Sawy R, Hart P, Lawson S, Letemendia FJJ, Surridge DHC, Wilson DL (1980) Cortical evoked potentials and auditory decision times in diabetics. Prog Brain Res 54: 516–521
23. Donald MW, Bird CE, Lawson JS, Letemendia FJJ, Monga TN, Surridge DH, Varette-Cerre P, Williams DM, Williams DML, Wilson DL (1981) Delayed auditory brain stem responses in diabetes mellitus. J Neurol Neurosurg Psychiatry 44: 641–644
24. Fedele D, Martini A, Cardone C, Comacchio F, Bellavere F, Molinari G, Negrin P, Crepaldi G (1984) Impaired auditory brainstem evoked responses in insulin-dependent diabetic subjects. Diabetes 33: 1085–1089
25. Martini A, Comacchio F, Molinari G, Fedele D, Crepaldi G (1985) Auditory brain stem evoked responses as a function of stimulus repetition rate in diabetes mellitus. Adv Audiol 3: 131–140
26. Martini A, Comacchio F, Fedele D, Crepaldi G, Sala O (1987) Auditory brainstem evoked responses in the clinical evaluation and follow-up of insulin-dependent diabetic subjects. Acta Otolaryngol (in press)
27. Garland H, Tverner D (1953) Diabetic myelopathy. Br Med J i: 1405–1408
28. Slager UT (1978) Diabetic myelopathy. Arch Pathol Lab Med 102: 467–469
29. Logothetis J, Baker AB (1963) Neurologic manifestations in diabetes mellitus. Med Clin North Am 47: 1459–1466
30. Griggs DE, Olsen CW (1937) Changes in spinal cord in diabetes mellitus. Arch Neurol Psychiatry 38: 564–571

31. El-Negamy E, Sedgwick EM (1979) Delayed cervical somatosensory potentials in cervical spondylosis. J Neurol Neurosurg Psychiatry 42: 238–241
32. Eisen A, Odusote K (1980) Central and peripheral conduction times in multiple sclerosis. EEG Clin Neurophysiol 48: 253–265
33. Strenge H, Hedderich J (1982) Age-dependent changes in central somatosensory conduction time. Eur Neurol 21: 270–276
34. Gupta RP, Dorfman LJ (1981) Spinal somatosensory conduction in diabetes. Neurology 31: 841–845
35. Cracco J, Castells S, Mark E (1984) Spinal somatosensory evoked potentials in juvenile diabetes. Ann Neurol 19: 55–58
36. Thomas PK, Eliasson SG (1975). Diabetic neuropathy. In: Dyck PJ, Thomas PK, Lambert EH (eds) Peripheral neuropathy. Saunders, Philadelphia, pp 965–981
37. Canal N, Comi G, Saibene V, Musch B, Pozza G (1978) Relationship between peripheral and autonomic neuropathy in insulin dependent diabetes: a clinical and instrumental evaluation. In Canal N, Pozza G (eds) Peripheral neuropathies. Elsevier/North-Holland Biomedical Press, Amsterdam, pp 247–255
38. Spritz N (1978) Nerve disease in diabetes mellitus. Med Clin North Am 62: 787–798
39. Ward JD, Barnes CG, Fisher DJ (1971) Improvement in nerve conduction following treatment in newly diagnosed diabetes. Lancet i: 428–431

Diabetic Complications: Early Diagnosis and Treatment
Edited by D. Andreani, G. Crepaldi, U. Di Mario and G. Pozza


# CHAPTER 15

# *Clinical Aspects of Peripheral Neuropathies in Diabetes*

N. CANAL and G. POZZA*
*Department of Neurology, *Clinic of Internal Medicine, University of Milan — Istituto Scientifico S. Raffaele, Milan, Italy*

Disturbances of the peripheral nervous system in diabetes are so common as to be considered, along with retinopathy and nephropathy, one of the major later complications of the disease. In the last 20 years sophisticated electroneurographic tests have allowed an assessment of disturbances in the peripheral nervous system which far surpasses simple clinical evaluation and allows the size of the phenomenon to be established. Furthermore, the tests allow the identification of diabetic patients who are asymptomatic but whose neurophysiological responses indicate an alteration in nerve function parameters (1). One might postulate that these patients with reversible subclinical neuropathy (Figure 1) may eventually develop fully expressed clinical neuropathy unless adequately treated.

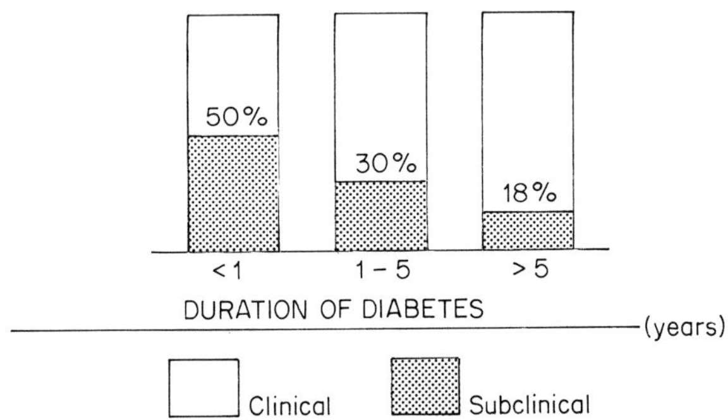


Figure 1. Relationship of prevalence of subclinical peripheral neuropathy of diabetes. From Canal et al. (2). Reproduced with permission of Casa Editrice 'Il Ponte'.

Diabetic neuropathy encompasses a variety of clinical pictures whose pathogenesis is probably multiple. Although there are many classifications, none of them is completely satisfactory; the one we would suggest was proposed by Brown and Asbury (3) (Table 1).

Table 1. Classification of diabetic neuropathies (modified from Brown and Asbury (3))

1. Distal symmetrical polyneuropathy
   - A. Mixed sensory–motor–autonomic neuropathy
   - B. Predominantly sensory neuropathy
   - C. Predominantly motor neuropathy
   - D. Predominantly autonomic neuropathy
2. Proximal symmetrical motor neuropathy ('diabetic amyotrophy')
3. Focal and multifocal neuropathies
   - A. Asymmetric proximal motor neuropathy
   - B. Cranial neuropathy
   - C. Intercostal and other mononeuropathies
   - D. Entrapment neuropathies

## CLINICAL FEATURES

### Motor Sensitive Symmetric Polyneuropathy

This is the most common form of peripheral nerve involvement (see ref. 4 for review). At first it may be subclinical, but it usually becomes clinically evident. Disturbances in sensitivity are the first to appear and are usually more marked than motor disturbances. In the initial stages these include paresthesia, dysesthesia, numbness and pain initially localized in the lower limbs, but with subsequent proximal diffusion in the trunk and upper limbs. As the disease advances objective deficit in sensitivity appears. In the form mainly involving the large diameter fibres, clinical features are loss of vibratory and joint sensation with absent tendon reflexes. Ataxia is evident and the clinical picture resembles that of tabes dorsalis (diabetic pseudotabes).

When the small fibres are mainly involved clinical symptoms are paresthesia, dysesthesia and pain. Paresthesia is an unpleasant sensation which presents itself as the absence of sensory stimuli; it gives a tingling sensation of pins and needles. Dysesthesia is an uncomfortable sensation provoked by inadequate stimuli: contact alone with clothes or blankets can give a burning sensation or deep pain. Sometimes cramps in the legs and feet occur at night. On examination a sensory loss is found mainly affecting pain and temperature sensitivity with a stocking and glove distribution, while deep sensation may be unaffected and tendon reflexes present. Motor disturbances are less important than sensory ones and are mainly localized in the small muscles of the hands and feet; muscle wasting sometimes occurs.

### Acute Painful Neuropathy

This is characterized by the sudden onset of burning pain localized in the extremities of the limbs and is accompanied by marked weight loss due to severe metabolic decompensation (5). Objective sensitivity is slightly reduced or often unaffected. These symptoms may be alleviated over a period of a few months by correcting the metabolic disorders.

## Proximal Motor Neuropathy

Proximal motor neuropathy is also known as *diabetic amyotrophy* (6). Clinical examinations would suggest a lesion of the motor horn cells of the lumbosacral motor roots with a vascular or metabolic pathogenesis, although pathological studies have never established this. While the term diabetic amyotrophy was initially used to describe asymmetric pelvifemoral atrophy, its use should be confined to bilateral cases in order to avoid confusion with mononeuropathies. This disorder is characterized (7, 8) by marked weakness of pelvic girdle muscles and by a gradual onset (usually over a few days or weeks). At the beginning there is usually lancinating pain in the lumbosacral region, the thighs and the buttocks. Symptoms are bilateral but sometimes slightly asymmetrical. Although very rarely, the shoulder girdle may be involved. Hyposthenia is such that the patient may fall because of the extreme weakness of the femoral muscles. The weak muscles soon atrophy; in more than half the cases, diabetic amyotrophy is associated with symmetrical sensory motor neuropathy. The onset of this disease is often accompanied by notable weight loss and deterioration in metabolic control. Diabetic amyotrophy is usually found, though not always, in middle-aged or older diabetic patients. The muscles most affected are the quadriceps femoris, ileopsoas and the abductors of the thigh. Approximately one-third of patients suffer from disturbances in sensitivity. The outcome is favourable with recovery of the strength and muscular trophism in 80% of cases.

## Mononeuropathy and Multiple Neuropathy

These forms of neuropathy must be clearly distinguished from sensory symmetric polyneuropathy, not only because of their clinical characteristics but also because their pathogenesis is probably different. Metabolic factors would seem to play a less important role in this type of neuropathy while local factors, such as vascular factors or compression, seem to have more importance and are capable of causing focal lesions of a single nerve.

## Mononeuropathy of Cranial Nerves

The cranial nerves most often affected are the oculomotor nerves (particularly the third) and the facial nerve; uni- or bilateral paralysis of several cranial nerves is not uncommon (9). Neuropathies of the third nerve are manifested with acute painful ophthalmoplegia without autonomic involvement. As in other instances of mononeuritis of cranial nerves, pathogenesis is ischemic. As ischemia is mainly centrofascicular, the parasympathetic fibres situated in the peripheral part of the nerve are not involved; this explains why pupillary response remains unaffected.

Paralysis of the facial nerve is definitely more frequent among diabetic patients compared to the general population (10); more than 60% of all patients seen by doctors because of peripheral paralysis of the facial nerve are diabetic. The outcome of this neuropathy is usually favourable with complete remission within 3–6 months.

### Mononeuropathy of the Limbs

This usually affects the lower limbs while the upper limbs are rarely affected. Onset is nearly always acute and muscle weakness essentially involves the quadriceps femoris, the adductors of the thigh, the ileopsoas and buttocks asymmetrically; the latter aspect serves to distinguish this neuropathy from diabetic amyotrophy. The knee jerk is absent on the affected side. These clinical features are very similar to the ones described by Raff et al. (11) as ischemic mononeuropathy multiplex; it is very probable that the pathogenesis in this case can also be attributed to multiple ischemia of the lumbosacral plexus and the nerve roots. The outcome is benign with possible residual deficits.

### Susceptibility to Entrapment

Compression of nerve roots in anatomic tunnels (carpal tunnel, tarsal tunnel, etc.) is more common in the diabetic subject than in the general population (12). Approximately 9% (13) of diabetic patients show electrophysiological evidence of carpal tunnel syndrome against the 2% of the general population. Those diabetic subjects most often affected are women over 40 years of age (Figure 2); a pre-existent polyneuropathy is a predisposing factor.

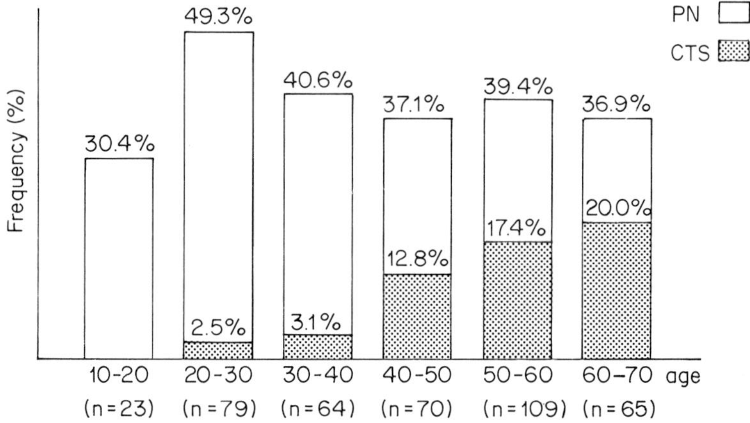


Figure 2. Prevalence of carpal tunnel syndrome (CTS) and peripheral symmetrical neuropathy (PN) as a function of age; number of patients in parentheses. From Comi et al. (12). Reproduced with permission of Elsevier Science Publishers.

The most frequent clinical feature is carpal tunnel syndrome which involves the median nerve; other possible places of entrapment are the cubital tunnel and Guyon's channel (ulnar nerve), the peroneal head (peroneal nerve) and the tarsal tunnel (posterior tibial nerve). These disturbances respond well to surgery, as in non-diabetic subjects.

### Insulin Neuritis

Onset of acute neuropathy soon after the beginning of insulin treatment was reported in 1933 by Caravati (14). Numerous successive observations have specified that this is a sensory motor polyneuropathy. It may also appear after treatment with oral hypoglycemic drugs (15). It would seem to be caused, not by the insulin itself, but by the abrupt metabolic changes brought about by insulin. Motor neuropathy has also been described in patients who have experienced repeated episodes of hypoglycemia due to insulinoma (16). The neuropathy subsides with the continuation of insulin therapy.

## AUTONOMIC NEUROPATHY

Autonomic failure is frequent in diabetic patients. It occurs in about 40% of cases of diabetes of more than 10 years standing (Figure 1) (17), but rises to about 50% if asymptomatic patients with altered tests of autonomic function are considered. Parasympathetic damage occurs earlier and is more severe than sympathetic modification (17) (Figure 3). Although clinical interest tends to be focused on cardiovascular disorders because of their poor prognosis, autonomic neuropathy may affect various organs and systems. We will describe the various clinical features these complications present (see ref. 18 for review).

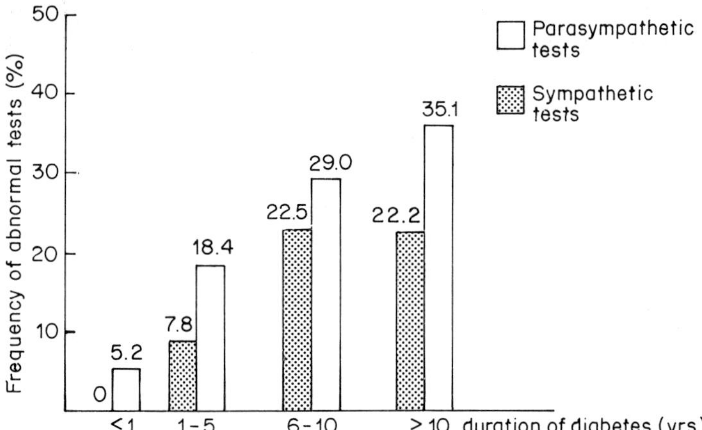


Figure 3. Relationship between the duration of diabetes and the frequency of abnormal cardiovascular tests in diabetic patients. From Canal and Comi (17).

## Genitourinary System

Vesical dysfunction often begins in an insiduous manner with increased intervals between voidings, weakness of the stream, postmicturition dribbling and a sensation of incomplete emptying of the bladder (19).

In an advanced phase there is evidence of increased residual urine with a distended, palpable bladder (suggesting an intra-abdominal turmour) and eventually overflow incontinence. Patients may at first be asymptomatic as bladder dysfunction is only shown up in abnormalities revealed by pyelography and cystometry. In the subsequent phase with marked urinary stasis, superimposed infection usually occurs, manifested by dysuria, urgency and frequency, and may develop into pyelonephritis and sometimes renal failure (20). A neurogenic bladder due to autonomic failure must be accurately distinguished from other clinical situations, such as prostatic hypertrophy, by diagnostic tests including cystometry, intravenous pyelography, uroflowmetry, EMG of perineal muscles and evoked potentials. Treatment, in addition to intermittent catheterization and chemiotherapy, includes cholinergic drugs and bladder neck resection.

### *Impotence*

Reduced or absent vis ergendi is a well-known complication in the diabetic patient (21). It occurs in 35–75% of diabetic males aged from 20 to 59 years. Deficiency in such a complex function may obviously be attributable to disturbances at various levels. One essential element for potency is an unaltered vascular situation, which is not always found in the diabetic patient. Although there are other possible factors, frequent autonomic failure in the diabetic patient has led to the conclusion that this may be the main cause of impotence. It should be differentiated from psychogenic impotence, which as a whole is the most common form of impotence reported to doctors. The various characteristics which allow us to differentiate between the types of impotence may be outlined as follows.

*Psychogenic impotence*: (1) has a sudden onset, often connected to serious emotional or physical events; (2) can be intermittent and may only occur in determinate situations; (3) may be limited to a specific partner; (4) nocturnal and erotically stimulated erection and ejaculations continue.

*Organic impotence*: (1) usually begins gradually, although it may be acute in periods of metabolic imbalance in the diabetic patient; (2) is persistent and progressive and is not connected to particular partners or circumstances; (3) no nocturnal erection or ejaculations occur; (4) libido is intact, at least at first.

The recording of penile tumescence during sleep is an important contribution to a differential diagnosis and shows absence or inadequacy of penile tumescence in the diabetic patient while it is adequate in psychogenic impotence (22). Diabetic impotence is not related to endocrine disturbances (prolactin, testosterone and gonadotropin levels are normal) (23), while it may be correlated to age, retinopathy, and autonomic neuropathy in other systems (cardiovascular system), even if, in many cases, it occurs in the absence of other signs or symptoms of peripheral nervous system involvement.

### *Retrograde Ejaculation*

This is another genital dysfunction caused by inadequate vegetative innervation (24). Normal propulsion of the sperm collected in the posterior urethra occurs with contraction of the bulbocavernosus muscle during orgasm and the simultaneous contraction of the internal vesical sphincter. If the latter is inadequate because of insufficient sympathetic outflow, the semen flows back into the bladder (and may be found in postcoital urine) and the orgasm occurs without any emission of semen. Although rare and without important consequences on a practical level, this may create considerable psychological problems and contribute to the diminished fertility seen among diabetic subjects.

## Gastrointestinal Tract

Although it is difficult to quantify the incidence of gastrointestinal disturbances (owing to a lack of bedside-specific diagnostic tests) they must be recognized in order to avoid them being misdiagnosed as surgical diseases, such as gastroduodenal ulcers, diverticulosis of the colon, etc.

*Esophageal motility* is often shown by instrumental tests (intra-esophageal manometry, cineradiography) to be slowed down because of the degeneration of either the preganglionic fibres of the vagus or of the esophageal nerves themselves (25). The symptoms are not very marked: modest dysphagia and retrosternal pain.

*Delayed emptying of the stomach* is a well-known clinical aspect of diabetes and is called 'gastoparesis diabeticorum' (26). Although this may be asymptomatic, in many cases it is manifested as anorexia, nausea, vomiting and a constant sense of fullness after meals. Even in patients who present no signs of gastric atonia, delayed emptying of the stomach may affect the absorption of food in an unpredictable way (especially carbohydrates and lipids). One consequence of the diminished secretion of acid is the well-known low incidence of peptic ulcers in the diabetic population (27).

### *Diarrhea*

This is probably the most common consequence of autonomic failure (28). Watery feces are often passed quite unsuspectingly, painlessly and preceded by moderate abdominal discomfort and intestinal rumbling. It frequently occurs at night and is associated with sphincteric incontinence. It is usually intermittent (episodes lasting hours or a few days and often followed by constipation) but may be continuous.

Autonomic pathogenesis is suggested also because of the similarities seen in vagotomized subjects, but the exact mechanism is not yet known. The most likely hypothesis is that the slowing down of the passage of food along the intestinal tract causes the bacterial flora to proliferate which in turn causes diarrhea, either directly or by causing the deconjugation of bile acids. This hypothesis is substantiated by the therapeutic action of broad-spectrum antibiotics and cholestyramine (a substance which forms insoluble complexes with bile salts).

### Cardiovascular System

Disturbances in the cardiovascular system have a greater overall effect in the diabetic subject than any other dysfunction and may threaten the actual survival of the patient (29). While the disturbances may be asymptomatic they can become clinically manifest both under certain physiological conditions (greater demand, for example, during physical exercise) and during emergency situations (stress, anesthesia, etc.).

*Postural hypotension* is certainly the most well-known consequence of autonomic failure (17). In actual fact, at least in its more serious clinical expression, it occurs quite late in the disease and quite seldom. The change from a reclining position to an upright one involves the accumulation of a certain amount of blood in the lower limbs and in the splanchnic region, and a decrease in cardiac output. The subsequent lowering of the blood pressure is, in normal subjects, compensated by an increase in the sympathetic output to the heart and the peripheral arteries caused by the carotid sinus reflex and the aortic baroreceptors. The lack of sympathetic outflow leads to a fall in blood pressure (both systolic and diastolic) which may reach levels below 70 mmHg or even be too low to be recorded. Tachycardia, which is often present in this situation, may be much lower or even absent. The fact that this is caused by sympathetic failure explains why it only appears at an advanced stage of the disease and that it is rarely serious. Clinical manifestation of this disturbance may be varied: nausea and vertigo, dizziness in the change from a reclining position to an upright one. The most serious cases involve momentary loss of consciousness where the patient has fallen and sustained fractures. As such episodes sometimes happen after insulin injection, they are at times wrongly attributed to hypoglycemia (30). It is not known exactly why they should occur: insulin may cause hypotension in normal subjects with autonomic failure. Postural hypotension is not due to hypoglycemia; it would seem to be due to the direct effect of the hormone on the heart and the peripheral vessels. Fractioning the daily dose of insulin is one of the first lines of treatment of postural hypotension (31). Beneficial effects have been obtained with the mineralocorticoid fludrocortisone (32) (0.1–0.4 mg/day), which increases plasma volume and which may have a direct effect on vascular tone. When edema occurs, as may be seen in heart failure or in nephrotic syndrome, orthostatic hypotension improves (32).

Parasympathetic denervation of the heart (which can occur before sympathetic failure) is sometimes manifested by *at rest tachycardia* (33) which is not modified in those situations during which there is usually an increase in heart rate (physical or mental exercise, arousal during sleep), or by the administration of certain drugs, such as atropine or propranolol. A higher incidence of *painless myocardial infarction* has been found in diabetic patients with autonomic neuropathy (34); this phenomenon has been described in terms of deficit in the parasympathetic afferents from the heart and was thought to be responsible for the sudden deaths which occur in diabetic patients. Recent studies, however, tend to relate sudden diabetic deaths to cardiorespiratory failure due to disturbances in the respiratory reflexes (29).

*Hypoglycemic unawareness* is the inability to give an adequate autonomic nervous response to a biohumoral stimulus, an instance of which is progressively lower glycemic levels (35). In normal subjects bradycardia and slight hypotension occur at first (the expression of increased parasympathetic outflow); subsequently tachycardia, pallor, sweating, caused by sympathetic outflow and increased secretion of catecholamine, occur, warning the patient of imminent hypoglycemia. All this is often absent in the diabetic patient with autonomic failure. Glucagon secretion, which is an efficient compensatory mechanism for hypoglycemia, is also reduced or absent in the diabetic patient with the subsequent rapid reduction in glycemic levels because of unbalanced exogenous or endogenous insulin. This clinical situation should be distinguished from that following postural hypotension.

## Thermoregulation

*Sweating abnormalities* are often described in diabetic subjects and are caused both by disorders in sympathetic innervation of the sweat glands and by disturbances in vasomotor reflexes. The typical clinical picture (36) includes hypohidrosis or anhidrosis in the lower limbs, but in more serious cases the lower trunk and the arms are involved as well. At the same time hyperhidrosis of the face and upper trunk occurs, which, according to some authors, is a compensatory mechanism for the decreased capacity of the lower part of the body to maintain stable thermoregulation. This sort of hyperhidrosis occurs in situations which involve an increase in body temperature (such as physical exercise, a warm bath, bed rest), and is independent from hyperglycemia from which it must be carefully distinguished. One peculiar clinical aspect of this is *gustatory sweating* which appears on the face and neck after eating spicy foods which normally excite salivation (37).

Thermoregulation may be found to be notably altered in diabetic patients with autonomic failure (38). This is due to sympathetic denervation of the skin arterioles which fail to respond adequately to body and environmental temperature changes. Changes in cutaneous temperature, which are particularly apparent in the lower limbs, may contribute to the formation of trophic ulcers which are characteristic of the diabetic foot (39).

## REFERENCES


1. Gilliat RW (1965) Clinical aspects of diabetic neuropathy. In: Cumings JN, Kremer M (eds) Biochemical aspects of neurological disorders. Blackwell, Oxford, pp 117–142
2. Canal N, Comi G, Saibene V, Musch B, Pozza G (1978) The relationship between

peripheral and autonomic neuropathy in insulin dependent diabetes: a clinical and instrumental evaluation. In: Canal N, Pozza G (eds) Peripheral neuropathies. Elsevier North-Holland, Amsterdam pp 247–255
3. Brown MJ, Asbury AK (1984) Diabetic neuropathy. Ann Neurol 15: 2–12
4. Thomas PK, Eliasson SG (1984) Diabetic neuropathy. In: Dyck PJ, Thomas PK, Lambert EH, Bunge R (eds) Peripheral neuropathy, second edition. W B Saunders, Philadelphia, pp 1773–1810
5. Archer A, Watkins PJ, Thomas PK, Sharma AK, Payan J (1983) The natural history of acute painful neuropathy in diabetes mellitus. J Neurol Neurosurg Psychiatry 46: 491–499
6. Garland H, Taverner D (1953) Diabetic amyotrophy. Br Med J i: 1405
7. Asbury AK (1977) Proximal diabetic neuropathy. Ann Neurol 2: 179
8. Chokroverty S (1982) Proximal nerve dysfunction in diabetic proximal amyotrophy: electrophysiology and electron microscopy. Arch Neurol 39: 403–407
9. Justin-Besancon L, Cornet A, Contamin F, Guerre J, Bignon J (1963) Atteinte aigue bilatérale et partiellement réversible de plusieurs peines crâniennes chez un diabétique ayant présente sept ans auparavant une atteinte encéphalique aigue réversible. Bull Soc Med Hop Paris 114: 985
10. Korczyn AD (1971) Bell's palsy and diabetes mellitus. 1: 108
11. Raff MC, Sangalan GV, Asbury AK (1968) Ischemic mononeuropathy multiplex associated with diabetes mellitus. Arch Neurol 18: 487–499
12. Comi G, Lozza L, Galardi G, Chilardi MF, Medaglini S, Canal N (1985) Presence of carpal tunnel syndrome in diabetics: effects of age, sex, diabetes duration and polyneuropathy. Acta Diabetol Lat 22: 259–262
13. Mulder DW, Lambert EH, Barton JA, Sprague RG (1961) The neuropathies associated with diabetes mellitus: a clinical and electromyographic study of 103 unselected diabetic patients. Neurology 11: 275–284
14. Caravati CM (1933) Insulin neuritis: a case report. Virginia Med Monthly 59: 745
15. Ellenberg M (1959) Diabetic neuropathy precipitated by diabetic control with tolbutamide. J Am Med Assoc 169: 1755–1757
16. Mulder DW, Bastron JA, Lambert EH (1956) Hyperinsulin neuropathy. Neurology 6: 627–635
17. Canal N, Comi G (1983) Instrumental and clinical features of autonomic involvement in peripheral neuropathies. In: Clinical and biological aspects of peripheral nerve diseases. Alan R Liss, New York, pp 149–160
18. Clarke BF, Ewing DJ, Campbell IW (1979) Diabetic autonomic neuropathy. Diabetologia 17: 195–212
19. Ellenberg M (1966) Diabetic neurogenic vesical dysfunction. Arch Intern Med 117: 348–354
20. Buck AC, Reed PI, Siddiq YK, Chisholm GD, Fraser TR (1976) Bladder dysfunction and neuropathy in diabetes. Diabetologia 12: 251–258
21. Comi G, Pescatori D, Bossi A, Fusi MG, Toussoun J, Pozza G (1982) Clinical and instrumental diagnosis of autonomic neuropathy in insulin dependent diabetes. Acta Diabetol Lat 19: 577
22. Karacan I, Scott FB, Salis PJ, Attia SL, Ware JC, Altinel A, Williams RI (1977) Nocturnal erections, differential diagnosis of impotence and diabetes. Bibl Psychiatry 12: 373–380
23. Kolodny RC, Kolodny FC, Kahan CB, Goldstein HH, Barnett DM (1974) Sexual dysfunction in diabetic men. Diabetes 23: 306–309
24. Ellenberg M, Weber H (1966) Retrograde ejaculation in diabetic neuropathy. Ann Intern Med 65: 1237–1246

25. Mandelstam P, Lieber A (1967) Esophageal dysfunction in diabetic neuropathy-gastroenteropathy. J Am Med Assoc 201: 582–586
26. Kassander P (1958) Asymptomatic gastric retention in diabetics (gastroparesis diabeticorum). Ann Intern Med 48: 797–812
27. Dotevall G (1959) Incidence of peptic ulcers in diabetes mellitus. Acta Diabetol Scand 164: 463–467
28. Katz LA, Spiro HM (1966) The gastrointestinal manifestions of diabetes. N Engl J Med 275: 1350–1361
29. Ewing DJ, Campbell IW, Clarke BF (1980) The natural history of diabetic autonomic neuropathy. Q J Med 49: 95–108
30. Page M, Watkins PJ (1976) Provocation of postural hypotension by insulin in diabetic autonomic neuropathy. Diabetes 25: 90–95
31. Palmer KT, Perkins CJ, Smith RBW (1977) Insulin approvated postural hypotension. Aust NZ J Med 7: 161–162
32. Campbell IW, Ewing DJ, Clarke BF (1976) Therapeutic experience with fludrocortisone in diabetic postural hypotension. Br Med J i: 872–874
33. Wheeler T, Watkins PJ (1973) Cardiac denervation in diabetes. Br Med J iv: 584–586
34. Campbell IW, Ewing DJ, Clarke BF (1978) Painful myocardial infarction in severe diabetic autonomic neuropathy. Acta Diabetol Lat 15: 201–204
35. Sussman KE, Crout JR, Marble A (1963) Failure of warning in insulin-induced hypoglycaemic reactions. Diabetes 12: 38–45
36. Goodman JI (1966) Diabetic anhidrosis. Am J Med 41: 831–835
37. Watkins PJ (1973) Facial sweating after food: a new sign of diabetic autonomic neuropathy. Br Med J i: 583–587
38. Moorhouse JA, Carter SA, Doupe J (1966) Vascular responses in diabetic peripheral neuropathy. Br Med J i: 883–888
39. Deanfield JE, Daggett PR, Harrison MJG (1980) The role of autonomic neuropathy in diabetic foot ulceration. J Neurol Sci 47: 203–210

Diabetic Complications: Early Diagnosis and Treatment
Edited by D. Andreani, G. Crepaldi, U. Di Mario and G. Pozza


CHAPTER 16

# *Current Management of Diabetic Autonomic Neuropathy*

D. FEDELE, F. BELLAVERE* and C. CARDONE*
*Department of Endocrinology, University of Palermo; *Department of Internal Medicine, University of Padua, Italy*

Over the last decade the attention of diabetologists has increasingly focused on an important complication of diabetes mellitus: autonomic neuropathy (AN). Although this complex pathology has been recognized since the 1940s (1, 2), it has only become a subject of growing interest since the seventies. This was probably due in part to the introduction of a new and simple methodological approach to the study of the autonomic control of the heart (3, 4) and in part to the discovery of a high mortality rate among diabetic patients affected by AN (5). Since the early 1980s, numerous studies demonstrating the widespread presence and early onset of this complication among diabetic patients have revised the previous concept of AN as an uncommon and late complication of diabetes (6–9). More recently another important question has been raised, namely the possible influence of AN on the onset and course of other diabetic complications such as nephropathy (10, 11), cardiopathy (12) and even the regulation of glucose homeostasis (13).

It is now generally agreed that, although the manifestations may vary, AN involves the regulatory systems of the whole body, producing varying degrees of dysfunction in all organs. In this context, we feel that the definition of AN formulated by ourselves some years ago is still valid: diabetic AN is a generalized dysfunction of the autonomic nervous system, of uncertain etiology and insidious onset, unpredictably and unevenly affecting the various areas of the body (14).

That AN is a generalized disorder has received frequent confirmation, notably in recent observations of cardiovascular reflex dysfunctions in diabetic patients with abnormal esophageal motility (15), delayed gastric emptying (16), pupillary dysreflexia (17, 18), augmented ocular tone (19) and abnormal neuroendocrine responses (20).

## DIAGNOSIS

In the past the diagnosis of AN was essentially based on the description of symptoms, but recent advances in medical technology have allowed a more reliable detection of pathological signs so that the diagnosis of AN is now supported by many organ-targeted instrumental aids. The reliability of these aids has been discussed in many recent papers (21–23).

### Cardiovascular System

The autonomic function of the cardiovascular system is now routinely explored with a battery of five simple and reliable tests, introduced in 1978 (5), which may be performed by an experienced technician in any health centre. Three of the tests are based on RR interval variations during Valsalva manoeuvre, deep breathing, and change of posture from lying to standing; the remaining two are based on blood pressure (BP) response to standing (fall in systolic BP) and to sustained handgrip (increase in diastolic BP). The evaluation of cardiovascular response to these tests is treated in detail elsewhere (23). A scoring system has also been proposed with a view to providing a simple means for the objective evaluation of autonomic impairment (24). Although this battery of tests has proved an extremely useful tool, reservations still exist about the validity of tests drawing a comprehensive diagnosis from the exploration of the two different parameters, RR interval and BP variation, which present differing degrees of sensitivity and specificity. Hence, the recent concept that diabetic patients with AN show an early parasympathetic impairment (e.g. impaired RR variation response to the Valsalva manoeuvre, deep breathing and lying to standing) followed by a less pronounced sympathetic impairment (e.g. impaired blood pressure response to standing or sustained handgrip) is plausible, but still requires confirmation. However, new tests designed to extract the maximum information from a single parameter (RR variation) have now been proposed. The characteristic patterns of RR variation after lying down have been studied as useful indicators of both parasympathetic and sympathetic function (25–27), and heart rate response to coughing (28) has been found to be a simple index of parasympathetic integrity. Further studies will be required to show the role and importance of these findings in the diagnosis of AN.

A new and interesting approach to the detection of parasympathetic impairment is 24-hour monitoring of the sudden beat-by-beat variations which have been shown to be a sensitive index of parasympathetic activity (29). The disadvantage of this method is that it requires sophisticated equipment, but it does appear to circumvent the problem of the 'hemodynamic component' that to some extent influences all the cardiovascular tests in common use. It is in fact known that patients with hemodynamic imbalance can show alterations in cardiovascular reflex tests not necessarily dependent on autonomic impairment (30). As it is well known that myocardial function and baroreceptor sensitivity decline with age, the diagnosis of

AN must obviously take the age of the subject examined into account (31–34), especially in the case of elderly patients (35, 36).

Some limiting conditions which may influence results should also be taken into account in the performance and evaluation of cardiovascular autonomic tests. The presence of heart failure or severe arrythmias will obviously hinder a correct interpretation. Abnormal cardiac response patterns may also be encountered in patients with valvular heart disease, hypertension or pulmonary disease (obstructive or emphysematous). Drugs such as $\beta$-blockers, digitalis, antihypertensives and antispasmodics will also provoke altered cardiac reflex responses. Finally, all cardiovascular tests should be performed with caution in patients with acute hemorrhagic retinopathy, coronary heart disease and cerebrovascular diseases.

## Gastrointestinal System

As mentioned above, the attention of most investigators engaged in the study of diabetic AN has focused on the cardiovascular system, largely because of the availability of reliable, simple and non-invasive tests based on precise and easily quantifiable parameters such as heart rate and blood pressure. The autonomic involvement of the gastrointestinal system is more difficult to determine given the complexity and relatively poor reproducibility of the tests in use. The diagnosis of gastrointestinal autonomic dysfunctions hence requires a greater reliance on subjective symptomatology (21) as they may be confused with other disorders not related to diabetes.

The best known autonomic dysfunctions of the enteric tract are the so-called gastroparesis diabeticorum (37) and diabetic diarrhoea. The first consists in delayed gastric emptying with loss of selective transit between solids and liquids causing a sensation of epigastric fullness and sometimes vomiting. Gastric emptying in diabetic patients has been studied with various techniques: barium meal (38), double scintiscanning (16, 39) and gastric impedence (40). This latter method may have a useful application in the study of gastroenteric AN as it is a non-invasive technique requiring relatively inexpensive equipment and gives fairly reliable results compared to traditional scintiscanning (41). Besides delayed emptying, gastric disturbances in AN are also characterized by reduced acid secretion due to vagal damage (42). This finding gives a more complicated picture of the co-existence of mechanical and biochemical disorders in the autonomic stomach. As both these functions are thought to be essential in meal absorption, and hence in metabolic regulation, we feel that efforts should be made to evaluate them together, possibly by means of a single procedure. In the case of diabetic diarrhoea, although this disorder is a well-known symptom of autonomic neuropathy, there are as yet no instrumental aids for differential diagnosis with other causes of diarrhoea. It is in fact not associated with malabsorption and manifests itself especially at night. The autonomic mechanism underlying this phenomenon is not yet understood. Recently reported success in treatment with clonidine (43) raises the hypothesis that diabetic diarrhoea may be caused by an $\alpha$-adrenergic receptor dysfunction in the gut.

A less well-known symptom of diabetic AN is constipation. A reduced postprandial colonic motility has been demonstrated (44) but this finding still awaits confirmation. Fecal incontinence may also occur in AN, and anorectal sensorimotor function has been shown to be impaired in patients with cardiac autonomic neuropathy (45).

A complete picture of the autonomic disturbances of the gastrointestinal tract must also include gallbladder and esophageal dysfunctions. Esophageal alterations, which have frequently been recorded in AN, consist in abnormal dilatation, reduced peristaltic pressure and the presence of tertiary contractions (15). These dysfunctions have no clearly defined symptomatology and in our opinion no certain clinical significance.

Although gallbladder dysfunction in diabetic AN was strongly hypothesized (21) some time ago, as far as we are aware there is still no definitive evidence in support of its inclusion among the autonomic disorders associated with diabetes mellitus.

## Urogenital System

Autonomic involvement of the urogenital system has two main manifestations: the so-called 'diabetic bladder' and impotence.

The neurogenic bladder in diabetes has a peculiar feature of sensory and parasympathetic motor denervation. Its classic symptomatology consists in insensitivity to urinary filling, atony of the detrusor, and the presence of residual urinary volume. As a consequence of the characteristic insensitivity the neurogenic bladder is generally asymptomatic until the onset of urinary infection and, in more severe involvement, renal failure. The frequency of the events occurring in such cases are well documented elsewhere (46, 47). Insensitivity to filling and bladder atony are detected by cystomanometry, a test available in most urological departments. However, both these disorders can be deduced from careful monitoring of micturition intervals and with uroflowmetry. This latter is a simple, non-invasive technique, but caution is obviously required in the interpretation of results in view of other possible causes of dysuria such as bladder neck stenosis. The presence of residual volume may also be detected with ultrasound scanning (48).

Much has been written about impotence in diabetes. In spite of this, the role and importance of AN in this disorder is not yet clear. It has been reported that impotence is an early symptom of AN (24). The most common form of diabetic impotence is incomplete erection. A minor form manifests as retrograde ejaculation, allowing some sexual activity but not insemination (49). In the diagnosis of diabetic neurogenic impotence, all other possible causes of the disorder must be excluded, and, as a consequence, diagnosis can be uncertain (50). A careful recording of anamnestic data together with instrumental aids, such as the nocturnal study of penile tumescence (51) and the more recently adopted intrapenile injection of papaverine, may be useful in the determination of organic causes of non-erectile impotence. Retrograde ejaculation is demonstrated by the finding of a large number of spermatozoa in centrifuged urine after sexual intercourse.

The incidence of impotence in diabetes is known to be high with estimates ranging from 28% to 58%. However, it is possible that neurogenic impotence is not as widespread as was once thought (52). It should also be borne in mind that impotence in diabetic patients may also be caused by vascular dysfunctions. However, diabetic impotence does not appear to have an endocrine basis (53).

### The Ocular System

Pupillary abnormalities are well-known signs of autonomic dysfunction. They have been noted since the 1930s (1, 2) and in more recent years a reduction in pupillary diameter has been described (54). Provocative tests using pupillography have shown a blunted pupil adaption to dark in diabetic patients (55, 56). A simple test of pupil motility using a slit-lamp stimulus has been described and has demonstrated a reduced number of pupil size oscillations in diabetic patients with generalized AN (18). A new and interesting approach to the study of autonomic dysfunction in the ocular system uses the evaluation of ocular tone. The association between glaucoma and diabetes mellitus has been noted for some time, but the existence of a close correlation between diabetic AN and ocular hypertone has been demonstrated only in more recent years (19). This suggests a new and important aspect of autonomic involvement of the eye in diabetes.

### Endocrine System

Endocrine system activity is known to be strongly affected by that of the autonomic nervous system. Recent literature shows a considerable interest in this complex problem in view of the potential importance of this link for the maintenance of glucose homeostasis (13). Despite the many discrepancies in the evidence that has so far emerged, some basic findings appear to be consolidated:

1. The release of some hormones and neuropeptides, including glucagon, somatostatin, pancreatic polypeptide (PP), epinephrine (E), norepinephrine (NE) and gastric inhibitory polypeptide (GIP), is reduced in diabetic patients with AN.
2. Some of these hormones and peptides, such as PP and NE, may be effective markers of AN.

It has been known for some time that glucagon release is reduced in diabetic patients with AN (57), but the action of the autonomic nervous system on this hormone is difficult to determine given its complex kinetics, which are often altered even in diabetic subjects without AN. The demonstrable influence of the autonomic dysreflexia in reduced release of PP (20, 58), somatostatin (59) and GIP (60) is somewhat clearer, but does not appear to have practical consequences for metabolic equilibrium in the diabetic patient with AN.

The behaviour of NE and E in the diabetic patient with AN has, however, given rise to considerable interest in view of the fundamental contribution of both substances (particularly E) to glycemic equilibrium. The reduced response of E to hypoglycemia found in patients with AN (22, 61) has given rise to speculations about the possible role of AN in altered insulin counterregulation (13, 62), although this may also be attributed to other mechanisms (63). It is hence very important to identify the presence of any autonomic damage, particularly in the course of intensive insulin treatment, in order to reduce the possibility of hypoglycemic crises, the consequences of which may be especially severe in AN patients who are prone to hypoglycemic unawareness (21).

PP assay after mixed meal (20), physical stress (22) or hypoglycemia (62) has been found to be an excellent index of neuroendocrine autonomic damage. A more accurate identification of sympathetic autonomic damage may be obtained by NE assay after postural change (lying to standing), physical exercise (22) or intravenous antiacetylcholinesterase stimulus, while the response of NE to hypoglycemia remains controversial. However, given the existence of a good correlation between the neuroendocrine responses of PP, NE and non-invasive cardiovascular tests (20), the latter may be considered a sufficient index for the detection of more widespread parasympathetic and sympathetic autonomic damage.

## THERAPY

The treatment of the various forms of AN is still today largely symptomatic. As the etiology of AN is not clear, the identification of a general treatment is extremely problematic. The administration of aldose reductase inhibitors has had varying degrees of success and the efficacy and side-effects of these drugs are still under evaluation. Our experience suggests that a valid treatment is careful management of metabolic control. This has been shown to give a slight improvement of symptomatology and a small but significant short- and medium-term improvement in cardiovascular autonomic reflexes (64). More recently it has been suggested that captopril may be useful in the treatment of vagal autonomic neuropathy (65), although its efficacy is limited to the cardiovascular apparatus. This interesting proposal requires further confirmation. In the case of gastrointestinal AN the use of metoclopramide has excited some interest: this drug has been shown to improve both gastric emptying and colonic motility (66).

The use of drugs in the treatment of the diabetic bladder has met with little success, and the best advice remains controlled micturition with suprapubic hand pressure every 4–6 hours.

Impotence in diabetes may be ameliorated by the intrapenile injection of papaverine which may provoke a controlled erection for about 15 minutes. In subjects in whom this drug is not effective or gives rise to untoward effects (namely men affected by postural hypotension, headache, cerebral angiopathy, etc.) the only solution is a preferably semirigid penile implant under strict urological follow-up.

## REFERENCES


1. Jordan WR (1936) Neuritic manifestation in diabetes mellitus. Arch Intern Med 57: 307–366
2. Rundles RW (1945) Diabetic neuropathy. General review with report of 125 cases. Medicine 24: 111–160
3. Wheeler T, Watkins PJ (1973) Cardiac denervation in diabetes. Br Med J 4: 584–586
4. Ewing DJ (1978) Cardiovascular reflexes and autonomic neuropathy. Clin Sci 55: 321–327
5. Ewing DJ, Campbell IW, Clarke BF (1980) The natural history of diabetic autonomic neuropathy. J Med 193: 95–108
6. Ewing DJ (1984) Cardiac autonomic neuropathy. In: Jarrett RJ (ed) Diabetes and heart disease. Elsevier Biomedical Press, Amsterdam pp 99–132
7. Young RJ, Ewing DJ, Clarke BF (1983) Nerve function and metabolic control in teenage diabetics. Diabetes 32: 142–147
8. Sundkvist G, Lilja B (1985) Autonomic neuropathy in diabetes mellitus. A follow-up study. Diabetes Care 4: 529–534
9. Bellavere F, Bosello G, Cardone C, Girardello L, Fedele D (1985) Evidence of early impairment of cardiovascular reflexes in insulin dependent diabetics without autonomic symptoms. Diabete Metab 11: 152–156
10. Lilja B, Nosslin B, Bergstrom B, Sundkvist G (1985) Glomerular filtration rate, autonomic nerve function, and orthostatic blood pressure in patients with diabetes mellitus. Diabetes Res. 2: 179–181
11. Wincour PH, Dhar H, Anderson DC (1986) The relation between autonomic neuropathy and urinary sodium and albumin excretion in insulin treated diabetics. Diabetic Med 3: 436–440
12. Bellavere F, Ferri M, Guarini L, Piccoli R, Bax G, Cardone C, Fedele D (1987) Prolonged QT period in diabetic autonomic neuropathy. A possible role in sudden cardiac death. Br Heart J (in press)
13. Cryer PE (1986) The metabolic impact of autonomic neuropathy in insulin dependent diabetes mellitus. Arch Intern Med 146: 2127–2129
14. Bellavere F, Bosello G, Fedele D (1982) Malattia diabetica e sistema nervoso autonomo. Giorn Ital Diabet 2: 303–315
15. Channer KS, Jackson PC, O'Brien (1985) Oesophageal function in diabetes mellitus and its association with autonomic neuropathy. Diabetic Med 2: 378–382
16. Wright RA, Clemente R, Wathen R (1985) Diabetic gastroparesis: an abnormal gastric emptying for solids. Am J Med Sci 289: 240–242
17. Pfeifer MA, Cook D, Brodsky J, Tice D, Parrish D, Reenan A, Halte JB, Porte D Jr (1982) Quantitative evaluation of sympathetic and parasympathetic control of iris function. Diabetes Care 5: 518–528
18. Martyn CN, Ewing DJ (1986) Pupil cycle time—a simple way of measuring an autonomic reflex. J Neurol Neurosurg Psychiatry 49: 771–774
19. Clark CV, Mapstone R (1985) Autonomic neuropathy in ocular hypertension. Lancet ii: 185–187
20. Ewing DJ, Bellavere F, Reimersma DF, Espi DM, McKibben KD, Clarke BF, Buchanan RA (1986) Correlation of cardiovascular and neuroendocrine tests of autonomic function in diabetes. Metabolism 35: 349–353
21. Clarke BF, Ewing DJ, Campbell IW (1979) Diabetic autonomic neuropathy. Diabetologia 17: 195–212
22. Hilsted J (1982) Pathophysiology in diabetic autonomic neuropathy: cardiovascular hormonal and metabolic study. Diabetes 31: 730–737

23. Ewing DJ, Clarke BF (1986) Autonomic neuropathy: its diagnosis and prognosis. Clin Endocrinol Metab 15: 855–887
24. Bellavere F, Bosello G, Fedele D, Cardone C, Ferri M (1983) Diagnosis and management of diabetic autonomic neuropathy. Br Med J 287: 61
25. Bellavere F, Ewing DJ (1982) Autonomic control of the normal immediate heart rate response to lying down. Clin Sci 62: 57–64
26. Rodrigues EA, Ewing DJ (1983) Immediate heart rate response to lying down: simple test for cardaic parasympathetic damage in diabetes. Br Med J 287: 800
27. Bellavere F, Cardone C, Ferri M, Guarini L, Piccoli A, Fedele D (1987) Standing to lying heart rate variation: a simple test in the diagnosis of diabetic autonomic neuropathy. Diabetic Med 4: 41–43
28. Cardone C, Bellavere F, Ferri M, Fedele D (1987) Autonomic mechanisms in the heart rate response to coughing. Clin Sci 72: 55–60
29. Ewing DJ, Neilson JMM, Travis P (1984) New method for assessing cardiac parasympathetic activity using 24 hour electrocardiograms. Br Heart J 52: 396–402
30. Levin AB (1966) A simple test of cardiac function based upon heart rate changes induced by Valsalva manoeuvre. Am J Cardiol 18: 90–99
31. Kalbfleisch JH, Reinke A, Porth CJ, Ebert TJ, Smith JJ (1977) Effect of age on circulatory response to postural and Valsalva tests. Proc Soc Exp Biol Med 156: 100–103
32. Pfeifer MA, Weimberg CR, Cook D, Best JD, Reenan A, Halter JB (1983) Differential changes of autonomic nervous system function with age in man. Am J Med 75: 249–258
33. Bergstrom B, Lilja B, Rosberg K, Sundkvist G (1986) Autonomic function tests. Reference values in healthy subjects. Clin Phys 6: 523–528
34. Kaijser L (1986) Autonomic function tests—need for standardization? Clin Phys 6: 475–479
35. Crepaldi G, Cardone C, Feruglio M, Maggi S, Marchetti GP, Bellavere F, Fedele D (1985) Age-related changes of the cardiovascular reflex function. XIII International Congress of Gerontology, New York.
36. Robinson B, Johnson RH, Lambie DG, Palmer KT (1983) Do elderly patients with an excessive blood pressure on standing have evidence of autonomic failure? Clin Sci 64: 587–591
37. Kassander P (1958) Asymptomatic gastric retention in diabetics (gastroparesis diabeticorum). Ann Intern Med 48: 797–812
38. Taub S, Mariani A, Barkin JS (1979) Gastrointestinal manifestation of diabetes mellitus. Diabetes Care 2: 437–447
39. Campbell IW, Heading RC, Ewing DJ, Buist TAS, Tothill P, Clarke BF (1977) Gastric emptying in diabetic autonomic neuropathy assessed by a double isotope scanning technique. Gut 18: 462–467
40. Gilbey SG, Sutton RA, Thompson S, Watkins PJ (1985) A new simple non-invasive method for assessing gastric emptying and its application in diabetic autonomic neuropathy. Diabetic Med 2: 510a
41. Sutton JA, Thompson S, Sobnack R (1985) Measurement of gastric emptying rates by radioactive isotope scanning and epigastric impedance. Lancet i: 898–900
42. Buysschaert M, Donkier J, Dive A, Ketelslegers JM, Lambert AE (1985) Gastric acid and pancreatic polypeptide to sham feeding are impaired in diabetic subjects with autonomic neuropathy. Diabetes 34: 1181–1185
43. Fedorak RN, Field M, Chang EB (1985) Treatment of diabetic diarrhoea with clonidine. Ann Intern Med 102: 197–199
44. Battle WM, Snape WJ, Alavi A, Cohen S, Braunstein S (1980) Colonic dysfunction in

diabetes mellitus. Gastroenterology 79: 1219–1222

45. Lejeune D, Melange M, Daumerie C, Buysschaert M, Vanheuverzwijn R (1986) Contribution of anorectal manometry and ECG to the diagnosis of diabetic autonomic neuropathy. Gastroenterol Clin Biol 10: 554–557
46. Frimodt-Moller C (1980) Diabetic cystopathy: epidemiology and related disorders. Ann Intern Med 92: 318–321
47. Bradley WE (1980) Diagnosis of urinary bladder dysfunction in diabetes mellitus. Ann Intern Med 92: 323–326
48. Beylot M, Marion D, Noel G (1982) Ultrasonic determination of residual urine in diabetic subjects: relationship to neuropathy and urinary tract infection. Diabetes Care 5: 501–505
49. Ellenberg M, Weber H (1966) Retrograde ejaculation in diabetic neuropathy. Ann Intern Med 65: 1237–1245
50. McCulloch DK, Young RJ, Prescott RJ, Campbell IW, Clarke BF (1984) The natural history of impotence in diabetic men. Diabetologia 26: 437–440
51. Schiavi RC, Fischer C, Quadland M, Glover A (1985) Nocturnal penile tumescent evaluation of erectile function in insulin-dependent diabetic men. Diabetologia 28: 90–94
52. Watkins PJ, Edmonds ME (1983) Clinical presentation of diabetic autonomic failure. In: Bannister R (ed) Autonomic failure. A textbook of clinical disorders of the autonomic nervous system. Oxford University Press, Oxford, pp 337–370
53. Lester E, Grant AJ, Woodroffe FJ (1980) Impotence in diabetic and non-diabetic outpatients. Br Med J iii: 354
54. Hreidarsson AB (1982) Pupil size in insulin dependent diabetes. Relationship to duration, metabolic control and long term manifestations. Diabetes 31: 442–448
55. Hreidarsson AB (1979) Pupil motility in long term diabetes. Diabetologia 17: 145–150
56. Smith SA, Smith SE (1983) Reduced pupillary light reflexes in diabetic autonomic neuropathy. Diabetologia 24: 330–332
57. Maher DT, Tanenberg RJ, Greenberg BZ, Hoffman JE, Doe RP, Goetz FC (1977) Lack of glucagon response to hypoglycemia in diabetic autonomic neuropathy. Diabetes 26: 196–200
58. Krarup T, Shwartz TW, Hilsted J, Madsbad S, Verlaege O, Sestoft L (1979) Impaired response of pancreatic polypeptide to hypoglycemia: an early sign of autonomic neuropathy in diabetes. Br Med J ii: 1544–1546
59. Fernandez-Castaner M, Webb S, Levy I, Rios M, Casamitjana R, Bergua M, Figuerola D, Rivera F (1985) Somatostatin and counterregulatory hormone responses to hypoglycaemia in diabetics with and without autonomic neuropathy. Diabete Metab 11: 81–86
60. Levitt NS, Vinik AI, Child TP (1980) Glucose-dependent insulin-releasing peptide in non insulin-dependent maturity onset diabetes: effects of autonomic neuropathy. J Clin Endocrinol Metab 51: 254–258
61. Hoeldtke RD, Boden G, Shuman CR, Owen OE (1982) Reduced epinephrine secretion and hypoglycaemia unawareness in diabetic autonomic neuropathy. Ann Intern Med 96: 459–462
62. White NH, Gingerich RL, Levadosky LA, Cryer PE, Santiago JV (1985) Plasma pancreatic polypeptide response to insulin induced hypoglycaemia as a marker for defective glucose counterregulation in insulin–dependent diabetes mellitus. Diabetes 34: 870–875
63. Bolli GB, De Feo P, Compagnucci P, Caterchini MG, Angeletti G, Santeusanio F, Brunetti P, Gerich JE (1983) Abnormal glucose counterregulation in insulin-dependent diabetes mellitus; interaction of anti-insulin antibodies and impaired glucagon and epinephrine secretion. Diabetes 32: 134–141

64. Fedele D, Bellavere F, Cardone C, Ferri M, Crepaldi G (1985) Short and long term continuous insulin infusion system treatment in patients with autonomic diabetic neuropathy. Horm Metab Res 17: 410–413
65. Moore MV, Jeffcoate WJ, MacDonald IA (1986) Inprovement in diabetic autonomic neuropathy induced by captopril. EASD 22 Annual Meeting Rome 16–20 September
66. Snape WJ, Battle WM, Schwartz SS (1982) Metoclopramide to treat gastroparesis due to diabetes mellitus. A double blind controlled trial. Ann Intern Med 96: 444–446

Diabetic Complications: Early Diagnosis and Treatment
Edited by D. Andreani, G. Crepaldi, U. Di Mario and G. Pozza


CHAPTER 17

# *Vascular and Neural Damage in the Diabetic Foot*

J. D. WARD
*Royal Hallamshire Hospital, Sheffield, UK*

Consideration will be given to three important features of the diabetic foot:

1. Obstructive arterial vascular disease (arteriosclerosis).
2. Primary nerve damage, both somatic and autonomic.
3. The important functional neurovascular interaction leading to arteriovenous shunting.

In addition, in practical terms the application of knowledge in all of these areas to clinical management and prevention of foot problems will be reviewed. Indeed in some instances one single factor may be dominant and therapy obvious, but on many occasions there will be a complex mixture of factors all of them at an advanced state of pathology which may result in therapy being less effective. Therefore, at all times in viewing problems of the diabetic *prevention* should be a primary aim. At the same time attempts should be made to minimize progress of vessel or nerve damage by means of satisfactory control of blood glucose and lipid metabolism, avoidance of smoking and possibly in the future the use of drugs which interfere with tissue abnormalities and pathology, for example aldose reductase inhibitors minimizing peripheral nerve damage.

## OBSTRUCTIVE ARTERIAL VASCULAR DISEASE

In both Type 1 and Type 2 diabetes the incidence and severity of arteriosclerosis is increased compared to the non-diabetic population, and moreover the disease is more widespread, occurring particularly badly below the level of the knee. Severe vascular calcification is often present and on radiographs of the foot it is common to see calicified outlines of vessels. As a result of this calcification and rigidity of vessels the doppler ultrasound measurement of ankle pressure index (API) may be falsely high when there is indeed major obstruction to forward flow. It is of interest that often in very obvious ischemia of the leg and foot in diabetes, pain—even in the presence of an ischemic ulcer—is not always severe indicating the common co-existence of major vessel disease and nerve damage.

There is no satisfactory metabolic explanation of vascular calcification in diabetes. It has been suggested that primary disease of sympathetic fibres leads to degeneration of the medial layers of major vessels and subsequent calcification (1).

The diabetic subject with peripheral vascular disease should be offered the same investigative procedures as the non-diabetic subject—API with doppler ultrasound and arteriography. Surgical treatment will often be possible but, because of the distal nature of the disease with heavy vascular calcification, the outcome in diabetes is not so satisfactory as in the non-diabetic subject. The efficacy of balloon angioplasty for local proximal and possibly distal lesions is being studied, but it is not clear whether this procedure has a place in diabetes. Surgical reconstruction should be offered in suitable cases and some attempts have been made to reconstruct the more peripheral vessels by the use of microsurgery (2).

So-called peripheral vasodilator drugs have no place in arteriosclerotic disease, there being no trials showing any benefit of such agents. Regrettably the natural history of progression to local ischemia of part of the foot (often precipitated by a small pressure sore or abrasion) is to total foot and then limb ischemia and then amputation.

## PRIMARY NERVE DAMAGE

In subjects with significant foot problems, such as ulceration, there is a marked degree of peripheral nerve damage, both of somatic nerve fibres and of the autonomic nervous system. It seems likely that the first fibres to be damaged are the small fibres that are important in establishing the sympathetic system; this probably occurs some time before large fibre loss, axonal degeneration and demyelination. With the establishment of more obvious peripheral nerve damage there is undoubted sympathetic dysfunction (3), and such small fibre loss probably has a major part to play in the production of arteriovenous shunting (see the following section).

As a result of somatic peripheral nerve damage, mainly involving large fibres, axon and myelin sheaths, the following features appear;

(1) Painful sensory symptoms—with tingling, cramps, shooting pains and hyperesthesia; but
(2) There is also *lack of pain* often with complete anesthesia of the foot. In some subjects at the same time painful sensory symptoms are appreciated—the painful, painless foot.
(3) Very significant muscle weakness and wasting in the foot leading to an abnormal posture with clawed toes and dropped metatarsal heads. As a consequence of this, the normal tone of the foot is lost and weight is not spread equally over

a number of areas of the foot. Areas of extremely high pressure (as high as 50 $kg/cm^2$) develop in one or two areas of the foot and under such pressure skin with a relatively poor blood supply is likely to break down, assisted by friction and stress.

Damage to sympathetic nerve fibres (small fibres) leads to poor skin nutrition and a dry vulnerable skin which along with reduced subcutaneous tissue and stiffening of the foot arch, similar to that seen in the hands of long-standing diabetic subjects, makes breakdown and ulcer formation very likely. Infection of such lesions, although not a primary vascular or neurological event, is a major factor resulting in massive tissue destruction (4).

## THE NEUROVASCULAR INTERACTION (ARTERIOVENOUS SHUNTING)

Allowing for the fact that on many occasions a degree of obstructive arterial disease may be present and will presumably aggravate blood flow factors, this section will focus purely on the abnormal blood flow patterns in the 'neuropathic foot'. It is now well established that in such a foot (and leg) arteriovenous shunting is present (5–8). Such a neuropathic foot is warm, often 2–3°C warmer than room temperature, has an easily palpable and often visible dorsalis pedis pulse, and visible distended veins are seen in the foot and lower leg when the subject is lying flat (9). Doppler ultrasound studies reveal a sonogram indicative of fast forward blood flow, and samples from these distended veins reveal oxygenated venous blood. Moreover, in the neuropathic foot the volume of blood flow is increased (10).

The major reason for this abnormal flow and shunting of blood is sympathetic nerve failure, i.e. an autonomic neuropathy of the legs. A similar doppler sonogram and venous oxygenation of blood from foot veins have been demonstrated in non-diabetic subjects with quadriplegia (11). However, it is also possible that the abnormal metabolic state of diabetes itself contributes to increased flow and the fact that many peripheral small vessels in the foot are occluded may encourage return of blood by larger and more proximal channels.

Other effects of this sympathetic failure are the medial calcification of the vessels (1)—these rigid tubes further encouraging the fast forward flow of blood—and it has also been demonstrated that there is increased blood flow through the bones of the foot (12). The bones of the diabetic foot are often osteopenic with many fractures present in the metatarsals (13), and the combination of severely abnormal blood flow, increased bone flow, osteopenia and fractures causes the most advanced state of damage in the diabetic foot—the *Charcot foot*. In this condition there is gross destruction of bones around the midtarsal and ankle joints, with fractures, bony resorption and high isotope uptake. Fortunately, this clinical picture is rare. Further evidence for the important role of sympathetic dysfunction in the neuropathic foot is the return of the abnormal doppler sonogram to normal by coughing and other sympathetic stimuli and the resolution of the edema occasionally seen in severe neuropathy, along with improvement in the sonogram, following administration of ephedrine (14).

There are considerable abnormalities of the microcirculation in diabetes in general, not necessarily confined to subjects with obvious neuropathy (4). Vascular responses are often impaired and, using a heating probe with modified laser doppler, it has been shown that after minor thermal injury maximum skin blood flow was lower in subjects with diabetes (15), suggesting that, although in the neuropathic foot blood flow is fast and increased in larger vessels, the microcirculation to the skin and other tissues is impaired, i.e. that is the blood supply and nutrition of the skin are poor.

Arterial blood pressure may also have a significant part to play in subcutaneous flow for, in keeping with a stiff pressure passive microvascular bed, blood flow is increased or decreased in a linear relationship to the arterial blood pressure (16). It has been shown in these studies that autoregulation is basically impaired in diabetes during changes in blood pressure (17), and it is suggested by these authors that nerve damage is not a major factor in control of the skin blood flow autoregulation.

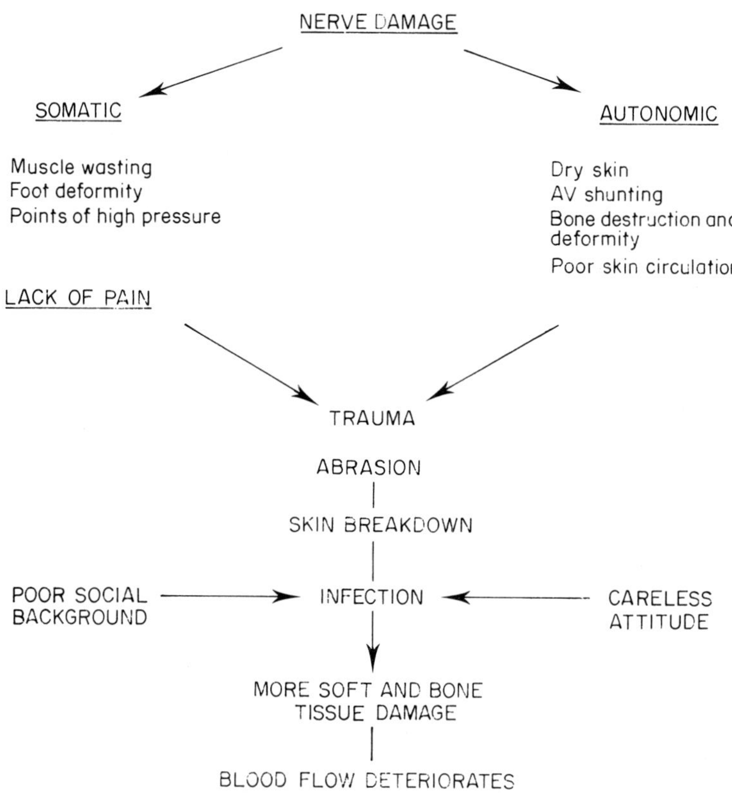


Figure 1. Factors involved in the development of a foot ulcer.

## DEVELOPMENT OF THE DIABETIC FOOT ULCER

Figure 1 lays out the factors involved in the development of a foot ulcer. This pathway is primarily involved in the development of the neuropathic ulcer, although some degree of obstructive arterial disease may be present. If a leg and foot is more frankly ischemic, breakdown of skin will heal less easily and often lead to further embarrassment to the circulation and a progression of ischemia to gangrene. Treatment once an ulcer is present consists of vigorous antibiotic therapy for any infection, expert chiropody assessment and treatment of the shape of the shoe and the suitability of foot-wear. If an ulcer is more advanced with tissue ischemia and infection, a combined medical and surgical assessment should be made to decide on the appropriateness of local or more major surgery. The warmer the foot with overt evidence of neuropathy, the more likely is local surgery to be successful in removing ischemic toes and frankly gangrenous and infected tissue. If clinical assessment indicates major vessel disease, especially with a poor API, then more major below- or above-knee amputation is likely.

## PREVENTION OF DIABETIC FOOT ULCERS

*Prevention* should be the major word used in a diabetic unit. The various factors leading to breakdown of skin and an ulcer have all been listed in this chapter and should be recognized by all of those working in the field of diabetes. Educational information on the basis of these known factors should then be passed on to the patients themselves. Such efforts are often limited and poorly organized, partly relating to the large numbers of people attending many clinics, or to a given community where many people do not attend established clinics. Thus, efforts should be made to *identify the vulnerable* and organize intensive educational and clinical support for them. It is possible to identify subjects who are very vulnerable to the possibility of foot ulceration at a simple clinical level with the construction of a vulnerability index based on the following factors:

(1) Symptoms of neuropathy.
(2) Past history of any foot ulcer.
(3) Presence of significant retinopathy or renal impairment.
(4) Clinical signs: (a) the warm deformed neuropathic foot or (b) the cold ischemic foot.
(5) Social and psychological factors, e.g. the elderly living alone with poor eyesight, or an apparently careless attitude towards foot care.

It is unlikely that sophisticated technical measurements are necessary in constructing this simple vulnerability index. Various machines for quantitating foot pressure and foot maps are not necessary. It is known that the vibration perception threshold correlates strongly with high foot pressure and the presence of foot ulceration, and the quantitative evaluation of seriously impaired vibration perception is likely to identify people who have already been assessed to be at risk. However, the systematic use of the measurement of vibration perception threshold in a diabetic clinic service at least ensures the simplest of facts, and that is that all people attending are requested at some time to remove their shoes and socks.

## SUMMARY

By the time significant nerve damage with a degree of major vessel disease is evident in the leg and foot in diabetes, subjects will certainly be at major risk of developing foot ulceration. With the exception of advanced ischemic vascular disease, if all the facts discussed in this chapter are appreciated and a clinical organization developed to implement their identification then it should be possible totally to avoid all significant foot ulceration in a given diabetic population.

## REFERENCES

1. Edmonds ME, Morrison N, Laws JW, Watkins PJ (1982) Medical arterial calcification and diabetic neuropathy. Br Med J 284: 928
2. LoGerfor FW (1986) Etiology, diagnosis and management of ischemia in the diabetic foot. Transplant Proc XVIII: 1605
3. Guy RJC, Clark CA, Malcolm PN, Watkins PJ (1985) Evaluation of thermal and vibration sensation in diabetic neuropathy. Diabetologia 28: 131
4. Connor H, Boulton AJM, Ward JD (eds) (1987) The foot in diabetes. John Wiley, Chichester
5. Scarpello JHB, Martin TRP, Ward JD (1980) Ultrasound measurement of pulse wave velocities in the peripheral arteries of diabetic subjects. Clin Sci 58: 53–57
6. Edmonds ME, Roberts VC, Watkins PJ (1982) Blood flow in the diabetic neuropathic foot. Diabetologia 22: 9
7. Boulton AJM, Scarpello JHB, Ward JD (1982) Venous oxygenation in the diabetic neuropathic foot: evidence of arteriovenous shunting. Diabetologia 22: 6
8. Ward JD (1982) The diabetic leg. Diabetologia 22: 141
9. Ward JD, Simms JM, Knight G, Boulton AJM, Sandler DA (1983) Venous distension in the diabetic neuropathic foot (physical sign of arteriovenous shunting). J R Soc Med 76: 1011
10. Archer AG, Robert VC, Watkins PJ (1984) Blood flow patterns in painful diabetic neuropathy. Diabetologia 27: 282–286
11. van Hoogen F, Brawn LA, Sherriff S, Watson S, Ward JD (1986) Arteriovenous shunting in quadriplegia. Paraplegia 24: 282–286
12. Watkins PJ, Edmonds ME (1982) Autonomic neuropathy: blood flow in the diabetic foot. In: Bostrom and Ljungstedt H (eds) Recent trends in diabetic research. Almqvist & Wiksell International, Stockholm, p 211
13. Cundy TF, Edmonds ME, Watkins PJ (1985) Osteopenia and metatarsal fractures in diabetic neuropathy. Diabetic Med 2: 461
14. Edmonds ME, Archer AG, Watkins PJ (1983) Ephedrine: a new treatment for diabetic neuropathic edema. Lancet i: 548
15. Rayman G, Williams SA, Spencer PD, Smagae LH, Wise PH, Tooke JE (1986) Impaired microvascular hyperaemic response to minor skin trauma in Type 1 diabetes. Br Med J 292: 1295–1298

16. Kastrup J, Mathiesen ER, Saurbrey N, Norgaard T, Parving HH, Lassen NA (1987) Effect of strict metabolic control on regulation of subcutaneous blood flow in insulin dependent diabetes. Diabetic Med 4: 30–36
17. Kastrup J, Norgaard T, Parving HH, Henriksen O, Lassen NA (1985) Impaired autoregulation of blood flow in subcutaneous tissue in long term Type 1 diabetic patients with microangiopathy. An index of arteriole dysfunction. Diabetologia 28: 711–717

Diabetic Complications: Early Diagnosis and Treatment
Edited by D. Andreani, G. Crepaldi, U. Di Mario and G. Pozza


CHAPTER 18

# *Diagnosis and Treatment of Autonomic Neuropathy of the Gastrointestinal Tract*

G. Menzinger and M. G. Felici
*Cattedra Malattie del Ricambio, 2nd University of Rome 'Tor Vergata', Italy*

Until recently it was thought that the gut was controlled by the central nervous system (CNS) through two efferent systems: the one (parasympathetic) mainly excitatory and the other (sympathetic) mainly inhibitory (1). The discovery of nerve fibres which are non-adrenergic and non-cholinergic has led to the identification of a third nervous system: the enteric nervous system (ENS) (1,2). The neurons of this system elaborate the information generated by gut sensory receptors and can directly activate the appropriate effector system; thus the ENS functions as a sort of visceral 'brain'.

On the other hand, it is now recognized that, contrary to a long-established opinion, a large proportion of vagus fibres are afferent. Many receptors, including stretch, touch, osmo- and chemoreceptors, are vagal. The relative afferent fibres synapse in the medulla in the region of the nucleus of the solitary tract; from here interneurons pass to the dorsal nucleus of the vagus nerve, from which vagal efferent fibres pass caudally and synapse in the ENS. The medulla is thus an important centre of interchange; the information reaching it from the gut may be directly relayed to the ENS and thus to the appropriate peripheral effectors (vagovagal reflex). On the other hand, messages reaching the medulla from higher CNS centres can modulate vagovagal reflexes; conversely, information reaching the medulla from the gut, besides being utilized to regulate effector activity in the gut, may be used by the higher CNS centres to regulate behavioural activity involving hunger and satiety.

It is important to recognize that, in this new formulation of neural control of intestinal activity, messages from the CNS through vagal and sympathetic fibres reach the appropriate effector not directly but through the modulation of the ENS. The activity of this system is mediated by the large number of regulatory peptides which have been identified in the ENS neurons, such as substance P, cholecystokinin

(CCK), vasoactive intestinal peptide (VIP) and others. It is uncertain if these peptides represent true neurotransmitters or are neuromodulators.

The incomplete knowledge of this very complex system, which has only recently been recognized, explains some of the difficulties in the interpretation of gastrointestinal responses to various stimuli and of the abnormalities observed in diabetic patients with and without autonomic neuropathy (AN).

It is relatively unusual for diabetic patients to complain of gastrointestinal symptoms due to AN; the major clinical syndromes are represented by gastroparesis diabeticorum, diarrhea, constipation and fecal incontinence (3). A larger number of patients recognize some abnormality when questioned specifically, and with the improvement of diagnostic techniques early abnormalities in gastrointestinal function are increasingly found in asymptomatic patients.

## ESOPHAGUS

Prolonged transit time and moderate dilatation of the esophagus has been documented by radiology (4) and delayed emptying of solids by a scintiscanning technique (5) which evaluates the transit time of a solid bolus prepared by adding $^{99m}$Tc macroaggregate albumin to cooking beef.

Manometric techniques show reduced tone of the lower sphincter (6) and a delay of esophageal peristalsis after swallowing, while there is an increase in spontaneous repetitive non-peristaltic contractions. Using this last technique an abnormal esophageal function was observed in diabetic patients with peripheral and autonomic neuropathy (6,7).

## STOMACH

The symptoms of gastric involvement include early satiety, bloating, abdominal pain, nausea and vomiting which may contain food ingested several hours earlier (3). Some patients vomit regularly while others have attacks of nausea for several days followed by vomiting and a transient improvement. In asymptomatic patients the barium meal often shows an increase in fasting residium, gastric dilatation, with reduced peristalsis, delayed emptying and atony of the duodenal bulb (8,9). In all of these patients glycemia is difficult to control and weight loss may occur. In insulin-dependent diabetic (IDD) patients frequent hypoglycemic attacks may occur due to unpredictably delayed absorption of nutrients.

There is a high incidence of gastroparesis in diabetic patients with AN (10), similar to that observed in vagotomized subjects. A vagal involvement in diabetic AN is confirmed by the reduction of gastric acid secretion, both basal and after vagal stimulation, e.g. using the insulin tolerance test (ITT) and sham-feeding (SF) (11,12).

Conventional techniques currently used to study gastric motility include evaluation of gastric electrical activity, or intraluminar pressures or both, recorded with perfused catheters or balloons.

In diabetic patients many electrical dysfunctions are observed. During fasting there is a significant reduction in migrating motor complexes (MMC); this is also observed in diabetic patients without symptoms of gastroparesis (13). There is also an alteration of antral motor activity, which is involved in the emptying of digestible solids.

A sensitive technique for the evaluation of gastric emptying is based on visualization, using a computer-assisted camera, of the radioactivity in the gastric area after a radiolabelled meal (10,14). $^{113}$In-labelled DTPA (diethyltriaminopentaacetic acid) is often used as a marker for the liquid component and $^{99}$Tc sulphur colloid as a marker for the solid component. A delay of solid but not of liquid emptying is commonly observed in diabetic patients (14).

Recently, a simple technique to evaluate gastric emptying after a normal meal without submitting the patients to unnecessary radiation has been developed using the application of real-time ultrasonography. While it is difficult to identify the various portions of the stomach, the gastric antrum is always easily recognizable and measurable, even in the presence of meteorism and obesity. Gastric emptying time is then based on the measurement of antral width before and after an ordinary mixed solid–liquid meal (15,16).

## GALLBLADDER

The high incidence of cholelithiasis in diabetic patients is well known. The cause of this association is not clear; an influence of overweight, dislipidemia, hepatomegaly and other factors is suggested, but none of these seem sufficient to explain the correlation.

Diabetic patients with AN show a higher prevalence of cholelithiasis (17). The same patients also show an enlarged and poorly contracting gallbladder. This could therefore be an important mechanism involved in cholelithiasis.

Real-time ultrasonography is a reproducible and accurate method for the quantitation of gallbladder contraction in humans. This method obviates the need for radiation exposure or intestinal intubation (17,18). The abnormalities in bladder contraction observed radiologically in diabetic patients have been confirmed using this method (Figure 1).

## DIARRHEA

Diarrhea can be one of the most troublesome gastrointestinal complications in diabetes mellitus. It is seen most frequently in young male diabetic patients with a history of poor diabetic control, AN and associated retinal and renal complications.

The diarrhea is characterized by frequent stools, of loose consistency and increased volume. Frequently the diarrhea is intermittent (at least 2–3 days per year), sometimes alternating with constipation; occasionally it may be severe and persistent and associated with nocturnal fecal incontinence (3). Sometimes there is no real diarrhea (the volume of stools is normal) and the frequency of stools may be the

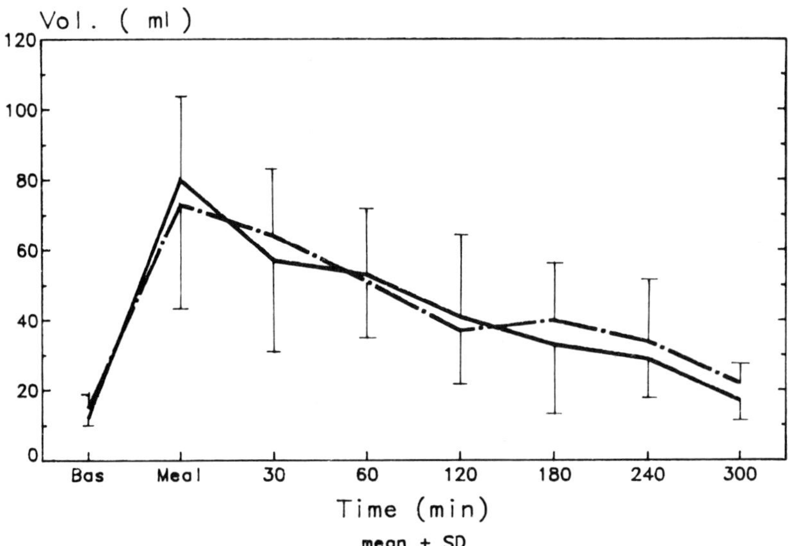


Figure 1. Gastric antrum volume in supine (—) and upright (– · –) positions in normal subjects ($n$ = 10)

expression of an isolated dysfunction of the anal sphincter.

The most popular explanation is that the diarrhea is a manifestation of AN. In fact diarrhea is frequent in patients with truncal vagotomy or sympathectomy and transit time through the small intestine is decreased both in these cases and in neuropathic diabetic patients.

Various abnormalities in the motility of the gut have been found in diabetic patients. The finding in some patients of a composite intestinal motility pattern (characterized by a marked reduction in frequency and amplitude of pressure activity with superimposed uncoordinated bursts), such as can be observed after celiac and mesenteric ganglionectomy (19) in dogs and in patients with postganglionic sympathetic lesions, suggests an involvement of not only cholinergic but also sympathetic gut innervation (13).

Recently a loss of adrenergic innervation in the intestinal mucosa has been shown in chronically diabetic rats, with defective stimulation of $\alpha 2$-receptors on enterocytes, resulting in impaired absorption of fluid and electrolyte from the lumen (20,21).

Other possible mechanisms, such as excessive bacterial growth, as a consequence of gastric and duodenal stasis, or bile salt malabsorption, have been suggested, but no evidence of bacterial overgrowth has been found in some studies and not all diabetic patients with diarrhea have steatorrhea (3).

The diagnosis of diabetic diarrhea at this time is justified only after the exclusion of other causes of diarrhea, such as celiac sprue (by examining jejunal biopsy), pancreatic insufficiency (pancreatic function tests) and bacterial overgrowth of the small intestine (quantitative bacterial culture of intestinal contents and breath analysis after oral administration of [ $^{14}CO_2$ ] xylose). Radiological findings are not specific.

## CONSTIPATION

Constipation is one of the most common, aspecific, gastrointestinal symptoms. It is typically intermittent and may alternate with diarrhea. There is a high prevalence of constipation in diabetic AN: up to 88% of diabetic patients with AN present this symptom (3). Manometric studies show a normal basal spike and motor activity in diabetic patients with constipation; while the response to meals is blunted in those without clinical constipation and absent in those with severe constipation. The response to meals is normalized after the parenteral injection of metoclopramide or neostigmine, suggesting an alteration in the neurohormonal response to the meal (13). With radiological studies it is possible to identify only the more severe abnormalities.

## FECAL INCONTINENCE

Fecal incontinence is a common but often unmentioned problem in diabetes; it is particularly common in diabetic patients with AN and in those with diarrhea. It was suggested that this disorder was caused by an abnormality of rectal afferent sensitive fibres, but recent manometric studies indicate that the cause of this complication is in fact a dysfunction of the internal anal sphincter (3,22).

## GASTROINTESTINAL HORMONES

There is clear evidence that the secretion of the hormones of the gastrointestinal axis, like the activity of the gastrointestinal system in general, is controlled by the autonomic nervous system (23,24) through an extensive network of cholinergic, adrenergic and peptidergic autonomic fibres identified in close proximity to the pancreatic islets (25) and gut endocrine cells. The response of these hormones to different stimuli may be an additional useful tool in the evaluation of the integrity of the autonomic nervous system.

### Motilin

Motilin, a hormone involved in the control of gastrointestinal motility, is mainly under vagal control (26). A marked elevation of basal motilin is observed in diabetic patients with AN. In normal subjects insulin hypoglycemia is followed by a reduction of motilin with a nadir at 20 minutes and a recovery phase reaching basal after 90 minutes. Diabetic patients with AN show a lower nadir and a delayed recovery phase after hypoglycemia, while diabetic patients without AN have a normal response (27,28).

### Somatostatin

Somastostatin modulates the function of many organs, such as gastric and pancreatic secretion etc. It is controlled by vagal and sympathetic innervation, and the influence of peptidergic neurons is also suggested (29).

In normal subjects an increase in somatostatin is observed after ITT and mixed meal. A reduced response of somatostatin to ITT and mixed meal is observed in diabetic patients with AN (30,31).

### Glucagon

Glucagon secretion is under the influence of cholinergic, adrenergic, peptidergic and purinergic nerves (25).

Mixed meal and ITT induce an increase in glucagon levels in normal subjects, whereas diabetic patients with AN have normal basal levels of glucagon with a reduced response after ITT. Non-insulin-dependent diabetic (NIDD) patients with AN have an exaggerated response to meals (32).

The report of a reduced response of glucagon to ITT in IDD (33) and possibly in NIDD patients without AN suggests, besides vagal damage, the presence of other mechanisms, such as an alteration of A-cell receptors to glucose (34,35).

### Gastric Inhibitory Polypeptide (GIP)

GIP seems to play an important role in the enteropancreatic release of insulin. It increases rapidly after a meal, with fat and glucose as major secretagogues (36).

Abnormalities in GIP secretion have been reported in diabetes mellitus. NIDD patients show basal and postprandial values of GIP which are lower compared to normal subjects. When these are divided into two groups with and without AN, it is found that the reduction of GIP response is only present in the group of patients with AN (37).

### Gastrin

Gastrin secretion is regulated by cholinergic and non-cholinergic intramural neurons (38). There is evidence to suggest both $\beta$- and $\alpha$-adrenergic modulation on gastrin secretion.

In normal subjects gastrin increases after ITT and mixed meal. Increased basal levels of gastrin have been reported in diabetic patients (pseudo Zollinger–Ellison Syndrome) (39). In diabetic patients with AN increased basal levels of gastrin coexist with a reduced response to ITT and an increased response to meals (40).

### Pancreatic Polypeptide

Pancreatic polypeptide (PP) is under the almost exclusive control of the vagus

(41,42), with extra vagal cholinergic modulation and a modest stimulatory influence of β-adrenergic fibres.

Protein-rich meal, SF and ITT (43,44) are the most important stimuli on PP secretion.

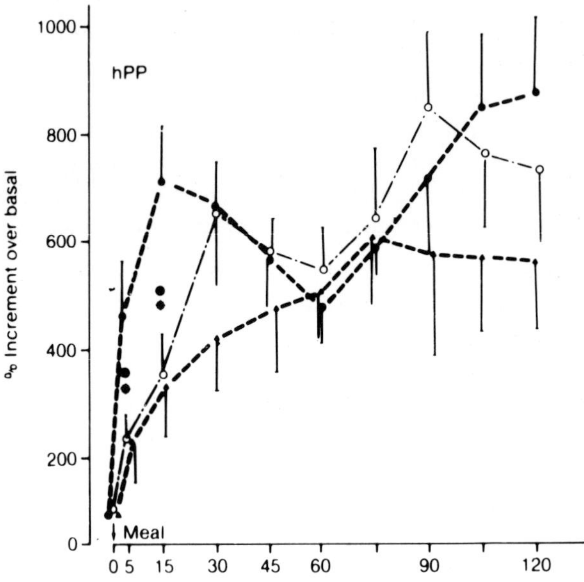


Figure 2. Percentage hPP increment over basal (mean ± SE) after a protein rich meal in 9 normal subjects (N: ●---●), 12 diabetic patients without autonomic neuropathy (WAN: o–·–o) and in 9 diabetic patients with autonomic neuropathy (AN: ▲__ __ __▲). N vs WAN $*p<0.05$; N vs AN $p<0.05$ (49).

Diabetic patients with AN have a markedly reduced response to ITT and to SF compared to normal subjects (12,44–47). In these patients the early 'cephalic' PP response to a protein-rich meal is also significantly reduced compared to normal subjects (47) (Figure 2). Some reduction of the 'cephalic' response (47), and also of the response to ITT, has been observed in diabetic patients without AN (48), indicating that the PP response to these stimuli may be an early indicator of damage to the autonomic nervous system.

The PP response to the above mentioned stimuli is probably the best indicator available of neuropathic involvement of the gastrointestinal parasympathetic fibres.

## TREATMENT

Though work in rats (49) indicates that a regression of lesions of intestinal neuron ganglia induced by experimental diabetes can be obtained by strict metabolic control through pancreas transplantation, at the present time no indication is available for an etiologic treatment of autonomic neuropathy of gastrointestinal tract in humans. Symptomatic treatment is considered below.

### Esophageal Dysfunctions

Symptoms relating to the esophagus are uncommon and are represented by heart burn, retrosternal discomfort and dysphagia. The treatment of esophageal disorders is often unsatisfactory. The drugs of choice are metoclopramide (14) and domperidone (5). After metoclopramide infusion there is an increased contractile activity that does not seem to be correlated with increased esophageal emptying. More recently, domperidone has been used which induces an improvement of symptoms without, however, an objective improvement of solid emptying (5).

### Stomach

Metoclopramide and domperidone represent the drugs of choice also in the treatment of gastroparesis diabeticorum (10,14,50).

Metoclopramide inhibits the CNS chemoreceptor trigger zone for vomiting and stimulates gastrointestinal peristaltic propulsive activity. Symptomatic relief occurs in the majority of patients with the use of either metoclopramide or domperidone, but this improvement is often transient.

### Diarrhea

Treatment of diabetic diarrhea is often unsatisfactory and many therapeutic trials with diet modification and the administration of cholestiramine, metoclopramide and antibiotic agents have all proved disappointing.

The recent report of the loss of adrenergic innervation of enterocytes has suggested treatment with an $\alpha 2$-agonist, clonidine. Preliminary data indicate a reduction in diarrhea (20,21).

### Constipation

Therapy for constipation is usually symptomatic, with administration of laxative, cathartics or enema. An improvement in constipation is observed in patients treated with metoclopramide. Other treatments, such as high fibre diets and ano-rectal myectomy, have not been extensively evaluated in diabetes.

### Fecal Incontinence

The pharmacological therapy for fecal incontinence has not been formally tested. Diphenoxilate with atropine is one of the commonest drugs used; it does not act on anal sphincter pressure, but as an anti-diarrhoic drug.

## REFERENCES

1. Wingate DL (1986) Neurophysiology of the gastrointestinal tract. In: Kern F, Blum BL (eds) The gastroenterology annual, third edition. Elsevier Science Publishers, Amsterdam
2. Wood JD (1984) Enteric neurophysiology. Am J Physiol 247 (Gastrointest Liver Physiol 10): G285
3. Feldman M, Schiller R (1983) Disorder of gastrointestinal motility associated with diabetes mellitus. Ann Intern Med 98: 378–384
4. Forgacs S, Keri L, Osvath J, Fabian I (1979) Oesophageal dysfunction in diabetes mellitus. Acta Diabetol Lat 16: 227–234
5. Maddern GJ, Horowitz M, Janienson GC (1985) The effect of domperidone in oesophageal emptying in diabetic autonomic neuropathy. Br J Clin Pharmacol 19: 441–444
6. Channer KS, Jackson PC, O'Brien et al. (1985) Oesophageal function in diabetes mellitus and its association with autonomic neuropathy. Diabetic Med 2: 378–382
7. Atkinson MJ, Hosking J (1983) Gastrointestinal complications of diabetes mellitus. Clin Gastroenterol 12: 633–650
8. Taub S, Mariani A, Barkin JSD (1979) Gastrointestinal manifestations of diabetes mellitus. Diabetes Care 2: 437–447
9. Zitomer BR, Gramm HF, Zozok GP (1986) Gastric neuropathy in diabetes mellitus: clinical and radiologic observation. Metabolism 17: 199–211
10. Campbell IW, Heading RC, Tothil P, Buist TAS, Ewing DJ, Clarke BF (1977) Gastric emptying in diabetic autonomic neuropathy. Gut 18: 462–467
11. Feldman M, Corbett DB, Ramsey EJ, Walsh JH, Richardson CT (1979) Abnormal gastric function in long standing insulin-dependent diabetic patients. Gastroenterology 77: 12–17
12. Buysschaert M, Donckier J, Dive A, Ketelsleger JM, Lambert AE (1985) Gastric acid and pancreatic polypeptide response to sham-feeding are impaired in diabetic subjects with autonomic neuropathy. Diabetes 34: 1181–1185
13. Camilleri M, Malagelada JR (1984) Abnormal intestinal motility in diabetics with gastroparesis syndrome. Eur J Clin Invest 14: 420–427
14. Loo FD, Palmer DW, Soergel KH, Kalbfleisher JH, Wood CM (1984) Gastric emptying in patients with diabetes mellitus. Gastroenterology 86: 485–491
15. Bolondi L, Bortolotti M, Santi V, Colletti T, Gaiani S, Labò G (1985) Measurement of gastric emptying time by real-time ultrasonography. Gastroenterology 89: 752–759
16. Ricci R, Bontempo A, La Bella A, De Tschudy A, Corazziari E (1987) Ultrasonography is a valuable method to assess the volume of gastric antrum. Gastroenterology (in press)
17. Marumo K, Hayashi M, Fujii S, Seki J, Wada M, Asia H (1981) Gallbladder function in diabetics with ultrasonography. JSUM Proc 38: 383
18. Vogelberg KU, Kubler HGW, Cicmir J, Rathmann W (1984) Gallenblasenkontraktilitat, Cholelithiasis und autonome Neuropathie bei Diabetes Mellitus. Dtsche Med Wochenschr 109: 1712–1715
19. Marlett JA, Code CF (1979) Effect of celiac and superior mesenteric ganglionectomy on interdigestive myoelectric motor complex in dogs. Am J Physiol 237: E432–436
20. Fedorak RN, Field M, Chang EB (1985) Treatment of diabetic diarrhea with clonidine. Ann Intern Med 102: 197–199
21. Chang EB, Fedorak RN, Field M (1986) Experimental diabetic diarrhea in rat. Intestinal mucosal denervation hypersensitivity and treatment with clonidine. Gastroenterology 91: 564–569
22. Schiller RL, Santa Ana CA, Schmulen C, Henedr RS, Harford WV, Fordtram JS (1982)

Pathogenesis of fecal incontinence in diabetes mellitus. Evidence for internal anal-sphinter dysfunction. N Engl J Med 307: 1667–1671

23. Vinik AI, Glowniak JV (1982) Hormonal secretion in diabetic autonomic neuropathy. NY State J Med 82: 871–886
24. Hilsted J, Madsbad S, Krarup T, Sestoft L, Christensen NJ, Tronier B, Galbo H (1981) Hormonal, metabolic, and cardiovascular responses to hypoglycemia in diabetic autonomic neuropathy. Diabetes 30: 626–633
25. Aherén B, Taborsky GJ Jr, Porte D Jr (1986) Neuropeptidergic versus cholinergic and adrenergic regulation of islet hormone secretion. Diabetologia 29: 827–836
26. Mitznegg R, Bloom RS, Christofides N, Besterman H, Domschke W, Wunsch E, Demlin L (1976) Release of motilin in man. Scand J Gastroenterol 11 (Suppl 39): 53–56
27. Funkoshi A, Glowniak J, Owyang C, Vinik AI (1982) Evidence for cholinergic and vagal non-cholinergic mechanism modulating plasma motilin-like immunoreactive. J Clin Endocrinol Metab 54: 1192
28. Achem-Karam SR, Funakoshi A, Vinik AI, Owyang C (1985) Plasma motilin concentration and interdigestive migrating motor complex in diabetic gastroparesis: effect of metoclopramide. Gastroenterology 88: 492–499
29. Glaser B, Vinik AI, Zoghlin G (1981) Truncal vagotomy abolishes the somatostatin response to insulin induced hypoglycemia in man. J Clin Endocrinol Metab 52: 823
30. Lucey MR, Wass JAH, Fairclough P, Webb J, Webb S, Medbak S, Rees LH (1985) Autonomic regulation of post prandial plasma somatostatin, gastrin and insulin. Gut 26: 683–688
31. Creutzfeldt W, Erbert R (1986) The enteroinsular axis. In: Go WL, et al. (eds) The exocrine pancreas: biology, pathobiology, and the disease. Raven Press, New York, pp 333–359
32. Levitt NS, Vinik I, Sive AA, Child P, Jackson WPU (1979) Studies on plasma glucagon concentration in maturity-onset diabetics with autonomic neuropathy. Diabetes 28: 1015–1021
33. Bolli GB, De Feo P, Compagnucci P, Cartechini MG, Angeletti G, Santeusano F, Brunetti P, Gerich JE (1983) Abnormal glucose counterregulation in insulin-dependent diabetes mellitus. Diabetes 32: 134–141
34. Adamson U, Lins PE, Efendic S, Hamberg B, Wajngot A (1984) Impaired counter regulation of hypoglycemia in a group of insulin-dependent diabetics with recurrent episodes of severe hypoglycemia. Acta Med Scand 216: 215–222
35. Bolli GB, Tsalikian E, Haymond MW, Cryer PE, Gerich JE (1984) Defective glucose counterregulation after subcutaneous insulin in non-insulin-dependent diabetes mellitus. J Clin Invest 73: 1532–1541
36. Jorde R, Amlanld PF, Burhol PG (1986) The priming effect of glucose on the gastric inhibitory polypeptide-induced insulin release. Scand J Gastroenterol 21: 47–50
37. Levitt NS, Vinik AI, Child PT (1980) Glucose-dependent insulin-releasing peptide in non-insulin-dependent maturity-onset diabetes: effects of autonomic neuropathy. J Clin Endocrinol Metab 51: 254
38. Schubert ML, Bitar KN, Makhlouf GM (1982) Regulation of gastrin and somatostatin secretion by cholinergic and non cholinergic intramural neurons. Gastroenterology 82: No 5, Part 2: (Abstract)
39. Owyang C, Vinik AI (1982) Diabetic pseudo Zollinger–Ellison syndrome. Gastroenterology No. 5, Part 2: (Abstract) 1144
40. Sasaki H, Nagulesparan M, Dubois A, Straus E, Samloff IM, Lawrence WH, Johnson GC, Siviers ML, Unger RH (1983) Hypergastrinemia in obese non-insulin-dependent diabetes: a possible reflection of high prevalence of vagal dysfunction. J Clin Endocrinol Metab 56: 744

41. Schwartz TW, Holst JJ, Fahrenkrug J, Lindkaer JS, Nielsen O, Rehfeld JF, Schaffalitzky de Muckadell OB, Stadil F (1978) Vagal cholinergic regulation of pancreatic polypeptide secretion. J Clin Invest 61: 781
42. Floyd JC, Fajans SS, Pek S, Chance RE (1977) A newly recognized pancreatic polypeptide: plasma levels in health and disease. Rec Prog Horm Res 33: 519
43. Schwartz TW, Rehfeld JF, Stadil F, Larsson LI, Moon N, Chance RE (1976) Pancreatic polypeptide response to food in duodenal ulcer patients before and after truncal vagotomy. Lancet i: 1102
44. Taylor IL, Feldman M, Richardson CT, Walsh JH (1978) Gastric and cephalic stimulation of human pancreatic polypeptide release. Gastroenterology 75: 432
45. Schwartz TW, Stendquist B, Olbe L (1978) Physiology of mammalian PP and the importance of vagal regulation. In: Bloom SR (ed) Gut hormones. Churchill Livingstone, Edinburgh, p 261
46. Levitt MS, Vinik AI, Sive AA, Van Tonders, Lund A (1980) Impaired pancreatic polypeptide response to insulin-induced hypoglycemia in diabetic autonomic neuropathy. J Clin Endocrinol Metab 50: 445
47. Gambardella S, Felici MG, Annibale B, Delle Fave GF, Jacoangeli F, Spallone V, Menzinger G (1986) Pancreatic polypeptide response to a protein-rich meal in diabetic patients with and without autonomic neuropathy. J Endocrinol Invest 9: 1
48. Histed J, Madsbad S, Kraruo T, Tronier B, Galbo H, Sestoft L, Schwartz TW (1982) No response of pancreatic hormones to hypoglycemia in diabetic autonomic neuropathy. J Clin Endocrinol Metab 54: 815
49. Schmidt RE, Plurad BS, Olack BJ, Scharp DW (1983) The effect of pancreatic islet transplantation and insulin therapy on experimental diabetic autonomic neuropathy. Diabetes 32: 532–540
50. Snape WJ, Bottle WM, Schwartz SS, et al. (1982) Metoclopramide to treat gastroparesis due to diabetes mellitus. A double blind controlled trial. Ann Intern Med 96: 444–446

Diabetic Complications: Early Diagnosis and Treatment
Edited by D. Andreani, G. Crepaldi, U. Di Mario and G. Pozza


CHAPTER 19

# *Treatment of Diabetic Somatic Neuropathies*

G. CREPALDI and D. FEDELE*
*Department of Internal Medicine, University of Padua; *Department of Endocrinology, University of Palermo, Italy*

Until a few years ago the treatment of neurological impairment in diabetic patients was a very difficult problem for both neurologists and diabetologists. Moreover, little was known about the factors involved in its etiopathogenesis and there was a lack of efficacious drugs to relieve the signs and symptoms of diabetic neuropathy. For this reason, in 1983 an editorial in *The Lancet* questioned if anything could be done for patients with diabetic neuropathy, or whether, after having diagnosed the complication, patients could only be commiserated with (1).

Fortunately over the past years the growing body of data relating to this very frequent late complication of diabetes has allowed a better understanding of its pathogenesis and, in particular, an improved and more proficient management of the neurological signs and symptoms.

Recently the role of hyperglycemia in diabetic neuropathy has been very clearly demonstrated (2). It has been highlighted as the most important etiological factor in the development of diabetic peripheral polyneuropathies. The latter conditions can in fact be classified as prevalently metabolic neuropathies, whereas mononeuropathies can be considered prevalently vascular neuropathies owing to the relevance of atherosclerosis and microangiopathy in their pathogenesis (3,4).

Experimental data have confirmed that the high plasma glucose levels in diabetic subjects can cause neural damage which both increases polyol pathway activity with nerve accumulation of sorbitol and fructose (5), and enhances the non-enzymatic glycosylation of nerve proteins (6,7).

Increased activity of the polyol pathway decreases the active concentration or synthesis of myoinositol in the nerve and negatively influences the $Na^+-K^+$-ATPase activity (2,8). The first causes impairment in nerve conduction velocity, followed by structural nerve damage (2).

Neural damage can be caused by the hyperglycosylation of both myelin and tubulin in the nerve. In 1986 Brownlee et al. (7), in the context of demonstrating the presence of advanced glycosylation end-products in the nerve, showed excessive trapping of immunoglobulins from myelin in the diabetic peripheral nerve, but not from myelin in the central nervous system. This difference has been related to the blood–brain barrier which prevents the passage of significant amounts of immunoglobulins from the plasma into the cerebrospinal fluid. Moreover, these data could explain the rare occurrence of symptoms of central neuropathy in diabetic subjects.

The relevance of metabolic factors in the pathogenesis of diabetic neuropathies justifies the importance of the improvement of metabolic control in the management of these diabetic complications.

In addition to new data on the pathogenesis of diabetic neuropathy, several controlled trials have recently shown the efficacy of some drugs in the treatment of diabetic neuropathy with an improvement of both signs and symptoms. The very promising results related to the use of these drugs, in particular tricyclics for pain and aldose reductase inhibitors and gangliosides for clinical signs, encourage us to be more optimistic regarding the future treatment of diabetic subjects affected by neuropathy.

## TREATMENT OF PAIN IN DIABETIC NEUROPATHY

In the treatment of diabetic neuropathy the physician must take into consideration the management of the symptoms, in particular of pain which in some cases can be severe causing acute suffering to the patient, and the treatment specifically addressed to the presumed cause of the disease.

Pain is a feature of both diabetic mononeuropathies and peripheral polyneuropathy. Pain starts suddenly in mononeuropathy and is often acute and asymmetrical; it spontaneously disappears after some weeks or months. On the other hand, pain in peripheral polyneuropathy starts insidiously, is often symmetrical, and can persist over many years, even if with a variable intensity.

Table 1 shows the measures and drugs reported to be efficacious in the treatment of pain in diabetic neuropathy.

### Blood Glucose Control

The improvement of metabolic control with the achievement of near normal daily blood glucose profiles is the first and most important step in control of diabetic patients with painful neuropathy. Insulin treatment may be indicated in non-insulin-dependent subjects, particularly if diet and oral hypoglycemic agents are inadequate to obtain the required normalization of blood glucose and glycosylated hemoglobin values. The relief of the painful symptoms is generally obtained after some weeks of good, stable metabolic control (9). Continuous subcutaneous insulin infusion (CSII) with micropumps can be very useful in some cases in which normal glucose values can not be obtained with conventional therapy. Recent data show that the

Table 1. Measures and drugs reported to be effective in the treatment of pain in diabetic neuropathy

—Blood glucose control
—Drug therapy
  (a) Simple analgesics: aspirin, paracetamol, etc.
  (b) Anticonvulsants: carbamazepine, phenytoin
  (c) Tricyclic antidepressants: imipramine, amitriptyline
  (d) Antidepressants: mianserin, trazodone
  (e) Phenothiazines: fluphenazine, chlorpromazine
  (f) Benzodiazepines: diazepam, clonazepam
  (g) Other drugs: amphetamines, lidocaine
  (h) Aldose reductase inhibitors
  (i) Gangliosides
—Dietary myoinositol intake
—Other measures
  (a) Careful exercise programmes
  (b) Transcutaneous nerve stimulation

improvement of metabolic control with CSII is effective in the management of pain in diabetic patients affected by painful neuropathy (10,11). These results confirm the observation that blood glucose levels can influence pain threshold and tolerance. In fact Morley et al. (12) showed a lower pain threshold and tolerance in diabetic patients compared to control subjects and hyperalgesia in normal subjects after glucose infusion. Moreover, the high blood glucose levels reduce the antinociceptive effect of morphine in animals (13). All these findings suggest that, as in animals, glucose could modulate opioid receptors in humans.

Indeed it was recently reported that 'whether or not these new observations are relevant to the routine management of painful neuropathy, any diabetic patient with symptomatic neuropathy should be offered the best blood glucose control that is achieveable' (14).

## Drug Therapy

Many drugs have been reported to induce some improvement in the painful symptoms of diabetic patients, but very few have had positive experimental reports with consistent double-blind trials. Simple analgesics such as aspirin (15), paracetamol and some non-steroidal anti-inflammatory drugs are generally reported to induce some benefit. Other more potent analgesics should be avoided in consideration of the long duration of the symptoms and the possible risk of addiction.

Data regarding the use of anticonvulsants, such as phenytoin (16–18) and carbamazepine (19,20) are contradictory and unsatisfactory.

The results obtained with tricyclic antidepressants alone, such as imipramine, amitriptyline and mianserin (21,22), or better still in combination with phenothiazines such as fluphenazine and chlorpromazine, seem to be more effective

(23,24). Recently Young and Clarke (25) studied 80 consecutive untreated patients with painful neuropathies inducing the relief of symptoms with simple analgesics in 9 cases, with imipramine in 43 (50–150 mg at night), with amitriptyline in 9 (50–150 mg), with mianserin in 6 (30–90 mg at night), and with fluphenazine (1–6 mg/day) or chlorpromazine (50–100 mg/day) in 8 patients. Pain was relieved with clonazepam (0.5–3 mg/day) in 2 patients, whereas pharmacotherapy had no effect on 3 subjects. The combination of amitriptyline (50–100 mg at night) with fluphenazine (1–5 mg/day) or chlorpromazine (50–100 mg daily) can be used in those patients who are unresponsive to antidepressants alone (23,25). Antidepressants and phenothiazines must be started cautiously at low doses and increased slowly. Side-effects, such as a dry mouth and exacerbation of autonomic symptoms, were reported after the administration of tricyclic antidepressants (25).

The mode of action of tricyclic antidepressants is still controversial, but they probably act both by improving the coexisting depression and by inhibiting serotonin uptake, thus blocking the serotonergic part of the central pain pathway (26). In fact a non-tricyclic antidepressant such as trazodone seems also to be effective on the symptoms of diabetic neuropathy, and this is probably related to the inhibition of serotonin (27). Recently Mendel et al. (28) reported a double-blind placebo-controlled trial in 6 diabetic patients treated with amitriptyline (75 mg orally at bedtime) and fluphenazine (1 mg three times daily) for 2 weeks. The pain relief observed was no greater than that obtained with placebo.

Drugs such as amphetamine (29) and lidocaine (30) have also been reported for pain relief in diabetic neuropathy but these findings have not been confirmed to date.

Both aldose reductase inhibitors (31,32) and gangliosides (33,34) have recently been shown to be effective in decreasing pain and symptoms in diabetic patients. Lastly, dietary supplement of myoinositol has also been reported to relieve pain and temperature perception in insulin-dependent diabetic subjects (35).

Other measures, such as cooling the feet (36), careful exercise programmes (37) and transcutaneous nerve stimulation (38), have been proposed but must still be experimentally demonstrated.

Table 2. Measures reported to be effective in the treatment of diabetic neuropathy

—Blood glucose control
—Aldose reductase inhibitors: alrestatin, sorbinil, Tolrestat, Statil
—Gangliosides
—Neurotrophic vitamins
—Dietary myoinositol intake
—Isaxonine

## SPECIFIC TREATMENT IN DIABETIC SOMATIC NEUROPATHY

The treatment specifically addressed to the supposed etiopathogenetic causes of diabetic neuropathy supported to date by experimental data consists in the near normalization of blood glucose levels and in the use of some drugs, such as aldose reductase inhibitors and brain gangliosides.

No documentation exists regarding the efficacy of neurotrophic vitamins in diabetic neuropathy, whereas clincial trials in humans have not confirmed data on the efficacy of dietary myoinositol supplementation in diabetic neuropathy (Table 2).

## Blood Glucose Control

The important role played by elevated blood glucose levels in the development of diabetic neuropathy can largely justify the attempts made to achieve optimum metabolic control in order to prevent or improve this very disabling complication of diabetes. Many uncontrolled (11,35,39–41) and controlled clinical trials (42,43) in the past years have supported, albeit with conflicting results (44), the efficacy of the near normalization of blood glucose levels in improving both symptoms and signs of diabetic peripheral neuropathy. Recently our results have shown that in insulin-dependent diabetic subjects with neuropathy CSII induced an improvement not only in the nerve motor conduction velocity but also in the cardiovascular responses to deep breathing, Valsalva manoeuvre and change of posture from lying to standing (41).

The data obtained from long-term clinical trials confirm the results reported by some authors after the start of insulin therapy in newly diagnosed diabetic subjects (45) or after the short-term normalization of blood glucose levels using an artificial pancreas (46,47).

## Aldose Reductase Inhibitors

The increased polyol pathway activity related to the higher blood glucose levels has been shown to induce an accumulation of sorbitol and fructose in tissues of non-insulin-dependent diabetics, with aldose reductase and sorbitol dehydrogenase enzymatic activities (5). The accumulation of these metabolic products of glucose has been related to the late complications of diabetes mellitus (5,48) and in particular to the development of ocular (49) and neurological complications. However, it has been postulated that inhibition of the aldose reductase activity blocking the accumulation of sorbitol in nerve could induce an improvement of neuropathy in diabetic subjects.

Alrestatin (AY-20,263) was the first aldose reductase inhibitor administered to patients with severe diabetic neuropathy. The results were negative in that there was no improvement in the objective evaluation (50,51) and, in particular, side-effects such as nausea and photosensitive skin rash occurred (51).

The aldose reductase inhibitor sorbitol has been studied extensively in vivo over the past few years. A few positive results on some symptoms of diabetic neuropathy have been reported by some authors (31,52,53), whereas the lack of a significant improvement was underlined by other studies (32,54). However, clinical trials have

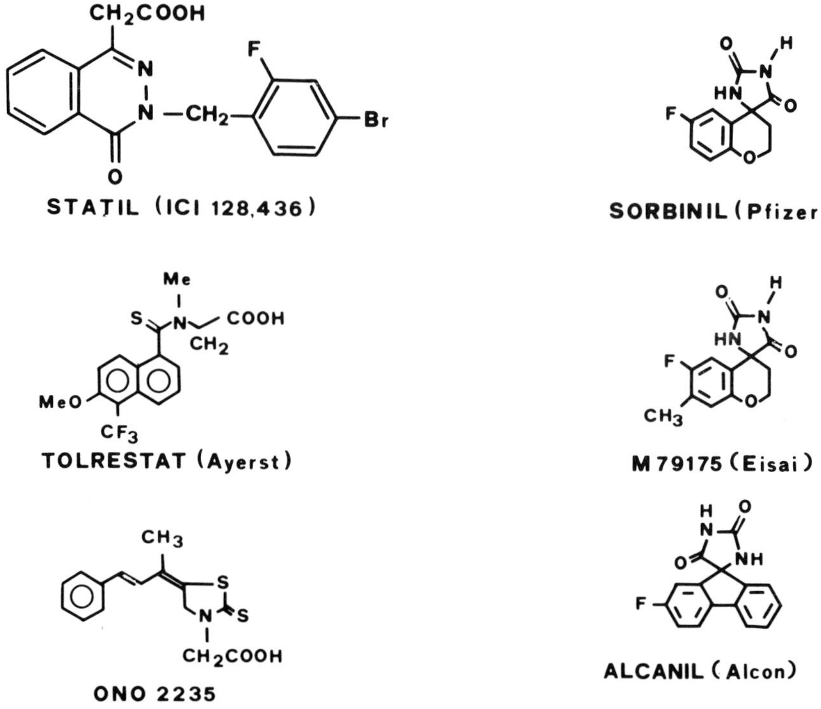

STATIL (ICI 128,436)

SORBINIL (Pfizer

TOLRESTAT (Ayerst)

M 79175 (Eisai)

ONO 2235

ALCANIL (Alcon)

Figure 1. The structure of some aldose reductase inhibitors.

documented the high incidence of side-effects and in some cases the appearance of Stevens–Johnson syndrome during treatment with sorbinil. Recently other aldose reductase inhibitors have become available for clinical experimentation (Figure 1). Tolrestat (55), Statil (56,57) and Ono 2235 (58) have been shown to be effective in animals in inhibiting aldose reducatase activity and improving eye and nerve damage. For this reason clinical trials are being carried out in the USA and European countries with Tolrestat (Ayerst) and Statil (ICI). If these drugs are demonstrated to have a better tolerability in vivo than alrestatin and sorbinil it is quite likely that in the near future there will be drugs available to treat diabetic neuropathy effectively. However, the question still remains whether or not the long-term inhibition of aldose reductase activity in the whole body can take place without causing side-effects in patients, in particular with regard to fructose-related functions such as reproduction. Fructose is of course very important in conditioning sperm motility (59).

## Gangliosides

Gangliosides are a class of glycosphingolipids that are normally present at neuronal membrane level where they play a very important role in neurotransmitter receptor

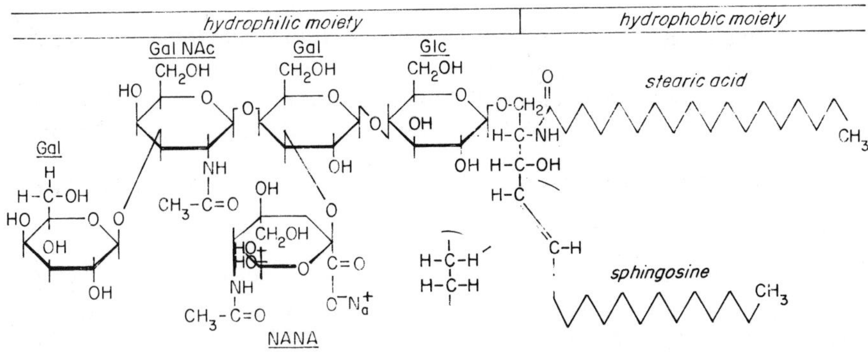


Figure 2. The structure of ganglioside $GM_i$. Glc = glucose, Gal = galactose, GalNAc = *N*-acetylgalactosamine, NANA = *N*-acetylneuraminic acid.

function. The ganglioside molecule is amphiphilic, i.e. it possesses both hydrophilic and hydrophobic parts (Figure 2), the structure being very important for its ultrastructural localization (60,61). Many experimental findings have shown that, after the administration of exogenous gangliosides, because of their high affinity to neuronal membranes they become stably inserted at the level of the neuronal membrane, causing important biophysical-functional modifications of the membrane properties. Data from animals in fact suggest that brain gangliosides enhance axonal sprouting, inducing rapid and correct reinnervation and a prompt functional recovery at the peripheral nerve and activating ($Na^+-K^+$)-ATPase with subsequent normalization of the ion pump and improvement in the nerve conduction velocity (62–65). These promising results have favoured the testing of gangliosides in the treatment of peripheral neuropathies including diabetic neuropathy with some positive results (60,61). After preliminary findings in uncontrolled, open studies (66,67), we performed a multicentre, double-blind controlled versus placebo study in 140 diabetic subjects with peripheral neuropathy (97 subjects with no or mild symptoms and 43 patients with frequent and severe symptoms). All subjects had an impairment of nerve conduction velocity in at least two of the four nerves evaluated (33,68,69). The results showed no change in metabolic parameters, but a significant improvement of symptoms and of some electrophysiological parameters, as well as a 'ganglioside preference' compared with placebo. The treatment period lasted 6 weeks with an intermediate wash-out period of 4 weeks, and consisted of daily intramuscular administration of 20 mg of gangliosides or of placebo. No side-effects were recorded during the trial.

Recently other controlled trials have confirmed these results, showing the positive effect of gangliosides (Cronassial, (Fidia) 20–40 mg daily) both on symptoms and on the objective signs and electrophysiological parameters of diabetic peripheral neuropathy (34,70–72). A multicentre randomized WHO study performed in four different countries (Italy, Portugal, China and Senegal) with 162 patients, using a daily dose of 40 mg of gangliosides for 16 weeks, gave further confirmation of the positive, even if sometimes small, effect of gangliosides in diabetic neuropathy.

To date more than two hundred million doses of gangliosides have been administered in 8 years to humans in many countries of the world and no side-effects have been recorded (60).

### Dietary Myoinositol Intake

The supposed role of the decrease in nerve myoinositol content in the pathogenesis of peripheral diabetic neuropathy (2,3) and positive experimental data in animals obtained after dietary myoinositol supplementation (33,73) were the basis for the proposal that this treatment could also be useful in humans. However, all human therapeutic trials with myoinositol have so far yielded largely negative results (33,74–77).

### Neurotrophic Vitamins

The 'antineuritic' vitamins—thiamine, pyridoxine and vitamin $B_{12}$—have been used in diabetics with peripheral neuropathy in the supposition that they might be useful, as in alcoholic and nutritional neuropathies. But a deficit of these vitamins has never been found in diabetic subjects. The supposed high blood levels of pyruvate, related to thiamine deficiency, were not confirmed and in particular were not correlated with neuropathy (78). After preliminary data showing some positive effects of pyridoxine in 10 diabetic subjects with neuropathy (79), a double-blind, placebo-controlled study in 18 subjects treated with 50 mg of pyridoxine three times a day for 4 months showed no differences in the results obtained after vitamin $B_6$ treatment compared to placebo (80). Moreover, it is useful to recall that high doses of pyridoxine can cause sensory neuropathy (81). Vitamin $B_{12}$ was also demonstrated to be ineffective in diabetic peripheral neuropathy (82). In conclusion, there are no experimental data to justify treatment of diabetic peripheral neuropathy with neurotrophic vitamins.

### Isaxonine

Experimental data in animals have demonstrated that isaxonine (*N*-isopropylamino-2-pyrimidine phosphate) accelerated nerve regeneration probably by stimulation of axonal sprouting (83) and therefore could be effective in the treatment of peripheral neuropathy. However, clinical trials have shown significant hepatic toxicity, with hepatitis in 28 of 100 000 patients (84) and this has led to the withdrawal of the drug from clinical studies.

## CONCLUSIONS

Increased knowledge regarding the etiopathogenetic factors of diabetic neuropathy and the availability of several drugs and of better metabolic control have permitted further developments in the treatment of peripheral neuropathies in diabetic subjects. The discordance and the frequently small evidence of findings obtained by the various clinical trials using all these drugs are probably related to the fact that the patients with clinical neuropathy recruited for these studies are generally subjects with a long duration of diabetes who therefore have irreversible tissue changes due to the accumulation of advanced glycosylation end-products (86). In fact peripheral neuropathy, like other late diabetic complications, is characterized by early functional reversible and late structural irreversible damage (87). It is likely that the various measures performed in the treatment of chronic diabetic neuropathy of long duration could induce only slight positive results related to the improvement of functional, but not structural, damage. For this reason only early preventive treatment in the preliminary stages of the disease could give better results. Today the efficacious prevention of neurological complications in diabetes can be obtained through the early and stable near normalization of blood glucose and glycosylated protein levels and eventually through the preventive administration of those drugs that are effective at nerve level.

## REFERENCES


1. Editorial (1983) Diabetic neuropathy. Where are we now? Lancet i: 1366–1367
2. Greene DA, Lattimer S, Ulbrecht J, Carroll P (1985) Glucose-induced alterations in nerve metabolism: current perspective on the pathogenesis of diabetic neuropathy and future directions for research and therapy. Diabetes Care 8: 290–299
3. Clements RS Jr (1979) Dabetic neuropathy—new concepts in its etiology. Diabetologia 28: 604–611
4. Johnson PC, Doll SC, Cromey DW (1986) Pathogenesis of diabetic neuropathy. Ann Neurol 19: 450–457
5. Gabbay KH (1973) The sorbitol pathway and the complications of diabetes. N Engl J Med 288: 831–836
6. Vlassara H, Brownless M, Cerami A (1981) Non-enzymatic glycosylation of peripheral nerve protein in diabetes mellitus. Proc Natl Acad Sci USA 78: 5190–5192
7. Brownlee M, Vlassara H, Cerami A (1986) Trapped immunoglobulins on peripheral nerve myelin from patients with diabetes mellitus. Diabetes 35: 999–1003
8. Winegrad AI, Simmons DA, Martin DB (1983) Has one diabetic complication been explained? (Editorial). N Engl J Med 308: 152–154
9. Boulton AJM, Ward JD (1986) Diabetic neuropathies and pain. Clin Endocrinol Metab 15: 917–931
10. White NH, Waltman SR, Krupin T Santiago JH (1981) Reversal of neuropathic and gastrointestinal complications related to diabetes mellitus in adolescents with improved metabolic control. J Pediatr 99: 41–45
11. Boulton AJM, Drury J, Clarke, Ward JD (1982) Continuous subcutaneous insulin infusion in the management of painful diabetic neuropathy. Diabetes Care 5: 386–390
12. Morley GK, Mooradian AD, Levine AL, Morley JE (1984) Mechanisms of pain in diabetic peripheral neuropathy: effect of glucose on pain perception in humans. Am J Med 77: 79–82
13. Simon GS, Dewey WL (1981) Narcotics and diabetes. I: The effect of streptozotocin-induced diabetes on the antinoceptive potency of morphine. J Pharmacol Exp Ther 218: 318–321

14. Editorial (1985) Pain perception in diabetic neuropathy. Lancet i: 83–84
15. Ward JD, Armstrong WD, Preston FE, et al. (1981) Pain in the diabetic leg: a trial of aspirin and dipyridamole in diabetic neuropathy. Pharmacotherapeutica 2: 642–647
16. Ellenberg M (1968) Treatment of diabetic neuropathy with diphenylhydantoin. NY State J Med 68: 2653–2655
17. Saudek CD, Werns S, Reidenberg MM (1977) Phenytoin in the treatment of diabetic symmetrical polyneuropathy. Clin Pharmacol Ther 22: 196–199
18. Chadda VS, Mathur MS (1978) Double-blind study on the effects of diphenylhydantoin sodium on diabetic neuropathy. J Assoc Phys India 26: 403–406
19. Rull JA, Quibrera R, Gonzales-Millan H, Lozano-Castenada O (1969) Symptomatic treatment of peripheral diabetic neuropathy with carbamazepine: double-blind cross-over study. Diabetologia 5: 215–218
20. Chakrabarti AK, Samantaray SK (1976) Diabetic peripheral neuropathy: nerve conduction studies before and after carbamazepine therapy. Aust NZ J Med 6: 565–568
21. Turkington RW (1980) Depression masquerading as diabetic neuropathy. J Am Med Assoc 243: 1147–1150
22. Kwinesdal B, Malin J, Froland A, Gram LF (1984) Imipramine treatment of painful diabetic neuropathy. J Am Med Asoc 251: 1727–1730
23. Davis JL, Lewis SB, Gerich JE, Kaplan RA, Shultz TA, Wallin JD (1977) Peripheral neuropathy treated with amitriptyline and fluphenazine. JAMA 238: 2291–2292
24. Battla H and Siverblatt CW (1981) Clinical trial of amitriptyline and fluphenazine in diabetic peripheral neuropathy. South Med J 74: 417–418
25. Young RJ, Clarke BF (1985) Pain relief in diabetic neuropathy: the effectiveness of imipramine and related drugs. Diabetic Med 2: 363–366
26. Botney M, Fields HL (1983) Amitriptyline potentiates morphine analgesia by a direct action on the central nervous system. Ann Neurol 13: 160–164
27. Khurana RC (1983) Treatment of painful diabetic neuropathy with trazodone. J Am Med Assoc 250: 1392
28. Mendel CM, Klein RF, Chappel DA, et al. (1986) A trial of amitriptyline and fluphenazine in the treatment of painful diabetic neuropathy. J Am Med Assoc 255: 637–639
29. Masor N (1971) New usage for an old drug in diabetic neuropathy: value of amphetamines for symptomatic relieve. J Natl Med Assoc 63: 380–383
30. Kastrup J, Angel HR, Peterson P, Dejgard A, Hilsted J (1986) Treatment of chronic painful diabetic neuropathy with intravenous lidocaine infusion. Med J 292: 173
31. Jaspan J, Herold K, Maselli R, Bartkus C (1983) Treatment of severely painful diabetic neuropathy with an aldose reductase inhibitor: relief of pain and improved somatic and autonomic nerve function. Lancet ii: 758–762
32. Young RJ, Ewing DJ, Clarke BF (1983) A controlled trial of sorbinil, an aldose reductase inhibitor, in chronic painful diabetic neuropathy. Diabetes 32: 938–942
33. Crepaldi G, Fedele D, Tiengo A, et al. (1983) Ganglioside treatment in diabetic peripheral neuropathy: a multicenter trial. Acta Diabetol Lat 20: 265–276
34. Naarden A, Davidson J, Harris L, Moore J, De Felice S (1984) Treatment of painful diabetic polyneuropathy with mixed gangliosides. Adv Exp Med Biol 174: 581–592
35. Greene DA, Brown MD, Braunstein SN, Schwartz SS, Asbury AK, Winegrad I (1981) Comparison of clinical course and sequential electrophysiological tests in diabetes with symptomatic polyneuropathy and its implications for clinical trials. Diabetes 30: 139–143
36. Watkins PJ (1984) Pain and diabetic neuropathy. Lancet i: 168–169
37. Herbison GJ, Jaweed MM, Ditunno JF Jr (1983) Exercise therapies in peripheral neuropathies. Arch Phys Med Rehabil 64: 201–205
38. Campbell JN, Long DM (1976) Peripheral nerve stimulation in the treatment of

intractable pain. J Neurosurg 45: 692–699
39. Pietri A, Evile A, Raskin P (1980) Changes in nerve conduction velocity after six weeks of glucoregulation with portable insulin infusion pump. Diabetes 29: 668–671
40. Tolaymat A, Roque JL, Russo LS (1982) Improvement of diabetic peripheral neuropathy with the portable insulin infusion pump. South Med J 75: 185–188
41. Fedele D, Negrin P, Cardone C, et al. (1984) Influence of continuous subcutaneous insulin-infusion (CSII) treatment on diabetic somatic and autonomic neuropathy. J Endocrinol Invest 7: 623–628
42. Holman RR, White VM, Orde-Peckar C, et al. (1983) Prevention of deterioration of renal and sensory-nerve function by more intensive management of insulin-dependent diabetic patients. A two randomized prospective study. Lancet i: 204–208
43. Service FJ, Rizza RA, Doube JR, O'Brien PC, Dyck PJ (1985) Near normoglycaemia improved nerve conduction and vibration sensation in diabetic neuropathy. Diabetologia 28: 722–727
44. Service FJ, Doube JR, O'Brien PC, et al. (1983) Effect of blood glucose control on peripheral nerve function in diabetic patients. Mayo Clin Proc 58: 283–289
45. Ward JD, Fisher DJ, Barnes CG, Jessop JD (1971) Improvement in nerve conduction following treatment in newly diagnosed diabetics. Lancet i: 428–430
46. Golden M, Nudleman K, Myers G, Charles A (1980) Improvement in peripheral nerve function in diabetes after short-term treatment with an artificial pancreas. Diabetes 29: 58
47. Troni W, Carta Q, Cantello R, Caselle MT, Rainero I (1984) Peripheral nerve function and metabolic control in diabetes mellitus. Ann Neurol 16: 178–183
48. Kinoshita JH, Kador PF, Robison G, (1984) NIH conference: aldose reductase and complications of diabetes. Ann Intern Med 101: 82–84
49. Kinoshita JH, Fukushi S, Kador P, Merola LO (1979) Aldose-reductase in diabetic complications of the eye. Metabolism 28 (Suppl.): 462–464
50. Gabbay KH, Spack N, Loo S, Hirsch HJ, Ackil A (1979) Aldose reductase inhibition: studies with Alrestatin. Metabolism 28 (Suppl) 471–476
51. Haldelsman DJ, Turtle JR (1981) Clinical trial of on aldose reductase inhibitor in diabetic neuropathy. Diabetes 30: 459–464
52. Judzewitsch RG, et al. (1983) Aldose reductase inhibition improves nerve conduction velocity in diabetic patients. N Engl J Med 308: 119–125
53. Fagius J, Brattberg A, Jameson S, Berne C (1985) Limited benefit of treatment of diabetic polyneuropathy with an aldose reductase inhibitor: 1 24 week controlled trial. Diabetologia 28: 323–329
54. Lewin IG, O'Brien IAD, Morgan MH, Corrall RJM (1984) Clinical and neurophysiological studies with the aldose reductase inhibitor, sorbinil, in symptomatic diabetic neuropathy. Diabetologia 26: 445–448
55. Koglin L, Kincald J, et al. (1986) The aldose reductase inhibitor Tolrestat increases peripheral nerve conduction velocities and decreases neuropathic pain in patients with symptomatic, peripheral diabetic neuropathy. Diabetes 35 (Suppl 1): 118A
56. Tomlinson DR, Townsend J, Fretten P (1985) Prevention of defective axonal transport in streptozotocin-diabetic rats by treatment with Statil (ICI 128436), an aldose reductase inhibitor. Diabetes 34: 970–972
57. Stribling D, Mirrless DJ, Harrison HE, Earl DCN (1985) Properties of ICI 128436 a novel aldose reductase inhibitor, and its effects on diabetic complications in the rat. Metabolism 34: 336–344
58. Goto Y, et al. (1985) Clinical study of a new aldose reductase inhibitor (ONO 2235) in diabetic neuropathy. J Jpn Diabet Soc 28: 89–99
59. Kozak GP (1982) Diabetic neuropathies. In: Kozak GP (ed) Clinical diabetes mellitus.

WB Saunders, Philadelphia, pp 288–301
60. Samson JC (1986) Gangliosides (Cronassial) as therapeutic agents in peripheral neuropathies. Drugs Today 22: 73–107
61. Leeden RW, Yu RK, Rapport MM, Suzuki K (eds) (1984) Ganglioside structure, function, and biochemical potential. Adv Exp Med Biol 174: 1–649
62. Gorio A, Carmignoto G, Facci L, Finesso M (1980) Motor nerve sprouting induced by ganglioside treatment. Possible implications for gangliosides on neuronal growth. Brain Res 197: 236–241
63. Leon A, Facci L, Toffano G, Sonnino S, Tettamanti G (1981) Activation of $(Na^{+}K^{+})$ATPase by nanomolar concentrations of $GM_1$ ganglioside. J Neurochem 37: 350–357
64. Norido F, Cannella R, Gorio A (1982) Ganglioside treatment of neuropathy in diabetic mice. Muscle Nerve 5: 107–110
65. Gorio A, Marini P, Zanoni R (1983) Muscle reinnervation. III. Motoneuron sprouting capacity, enhancement by exogenous gangliosides. Neuroscience 8: 417–419
66. Pozza G, Saibene V, Comi G, Canal N (1981) The effect of gangliosides administration in human diabetic peripheral neuropathies. In: Rapport MM, Gorio A (eds) Gangliosides in neurological and neuromuscular function, development and repair. Raven Press, New York, pp 253–258
67. Montenero P, Marozzi G, Chiaromonte F (1983) Possibilità di impiego dei gangliosidi cerebrali nel trattamento della neuropatia diabetica periferica. Clin Ter 106: 169–174
68. Fedele D, Crepaldi G, Battistin L (1984) Multicentre trial on gangliosides in diabetic peripheral neuropathy. Adv Exp Med Biol 174: 601–606
69. Fedele D, Crepaldi G (1986) Glucose-induced alterations in nerve metabolism: a reply. Diabetes Care 9: 313
70. Horowitz SM (1984) Gangliosides (Cronassial) therapy in diabetic neuropathy. Adv Exp Med Biol 174: 593–600
71. Abraham RR, Abraham RM, Wynn V (1984) A double blind placebo controlled trial of mixed gangliosides in diabetic peripheral and autonomic neuropathy. Adv Exp Med Biol 174: 607–624
72. WHO Scientific activities WHO-OMS. (1985) Bull 63: 655–656
73. Green DA, De Jesus PV, Winegrad AI (1975) Effects of insulin and dietary myoinositol on impaired peripheral motor nerve conduction velocity in acute streptozoctocin diabetes. J Clin Invest 55: 1326–1336
74. Salway JG, Finnegan JA, Barnett D, et al. (1978) Effect of myoinositol on peripheral-nerve function in diabetes. Lancet ii: 1282–1285
75. Gregersen G, Borsting H, Theil P, Servo C (1978) Myoinositol and function of peripheral nerves in human diabetics. A controlled clinical trial. Acta Neurol 58: 241–246
76. Clements RR, Vourganti B, Kuba T, Oh SJ, Darnell B (1979) Dietary myoinositol intake and peripheral nerve function in diabetic neuropathy. Metabolism 28 (Suppl): 477–481
77. Gregersen G, Bertelsen B, et al. (1983) Oral supplementation of myo-inositol: effects on peripheral nerve function in human diabetics and on the concentration in plasma, erythrocytes, urine, and muscle tissue in human diabetic and normals. Acta Neurol Scand 67: 164–171
78. Thompson RHS (1965) Biochemical aspects of diabetic neuropathy. In: Cuming JN, Kremer M (eds) Biochemical aspects of neurological disorders, second series. Blackwell, Oxford
79. Jones CL, Gonzales V (1978) Pyridoxine deficiency: a new factor in diabetic neuropathy. J Am Podiatry Assoc 68: 646–653
80. Levin ER, Hanscom TA, et al. (1981) The influence of pyridoxine in diabetic peripheral

neuropathy. Diabetes Care 4: 606–609

81. Schanmberg H, Kaplan J, et al. (1983) Sensory neuropathy from pyridoxine abus. N Engl J Med 309: 445–448
82. Shuman CR, Gilpin SF (1954) Diabetic neuropathy: controlled therapeutic trials. Am J Med Sci 227: 612–618
83. Picot-Dechavassine M, Mira JC (1985) Effects of isaxonine on skeletal muscle reinnervation in the rat: on electrophysiologic evaluation. Muscle Nerve 8: 105–114
84. Le Quesne PM, Fowler CJ, Harding AE (1985) A study of the effects of isaxonine on vincristine induced peripheral neuropathy in man and regeneration following peripheral nerve crush in the rat. J Neurol Neurosurg Psychiatry 48: 93–99
85. Le Quesne PM (1987) Trophic factors and vitamin therapy. In: Dick PJ, Thomas PK, Asbury AK, Winegrad HT, Porte D Jr (eds) Diabetic neuropathy. WB Saunders, Philadelphia, pp 194–198
86. Brownlee M, Vlassara H, Cerami A (1984) Nonenzymatic glycosylation and the pathogenesis of diabetic complications. Ann Intern Med 101: 527–537
87. Winegrad AI (1987) Does a common mechanism induce the diverse complications of diabetes? Diabetes 36: 396–406

# Nephropathy

Diabetic Complications: Early Diagnosis and Treatment
Edited by D. Andreani, G. Crepaldi, U. Di Mario and G. Pozza


# CHAPTER 20

# *Diabetic Vascular Disease: An Integrated View*

J. R. WILLIAMSON, K. CHANG, R. G. TILTON, and C. KILO
*Department of Pathology, Washington University School of Medicine, St. Louis, Missouri, USA*

Complications of diabetic vascular disease are clearly the major cause of premature mortality among diabetic subjects today. In addition, diabetic vascular disease, together with neuropathy, is responsible for most of the increased morbidity associated with diabetes. Until relatively recently, however, there were virtually no clues as to the pathogenetic mechanisms that mediate diabetes-associated injury to vessels and nerves.

Clues to the nature of the metabolic imbalances responsible for nerve damage in diabetic rats preceded those for vascular damage. Stewart et al. (1) were the first to demonstrate that sorbitol levels are increased and myoinositol levels are decreased in the sciatic nerve of diabetic rats. Since then numerous investigators have linked these abnormalities to functional and structural alterations in sciatic nerve (of rats) which are virtually identical to those described in humans (reviewed by Greene et al. (2)). These structural and functional changes appear to be the consequence of reduced $Na^+-K^+$-ATPase activity resulting from impaired phosphatidylinositol turnover and activation of protein kinase C. Interestingly, rats fed on diets enriched with galactose develop nerve damage and cataracts indistinguishable from those observed in diabetic rats. Both glucose and galactose are reduced to their corresponding sugar alcohols by the enzyme aldose reductase which utilizes the cofactor NADPH as the source of hydrogen.

## CAPILLARY BASEMENT MEMBRANE THICKENING

Evidence that diabetic vascular disease is linked to similar metabolic imbalances has been much more difficult to demonstrate. The first studies implicating increased polyol metabolism in the pathogenesis of diabetic vascular disease were the morphometric investigations performed by Frank et al. (3) and Robison et al. (4) in which retinal capillary basement membrane thickening was induced in rats fed on diets enriched with galactose. The inclusion of sorbinil, an inhibitor of the enzyme aldose reductase, in the diet prevented the basement membrane thickening. More recently, Robison et al. (5) have reported that a second, structurally different aldose reductase inhibitor (tolrestat), also prevents galactose-induced retinal capillary basement membrane thickening in the rat; likewise, Chandler et al. (6) have reported that Alcon 1576 (another structurally different inhibitor of aldose reductase) prevents diabetes-induced increased retinal capillary basement membrane thickening. Thus, these observations all suggest that capillary basement membrane thickening, the ultrastructural hallmark of diabetic microangiopathy (7), is an aldose reductase linked phenomenon.

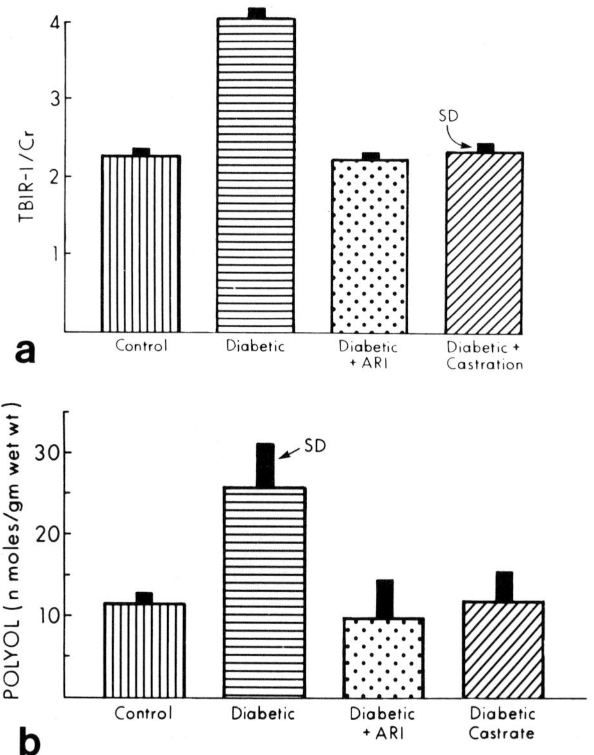


Figure 1. Effects of aldose reductase inhibitors (ARI) (sorbinil and tolrestat) included in the diet (to provide a daily dose of ~ 0.2 mmol/kg) and castration on diabetes-induced increases in $^{125}$I-labelled albumin permeation (a) and sorbitol levels (b) in new granulation tissue.

## INCREASED VASCULAR PERMEABILITY

The most characteristic functional abnormality in the vessels of poorly controlled human diabetic subjects is probably increased vascular permeability. It has been demonstrated in virtually every tissue examined, using a wide variety of tracer molecules (8). We have recently demonstrated highly significant increases in vascular permeability in the eyes (anterior uveal vessels, choriocapillaries, and retina), aorta, sciatic nerve, and new granulation tissue vessels in spontaneously diabetic female BB/W rats, in male rats with streptozotocin-induced diabetes, and in rats fed on galactose-enriched diets (8–10). These increases in vascular permeability are also prevented by several structurally different inhibitors of aldose reductase (9–11) (Figures 1a, 2a, 3a, and 4). Similarly, aldose reductase inhibitors normalize or markedly reduce diabetes-induced increases in tissue polyol levels in these same tissues (9–11).

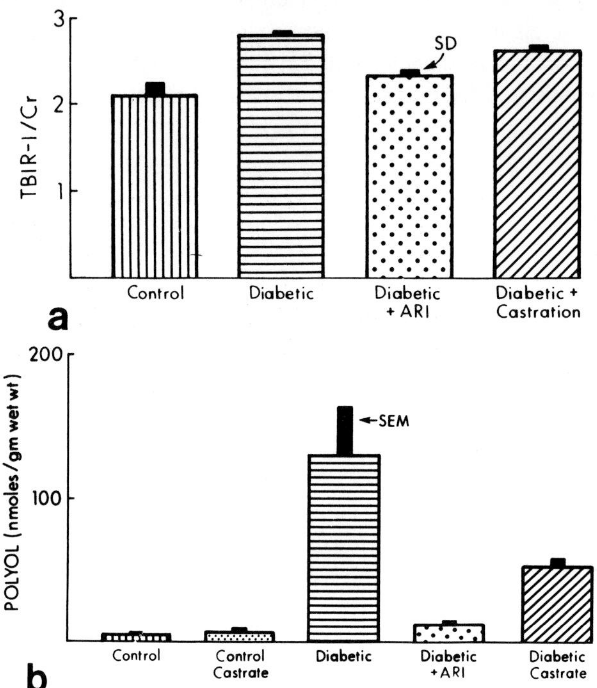


Figure 2. Effects of aldose reductase inhibitors (ARI) (sorbinil and tolrestat) included in the diet (to provide a daily dose of ~ 0.2 mmol/kg) and castration on diabetes-induced increases in $^{125}$I-labelled albumin permeation (a) and sorbitol levels (b) in retina.

The demonstration that $^{125}$I-labelled albumin permeation of the aorta is increased in diabetic rats of special interest since it suggests a mechanism which could explain the acceleration of atherosclerotic vascular disease in human diabetes. Thus, even individuals with relatively 'normal' levels of atherogenic plasma lipoproteins could leak increased amounts of such lipoproteins into the walls of the arteries.

In view of evidence that new vessels produced by neovascularization of the retina and the optic disc in poorly controlled human diabetic subjects are especially leaky and prone to hemorrhage (12,13), it is noteworthy that new subcutaneous vessels formed in response to an angiogenic stimulus in diabetic rats appear to be the most susceptible of any vessels examined to the effects of diabetes on vascular permeability (8). Furthermore, in view of the fact that these new vessels must be derived from connective tissue vessels in overlying skin or underlying muscle (fascia), it is noteworthy that vascular permeability is altered minimally, if at all, in these tissues at points remote from the site of angiogenesis. These findings suggest that angiogenesis in the diabetic milieu gives rise to vessels which are, in turn, especially susceptible to diabetes-induced injury. An important implication of these observations and the latter interpretation is that proliferative vascular responses to injury caused by risk factors for atherosclerosis, including hypertension, hypercholesterolemia, cigarette smoking, immune injury, etc., may result in vessels which are more susceptible to diabetes-induced injury, thereby accounting for the well known acceleration of diabetic vascular disease by these risk factors.

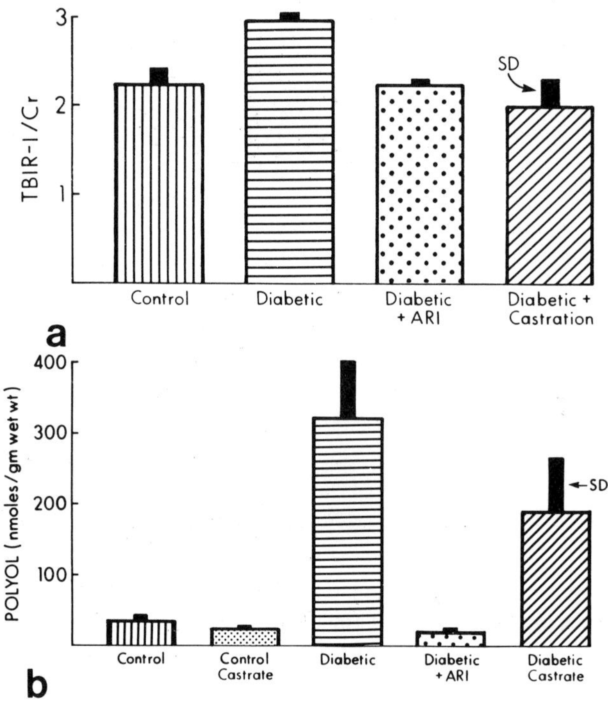


Figure 3. Effects of aldose reductase inhibitors (ARI) (sorbinil and tolrestat) included in the diet (to provide a daily dose of ~ 0.2 mmol/kg) and castration on diabetes-induced increases in $^{125}$I-labelled albumin permeation (a) and sorbitol levels (b) in sciatic nerve.

## HEMODYNAMIC CHANGES

Hemodynamic changes, including increased blood flow in the retina (and other

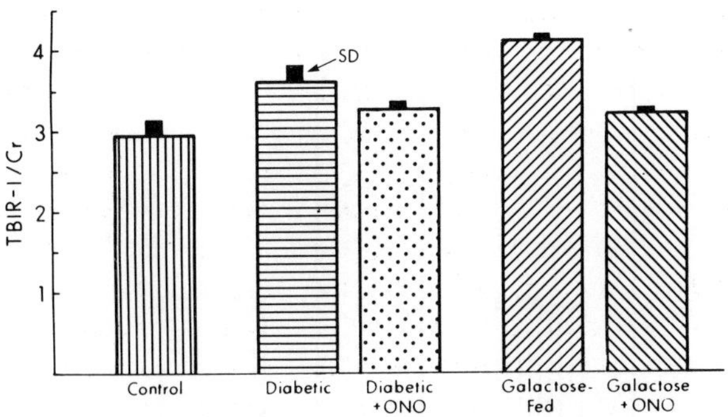


Figure 4. Effect of an aldose reductase inhibitor (Ono 2235) included in the diet (to provide a daily dose of ~ 0.16 mmol/kg) on increased $^{125}$I-labelled albumin permeation in the aorta induced by diabetes of 3 weeks' duration or by a galactose-enriched diet (fed for 3 weeks).

tissues) and increased glomerular filtration rate in the kidney, have been described by many investigators in diabetic humans and experimental animals (reviewed by Parving et al. (14)). These changes are prevented and/or normalized by improved glycemic control. We have recently found that diabetes-induced increases in blood flow (in rats) in the eye (anterior uvea, choroid, retina, and optic nerve) and in sciatic nerve are markedly reduced or normalized by several structurally different inhibitors of aldose reductase (15). Blood flow to the brain was not increased in these diabetic rats. These same aldose reductase inhibitors also prevent diabetes-induced increases in glomerular filtration rate and in albumin permeation of the kidney (9) (Figure 5). These findings are consistent both with the observation of Goldfarb et al. that sorbinil- and myoinositol-supplemented diets normalize glomerular filtration rate in diabetic rats (16), and with the evidence that sorbinil normalizes diabetes-induced reductions in $Na^+-K^+$-ATPase activity and elevated polyol levels in isolated glomeruli obtained from diabetic rats (17,18).

Thus a growing body of evidence indicates that capillary basement membrane changes, hemodynamic alterations, and increased vascular permeability associated with diabetes are all linked to the increased metabolism of glucose to sorbitol and are prevented by inhibitors of aldose reductase which have no effect on plasma glucose levels.

## HORMONAL MODULATION OF DIABETIC VASCULAR DISEASE AND NEUROPATHY

Numerous investigators have reported that the frequency and severity of diabetic retinopathy are markedly increased in postpubertal compared with prepubertal Type 1 diabetic subjects with disease of comparable duration and severity (cited by Williamson et al. (9)); Krolewski et al. have observed the same trend for diabetic

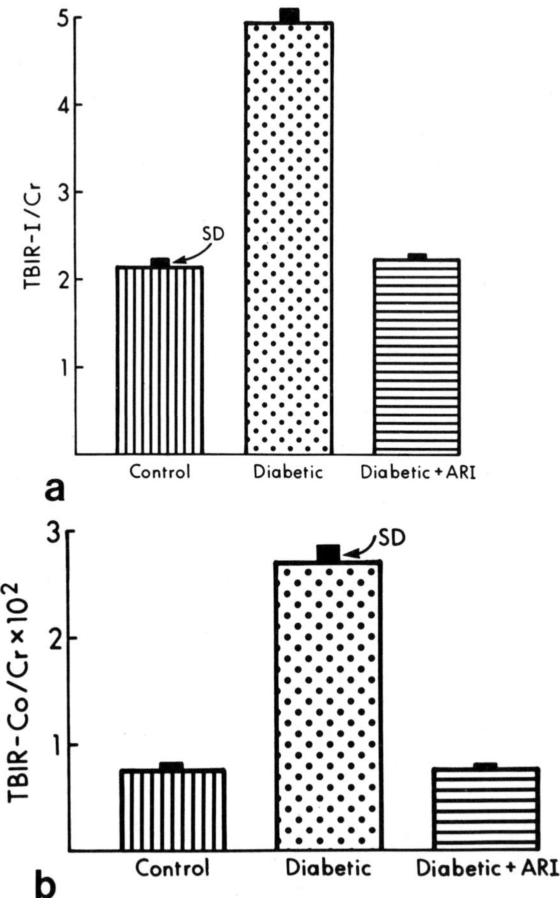


Figure 5. Effects of aldose reductase inhibitors (ARI) (sorbinil and tolrestat) included in the diet (to provide a daily dose of ~ 0.2 mmol/kg) on diabetes-induced increased permeation of the kidney by $^{57}$Co-EDTA (an index of glomerular filtration rate) (a) and $^{125}$I-labelled albumin (b). Tracer permeation was assessed 3 minutes after tracer injection.

nephropathy (19). In two independent studies (20,21), we have observed a highly significant correlation between glycemia and muscle capillary basement membrane thickening in postpubertal but not in prepubertal Type 1 diabetic subjects. These observations, together with the evidence that retinopathy and nephropathy are more common postpuberty than prepuberty, suggest that vascular glucose metabolism (by vessels affected by complications of diabetes) differs in pre- and postpubertal diabetic subjects.

In the study by Rogers et al. (21) we also observed a highly significant correlation between muscle capillary basement membrane thickening and bone age, independent of glycemia, in postpubertal diabetic subjects. In view of the evidence that bone age in postpubertal subjects with normal thyroid and pituitary function is primarily reflective of sex steroid production, these findings suggest the hypothesis that sex steroids may play an important role in modulating the vascular metabolism of glucose and the development of capillary basement membrane thickening, retinopathy, and nephropathy. The likelihood that sex steroids may also modulate diabetic neuropathy is suggested by the observation of Sosenko et al. (22) that an impaired vibratory perception threshold in Type 1 diabetic subjects is strongly correlated with glycemia postpuberty but not prepuberty.

Because of all of these observations implicating sex steroids in the pathogenesis of diabetic vascular disease and neuropathy, our group has examined the effects of castration on the increased changes in vascular permeability observed in male Sprague-Dawley rats with streptozotocin-induced diabetes (9,23). Castration reduces diabetes-induced vascular permeability increases in the retina (Figure 2a) and normalizes permeability in the sciatic nerve (Figure 3a) and in new granulation tissue vessels (Figure 1a). Castration also markedly reduces or normalizes polyol levels in these same tissues (Figures 1b, 2b, and 3b) without reducing plasma glucose levels (9,23).

These observations suggest the hypothesis that aldose reductase linked vascular permeability changes or increases associated with diabetes (and by inference, diabetic vascular disease in general) are strongly modulated by sex steroids. This hypothesis would explain the paucity of vascular complications and neuropathy in prepubertal Type 1 diabetic subjects. These observations and interpretations are consistent with the fact that aldose reductase was first described in the tissues of the male reproductive tract (24).

A growing body of evidence supports the likelihood that diabetic vascular disease and neuropathy in humans are also aldose reductase linked phenomena (25,26) and that polyol metabolism in diabetic humans is modulated by sex steroids (27). Red cell polyol levels in postpubertal Type 1 male diabetic subjects are twice those of prepubertal diabetic males with identical glycemia and $HbA_1$ levels. Similarly, even in non-diabetic subjects, polyol levels in red cells from postpubertal males are twice those of prepubertal males with identical glycemia.

## CONCLUSIONS

A considerable body of evidence indicates that the increased metabolism of glucose to sorbitol is of central importance in the pathogenesis of diabetic macroangiopathy, microangiopathy, and neuropathy. Hemodynamic changes in the eyes, sciatic nerve, and kidney, changes in vascular permeability in the eyes, kidney, aorta, sciatic nerve, and new vessels, and structural changes in retinal capillaries (all of which are equivalent to those described in human diabetic subjects) are prevented in diabetic animals by a variety of structurally different pharmaceutical agents which possess a common capacity to inhibit enzyme aldose reductase.

These findings suggest that metabolic imbalances linked to an increased flux of glucose through the polyol pathway result in the compromised functional and structural integrity of susceptible vessels and nerves. The development of the characteristic full-blown organ- and tissue-specific manifestations of diabetic vascular disease and neuropathy would be the consequence of superimposition of organ- and tissue-specific risk factors (independent of diabetes) on polyol-linked injury. Thus, increased permeability of arterial endothelium would permit increased permeation of atherogenic lipoproteins into the vessel wall which would in turn accelerate 'diabetic' atherosclerosis. Increased blood pressure will add to the increased blood flow and permeability changes in the eyes, to increased permeation of atherogenic lipoproteins into the arteries, and to increased glomerular filtration rate and albuminuria. Hypercholesterolemia would increase the concentration of atherogenic lipoproteins in plasma permeating arterial endothelium.

## REFERENCES

1. Stewart MA, Sherman WR, Kurien MM, Moonsammy GI, Wisgerhof M (1967) Polyol accumulations in nervous tissue of rats with experimental diabetes and galactosemia. J Neurochem 14: 1057–1066
2. Greene DA, Lattimer S, Ulbrecht J, Carroll P (1985) Glucose-induced alterations in nerve metabolism: current perspective on the pathogenesis of diabetic neuropathy and future directions for research and therapy. Diabetes Care 8: 290–299
3. Frank RN, Keirn RJ, Kennedy A, Frank KW (1983) Galactose-induced retinal capillary basement membrane thickening: prevention by sorbinil. Invest Ophthalmol Vis Sci 24: 1519–1524
4. Robison WG Jr, Kador PF, Akagi Y, Kinoshita JH, Gonzalez R, Dvornik D (1983) Retinal capillaries: basement thickening by galactosemia prevented with aldose reductase inhibitor. Science 221: 1177–1179
5. Robison WG Jr, Kador PF, Akagi Y, Kinoshita JH, Gonzalez R, Dvornik K (1986) Prevention of basement membrane thickening in retinal capillaries by a novel inhibitor of aldose reductase, tolrestat. Diabetes 35: 295–299
6. Chandler ML, Shannon WA, DeSantis L (1984) Prevention of retinal capillary basement membrane thickening in diabetic rats by aldose reductase inhibitors. Invest Ophthalmol Vis Sci 25: 159
7. Williamson JR, Kilo C (1983) Capillary basement membranes in diabetes. Diabetes 32 (Suppl 2): 96–100
8. Kilzer P, Chang K, Marvel J, Rowold E, Jaudes P, Ullensvang S, Kilo C, Williamson JR (1985) Albumin permeation of new vessels is increased in diabetic rats. Diabetes 34: 333–336
9. Williamson JR, Chang K, Tilton RG, Prater C, Jeffrey JR, Weigel C, Sherman WR, Eades DM, Kilo C (1987) Increased vascular permeability in spontaneously diabetic BB/W rats and in rats with mild versus severe streptozotocin-induced diabetes: prevention by aldose reductase inhibitors and castration. Diabetes (in press)
10. Chang K, Tomlinson M, Jeffrey JR, Tilton RG, Sherman WR, Ackermann KE, Berger RA, Cicero TJ, Kilo C, Williamson JR (1987) Galactose ingestion increases vascular permeability and collagen solubility in normal male rats. J Clin Invest (in press)
11. Williamson JR, Chang K, Rowold E, Marvel J, Tomlinson M, Sherman WR, Ackermann KE, Kilo C (1985) Sorbinil prevents diabetes-induced increases in vascular permeability but does not alter collagen crosslinking. Diabetes 34: 703–705

12. Norton E, Gutman F (1965) Diabetic retinopathy studied by fluorescein angiography. Ophthalmologica 150: 5–17
13. Kohner E, Dollery C, Paterson J, Oakley N (1967) Arterial fluorescein studies in diabetic retinopathy. Diabetes 16: 1–10
14. Parving HH, Viberti GC, Keen H, Christiansen JS, Lassen NA (1983) Hemodynamic factors in the genesis of diabetic microangiopathy. Metabolism 32: 943–949
15. Williamson JR, Chang K, Tilton RG, Allison W, Ashton T, Kilo C (1987) Increased ocular blood flow and $^{125}$I-albumin permeation in diabetic rats are aldose reductase-linked phenomena. (Abstract) (Submitted for publication)
16. Goldfarb S, Simmons DA, Kewrn E (1987) Amelioration of glomerular hyperfiltration in acute experimental diabetes by dietary myoinositol and by an aldose reductase inhibitor. (Abstract) Clin Res 34: 725A
17. Beyer-Mears A, Ku L, Cohen MP (1984) Glomerular polyol accumulation in diabetes and its prevention by oral sorbinil. Diabetes 33: 604–607
18. Cohen MP, Dasmahapatra A, Shapiro E (1985) Reduced glomerular sodium/potassium adenosine triphosphatase activity in acute streptozotocin diabetes and its prevention by oral sorbinil. Diabetes 34: 1071–1074
19. Krolewski A, Warram J, Christlieb A, Busick E, Kahn C (1985) The changing natural history of nephropathy in type 1 diabetes. Am J Med 78: 785–794
20. Sosenko JM, Miettinen OS, Williamson JR, Gabbay KH (1984) Muscle capillary basement membrane thickness and long-term glycemia in type 1 diabetes. N Engl J Med 311: 694–698
21. Rogers DG, White NH, Santiago JV, Miller JP, Weldon VV, Kilo C, Williamson JR (1986) Glycemic control and bone age are independently associated with muscle capillary basement membrane width in diabetic children after puberty. Diabetes Care 9: 453–459
22. Sosenko JM, Boulton AMJ, Kubrusly DB, Weintraub JK, Skyler JS (1985) The vibratory perception threshold in young diabetic patients: associations with glycemia and puberty. Diabetes Care 8: 605–607
23. Williamson JR, Rowold E, Chang K, Marvel J, Tomlinson M, Sherman WR, Accermann KE, Berger RA, Kilo C (1986) Sex steroid dependency of diabetes-induced changes in polyol metabolism, vascular permeability and collagen crosslinking. Diabetes 35: 20–27
24. Hers H (1956) Le mécanisme de la transformation de glucose en fructose par les vésicules séminales. Biochim Biophys Acta 22: 202–203
25. Cogan DG, Kinoshita JH, Kador PF, Robison G, Datilis MB, Cobo M, Kupfer C (1984) Aldose reductase and complications of diabetes. Ann Intern Med 101: 82–91
26. Cunha-Vaz JG, Mota CC, Leite EC, Abrue JR, Ruas MA (1986) Effect of sorbinil on blood–retinal barrier in early diabetic retinopathy. Diabetes 35: 574–578
27. Rogers DG, Deren S, Sherman WR, White NH, Santiago JV, Kilo C, Williamson JR (1986) Sex and puberty-related differences in red blood cell polyol levels (RBC-P) in type 1 diabetics. (Abstract) Diabetes 35 (Suppl 1): 105A

Diabetic Complications: Early Diagnosis and Treatment
Edited by D. Andreani, G. Crepaldi, U. Di Mario and G. Pozza


CHAPTER 21

# *The Evolution of Diabetic Nephropathy*

M. W. STEFFES, J. M. BASGEN and S. M. MAUER
*Departments of Laboratory Medicine and Pathology and Pediatrics, Medical School University of Minnesota, Minneapolis, Minnesota, USA*

Diabetic nephropathy occurs as a frequently lethal complication in patients with either Type 1, Type 2, or secondary diabetes mellitus (1). There is very good evidence in animals that nephropathy, as exemplified by glomerular lesions, emanates from metabolic alterations of the underlying disease (2). In people this relationship has been demonstrated most clearly in observations made on identical twins discordant for Type 1 diabetes (3). Also, other workers have implicated glycemic control in affecting the development of some changes encompassing diabetic nephropathy and retinopathy (4,5).

Functionally diabetic nephropathy first becomes manifest with hyperfiltration and microalbuminuria, present in poorly controlled patients or after strenuous exercise. An extended period of elevated glomerular filtration rate follows and may accompany (in those patients at risk for renal failure) rising microalbuminuria (6). Eventually if the patient experiences end-stage renal failure, the triad of clinical diabetic nephropathy (falling glomerular filtration rate, hypertension, and overt proteinuria) will begin to develop and progress inexorably. These functional changes caused by diabetes evolve over several years finally to a stage of marked diminution in renal function, wherein the renal disease itself may accelerate the demise of the kidney; and, without transplantation, the patient will die or face hemodialysis. Morphologically one can detect glomerular basement membrane widening within the first 2 years of diabetes mellitus, followed within approximately 5 years of disease by a detectable expansion of the mesangium. In patients who do not experience clinical diabetic nephropathy, these two morphologic lesions either advance very slowly or reach a stage from which they do not progress at all. In other patients mesangial expansion impinges upon and affects other structures in the glomerulus leading to the dramatic changes seen with a falling glomerular filtration rate, hypertension, and proteinuria. In the following sections we will illustrate those changes occurring in glomerular structures, to depict morphologically the pathogenesis of diabetic renal disease.

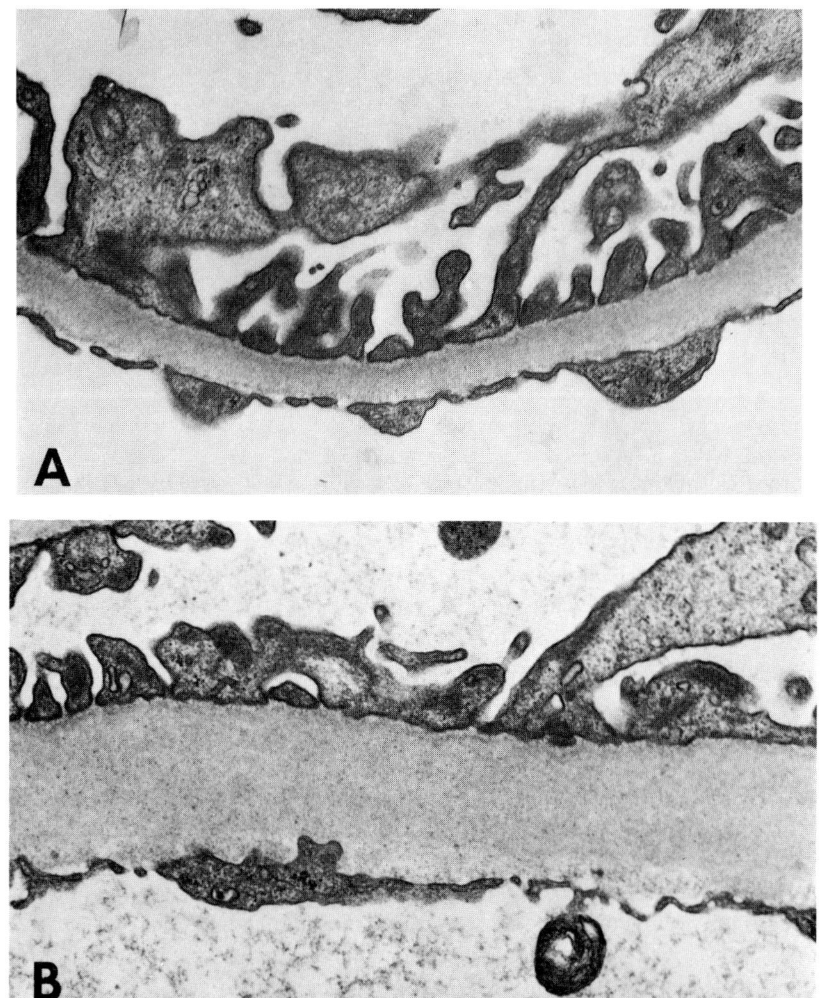


Figure 1. A: glomerular basement membrane in a normal person. B: the widening of the glomerular basement membrane in a diabetic patient; an example of the significant change occurring with diabetic nephropathy. Both electron micrographs at × 18 000.

## Glomerular Basement Membrane

The glomerular basement membrane presents a readily definable and easily measurable structure within the glomerulus. It is integral to the filtration barrier, at least in part through the presence of negatively charged proteoglycans within its matrix (7). The capacity to measure its width consistently and efficiently, as established by Gundersen, Østerby and colleagues, has demonstrated the early widening of the glomerular basement membrane within the first 2 years of exposure of the human kidney to the diabetic environment (8,9). The membrane then appears to widen variably as nephropathy advances in diabetic patients (Figure 1). Nevertheless, the widening of the glomerular basement membrane, per se, does not seem to influence directly the changes in renal function occurring in advanced (leading to end-stage) diabetic nephropathy. Although most patients with end-stage diabetic nephropathy will possess substantially widened glomerular basement membranes, there is no correlation between widening of the glomerular basement membrane and either the falling glomerular filtration rate, the presence of overt proteinuria, or hypertension (10).

In experimental animals, glomerular basement membrane is also a readily measured indicator of early diabetic glomerular disease. In the elegant experiments of Rasch (11,12) its widening was prevented by the initial application of intensive insulin therapy. In contrast, our experiments with islet transplantation after 7 months of diabetes failed to reverse the established widening of the glomerular basement membrane. Rather, the glomerular basement membrane continued to thicken at a rate established during the initial exposure to the diabetic environment (13). Interestingly, islet transplantation successfully reversed albuminuria (14) and the expansion of the mesangium (15). The dichotomy between the widened glomerular basement membrane and its inability to undergo reversal, contrasted with the response of the functional measure (i.e. albuminuria), also suggests that the width of glomerular basement membrane, per se, does not affect the level of albuminuria.

## THE MESANGIUM

The glomerular mesangium comprises cells and a matrix of proteins that lie between and give substantial support to the complex network of glomerular capillaries. The presence of contractile proteins in mesangial cells and their ability either to phagocytize or otherwise cause the elimination of entrapped proteins from the glomerular capillary network through the juxtaglomerular apparatus indicate a central role of the mesangium in renal function. Speculatively the mesangium may serve importantly as the intraglomerular regulator of flows and pressures as well as the functional entity to maintain a cleanly functioning glomerular filtration apparatus. With respect to diabetes mellitus and its attendant renal disease, the glomerular mesangium is central to understanding its early development and later the marked progression of clinical diabetic nephropathy, followed by end-stage renal failure. As stated above, the mesangium expands within 6–9 months of diabetes in rats made diabetic with streptozotocin and can be prevented with excellent metabolic control or reversed following islet transplantation (15,16). The duration of this early resiliency and its response to disease have not been clearly defined either in animals or in man (Figure 2). By morphometric measurements one can generalize that all

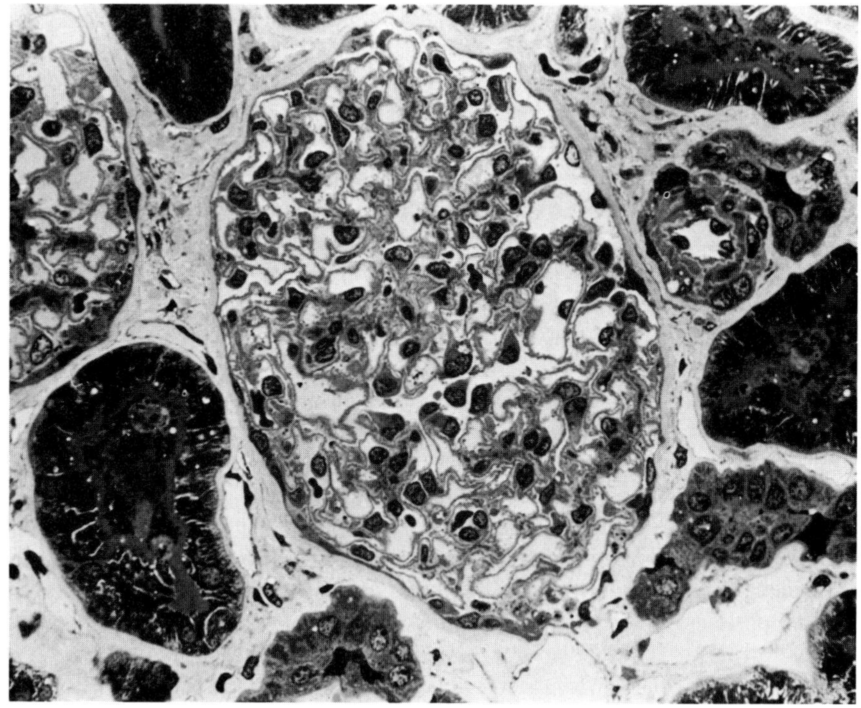

Figure 2. Glomerulus with a normal-appearing mesangium 1 month after the onset of Type 1 diabetes mellitus in a 15-year-old girl. In man readily detectable expansion of the mesangium can be found after 5 years of disease. Light micrograph at × 600.

patients with Type 1 diabetes mellitus will have changes referrable to diabetic nephropathy; i.e. widening of the glomerular basement membrane (3,8). The expansion of the mesangium follows (Figure 3), which in man can be minimal (essentially nondetectable except in identical twins discordant for Type 1 diabetes (3)) or marked leading to renal failure (Figure 4) (10).

The capacity to illustrate the changes in the mesangium of the diabetic subject is limited by the tools currently available to measure the volume fraction or total expanse of this arborizing structure. Nevertheless, the opportunity to study this lesion in many patients with a spectrum of disease has allowed us to make inferences as to the nature of the lesion of the mesangium in diabetic nephropathy and its dramatic influence upon other structures in the glomerulus and thereby upon the development of significant diabetic renal disease (Figures 2–4). The early expansion of the mesangium, potentially reversible as shown by the rat experiments (see above), may continue at a slow rate over the life of the patient with Type 1 diabetes whose kidneys do not progress to end-stage renal failure. The relationship of this stability of the mesangium and the efficacy of metabolic control has not been studied prospectively

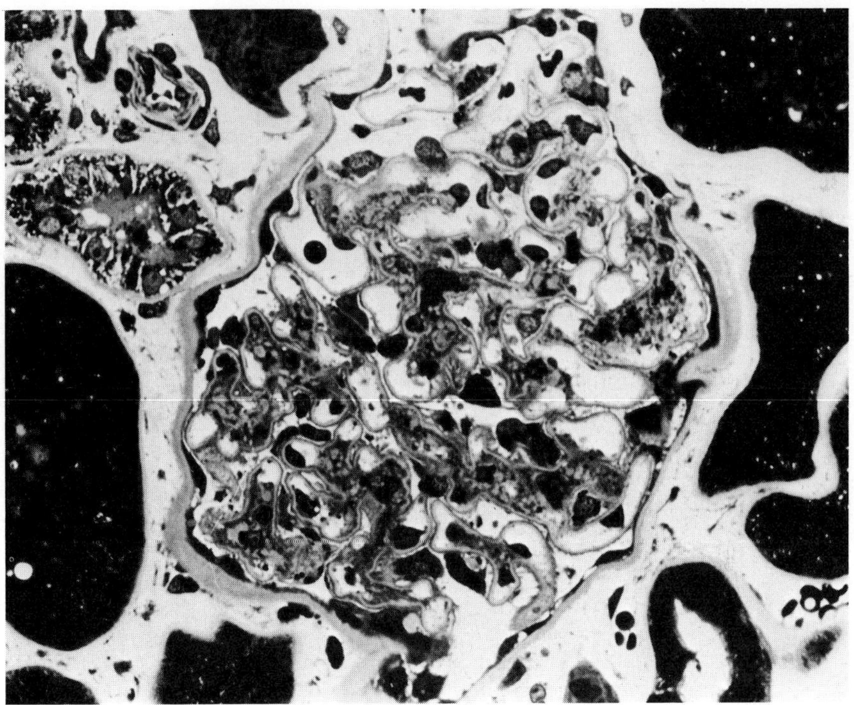

Figure 3. A glomerulus with a moderate expansion of the mesangium after 12 years of Type 1 diabetes mellitus in a 25-year-old woman. Light micrograph at × 600.

in man. Yet, the experiments in animals implicate strongly the role of metabolic control in affecting the development of mesangial expansion (15). Additionally, epidemiologic studies in man have signaled the level of control (albeit retrospectively attained) as strongly affecting the development of glomerular disease (and thereby inferentially influencing the progression of mesangial pathology) (1,17). By contrasting these separate studies (1,10,17) one can relate the diminution of renal function leading to failure with a progressive, diffuse (and sometimes nodular) glomerular nephropathy represented by an expanded mesangium occupying a substantial (one-third or greater) volume of the glomerular tuft (Figure 4). In other words, at end-stage renal disease in diabetes mellitus, individual glomeruli have either been occluded with hyalinization or are overcome by a progressive expansion of the glomerular mesangium.

The challenge to sort out the role of diabetes itself versus secondary factors related to the diabetic state (e.g. hemodynamic) has significant clinical importance. In addition to stressing optimal management in all patients with diabetes mellitus, the subset of patients for reasons other than diabetes relatively at risk to mesangial disease (and thus to end-stage diabetic nephropathy) must be identified. It is in this group of subjects that appropriate interventional strategies must be initiated to prevent abolition of renal function.

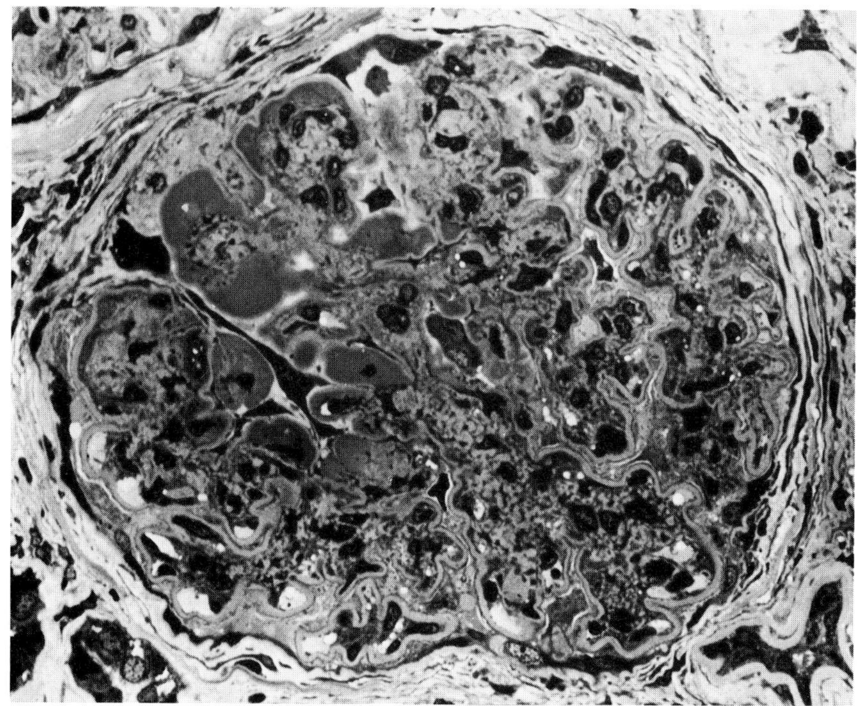

Figure 4. A glomerulus with marked and diffuse expansion of the mesangium obliterating many glomerular capillaries and their filtering surfaces after 19 years of Type 1 diabetes mellitus in a 26-year-old man. Light micrograph at × 600.

## ADVANCED, POTENTIALLY END-STAGE DIABETIC GLOMERULOPATHY

The progression of the lesions outlined above markedly affects renal function in diabetic patients. The triad of diabetic nephropathy (a falling glomerular filtration rate, microalbuminuria proceeding to overt proteinuria, and hypertension) mark the reaction of the kidney to marked reduction in functional renal mass. Potentially there are two lesions occurring in the diabetic kidney at this stage. One is a diffuse (sometimes nodular) expansion of the mesangium obliterating normal filtration function in the individual glomerulus. The expansion of the mesangium reduces the surface of the glomerular capillary available for filtration (10,18,19). It affects the slit pores of the epithelial podocytes, the areas of the membrane thought specifically to regulate glomerular filtration. Thus, in and of itself this marked expansion of the mesangium and its impingement upon capillary volume will reduce glomerular filtration. The rate at which the individual capillary may lose its capacity to filter the blood is dependent upon the actual size of the glomerus (and capillaries) as well as upon the volume of the glomerulus occupied by the mesangium (20). In other words, the same expansion of the mesangium in a large glomerulus will have a smaller effect upon capillary filtration surface than that expansion in a small glomerulus. In addition to the expansion of the mesangium and its reduction of glomerular function, a process of hyalinization of individual glomeruli may occur in the diabetic kidney. The hyalinization may arise from a process different from that leading to mesangial expansion. Further, this phenomenon occurs in a distribution which suggests that it results from an injury to the vascular supply of the kidney (21). If so, compromization of the larger vessels (potentially termed macroangiopathy) may be present in the end-stage diabetic kidney, at the time of a continuation of the microvascular (glomerular mesangium) lesion. Together these pathophysiologic developments may contribute to a steady decline in renal function and the clinical manifestations of end-stage diabetic nephropathy. Focal glomerulosclerosis occurs only rarely in the diabetic kidney in man (22). This alteration occurs in other human renal diseases and can be present in diabetic animal models with hyperfiltration. In animals the relation of these lesions to the diabetic state is beyond the scope of this paper.

## CONCLUSIONS

Within the first few months of disease in each diabetic patient diabetic glomerulopathy probably begins with fundamental biochemical lesions occurring within the glomerulus. These lesions become structurally manifest within the first 2 years of diabetes with a widening of the glomerular basement membrane followed at 5 years and later by an expansion of the mesangium. During the first decade of disease microalbuminuria becomes demonstrable; yet its relationship to morphologic lesions and their progression remains unclear. The mesangial expansion not only affects the volume of the mesangium and its structure within the glomerulus, but by nature of the limited volume of the glomerulus within which the mesangium can expand, that expanding mesangium can severely compromise the structure of glomerular capillaries as well as the surface of the glomerular capillaries available for filtration. Mesangial expansion coupled with the potentially separate process of hyalinization or total sclerosis of glomeruli can lead to marked changes in renal function, including a falling glomerular filtration rate, microalbuminuria rising to overt proteinuria, and hypertension. These functional and morphologic lesions are the hallmark of diabetic nephropathy and, carried to their conclusion, lead to renal failure and potentially the death of the patient. The factors contributing to this development, including glycemic control of diabetes as well as other non-diabetic related factors, must be elucidated and their effective contributions established. With clear pathophysiologic delineation of these lesions, therapeutic strategies affecting the development of diabetic nephropathy in a definitive way can be introduced.

## REFERENCES

1. Deckert T, Poulsen JE, Larsen M (1978) Prognosis of diabetics with diabetes onset before the age of thirty-one. I. Survival, causes of death, and complications. Diabetologia 14: 363–370
2. Steffes MW, Mauer SM (1984) Diabetic glomerulopathy in man and experimental animal models. Int Rev Exp Pathol 26: 147–175
3. Steffes MW, Sutherland DER, Goetz FC, Rich SS, Mauer SM (1985) Studies of kidney and muscle biopsies in identical twins discordant for Type 1 diabetes mellitus. N Engl J Med 312: 1281–1287
4. Pirart J (1978) Diabetes mellitus and its degenerative complications: a prospective study of 4400 patients observed between 1947 and 1973. Diabetes Care 1: 168–188, 252–263
5. Job D, Eschwege E, Guyot-Argenton C, Augry J, Tchobroutsky G (1976) Effect of multiple daily insulin injections on the course of diabetic retinopathy. Diabetes 25: 463–469
6. Viberti GC, Keen H (1984) The patterns of proteinuria in diabetes mellitus: relevance to pathogenesis and prevention of diabetic nephropathy. 33: 686–692
7. Klein DJ, Brown DM, Oegema TR (1986) Glomerular proteoglycans in diabetes. Diabetes 35: 1130–1142
8. Østerby R (1972) Morphometric studies of the peripheral glomerular basement membrane in early juvenile diabetes. I. Development of initial basement membrane thickening. Diabetologia 8: 84–92
9. Jensen EB, Gundersen HJG, Østerby R (1979) Determination of membrane thickness distribution from orthogonal intercepts. J Microsc 116: 19–33
10. Mauer SM, Steffes MW, Ellis EN, Sutherland DER, Brown DM, Goetz FC (1984) Structural-functional relationships in diabetic nephropathy. J Clin Invest 74: 1143–1155
11. Rasch R (1979) Control of blood glucose levels in the streptozotocin diabetic rat using a long-acting heat-treated insulin. Diabetologia 16: 185–190
12. Rasch R (1979) Prevention of diabetic glomerulopathy in streptozotocin diabetic rats by insulin treatment. Glomerular basement membrane thickness. Diabetologia 16: 319–324
13. Steffes MW, Brown DM, Basgen JM, Matas AJ, Mauer SM (1979) Glomerular basement membrane thickness following islet transplantation in the diabetic rat. Lab Invest 41: 116–118
14. Mauer SM, Brown DM, Basgen JM, Matas AJ, Steffes MW (1978) Effects of pancreatic islet transplantation on the increased urinary albumin excretion rates in intact and uninephrectomized rats with diabetes mellitus. Diabetes 27: 959–964
15. Steffes MW, Brown DM, Basgen JM, Mauer SM (1980) Amelioration of mesangial volume and surface alterations following islet transplantation in diabetic rats. Diabetes 29: 509–515
16. Rasch R (1979) Prevention of diabetic glomerulopathy in streptozotocin diabetic rats by insulin treatment. The mesangial regions. Diabetologia 17: 243–248
17. Krolewski AS, Warram JH, Christlieb AR, Busick EJ, Kahn CR (1985) The changing natural history of nephropathy in Type 1 diabetes. Am J Med 78: 785–794
18. Ellis EN, Steffes MW, Goetz FC, Sutherland DER, Mauer SM (1986) Glomerular filtration surface in type 1 diabetes mellitus. Kidney Int 29: 889–894
19. Ellis EN, Steffes MW, Chavers B, Mauer SM (1987) Observations of glomerular epithelial cell structure in patients with type 1 diabetes mellitus (submitted for publication)
20. Steffes MW, Ellis EN, Mauer SM (1986) Complications of diabetes mellitus and factors affecting their progression. Clin Chem 32: B54–B61
21. Horlyck A, Gundersen HJG, Østerby R (1986) The cortical distribution pattern of

diabetic glomerulopathy. Diabetologia 29: 146–150
22. Heptinstall RH (1983) Pathology of the Kidney. Little, Brown & Co, Boston/Toronto, pp 676–696

Diabetic Complications: Early Diagnosis and Treatment
Edited by D. Andreani, G. Crepaldi, U. Di Mario and G. Pozza


# CHAPTER 22

# *Non-Enzymic Glycation of Glomerular Basement Membrane: Biochemical and Immunological Modifications in Diabetic Nephropathy*

U. Di Mario, M. Sensi, P. Pozzilli and D. Andreani
*Cattedra di Endocrinologia 1, Clinica Medica 2, University of Rome 'La Sapienza', Italy*

The high proportion of patients developing diabetic nephropathy and eventually undergoing renal failure (1) rightly calls for great efforts to be made to discover the mechanisms involved in the pathogenesis of this complication. Research in diabetic nephropathy is hindered by the fact that the condition develops very slowly, is very difficult to study at regular intervals in vivo, and there are not yet equivalent animal models. Progress in this field therefore depends on the development of valid alternative experimental techniques with which to investigate the pathological mechanisms in conditions that simulate as closely as possible the in vivo situation.

It is evident, however, that no single in vitro experiment will be able to clarify all aspects of the complication. This is largely due to the fact that diabetic nephropathy has a complex etiology, as is clear from the other chapters included in this section. We shall therefore deal with the experimental study of one of the phenomena which is believed to contribute not only to the pathogenesis of nephropathy, but also to that of other diabetic complications: the post-translational, non-enzymic glycation of proteins. Although this reaction also occurs in normal conditions, the chronic hyperglycemia characteristic of diabetes mellitus has been associated with an increased non-enzymic glycation, and thus with an altered function of circulating proteins, such as hemoglobin (2–4), albumin (5–9) and low density lipoproteins (10–13). Longer-lived structural proteins, such as those of skin and tendon collagen, eye lens and peripheral nerve, are also affected, their excessive non-enzymic glycation being considered a contributory factor in the development of diabetic cataracts (14–16), collagen disease (17–21) and neuropathy (22,23).

The kidney is also affected by this process, since increased non-enzymic glycation of glomerular basement membrane (GBM) collagen has been reported both in the diabetic rat (24) and in diabetic man (25).

Among the pathomorphological characteristics of the diabetic kidney are a thickened GBM (26,27) and the presence of linear deposits of immunoglobulins, fibrin, complement factor C3 (28) and albumin (29) along the GBM. As the presence of immunoglobulins does not appear to be correlated to an active immunological process (30) the occurrence of non-immunological proteins is evidence of a secondary binding or trapping of proteins on the GBM. Such a phenomenon could be due to an altered chemical composition or indeed 'reactivity' of the GBM and/or the proteins themselves. As will be seen later, the non-enzymic glycation of GBM in diabetes might offer an explanation for these findings.

Unlike many other structures, the renal glomeruli are relatively easy to isolate and purify, and in this chapter we shall describe an experimental model employed to study the link between some of the pathomorphological glomerular changes and non-enzymic glycation.

## THE EXPERIMENTAL MODEL

### Isolation of Renal Glomeruli and Glomerular Basement Membrane

The technique to isolate either animal or human glomeruli was originally described by Greenspon and Krakower in 1950 (31). Since then several modifications and ameliorations have been introduced by various authors in order to produce purer populations of glomeruli (32,33).

The purifications of GBM, i.e. the removal of all glomerular cell components, is probably the most crucial step in the procedure. The method employed to destroy the cells could also affect the GBM in such a way that the results obtained and the conclusions reached might not have any relation to the situation in vivo.

At present, two techniques are employed to remove glomerular endothelial, epithelial, mesangial and blood cells. The first method uses ultrasound to disrupt the cell membranes (32); the second is based on the use of detergents (Triton X and deoxycholate) which selectively solubilize the various cell components (33). In our study human autopsy material was used, with the exclusion of kidneys from patients who had died of invasive diseases or renal pathology. A combination of the techniques described above was used for the preparation of GBM specimens (34). As shown in Figure 1, the GBM preparation obtained was free of cell contaminants.

### Non-Enzymic Glycation Reaction

The initial step in non-enzymic glycation consists of the attachment of the aldehyde (open) form of glucose to a protein N-terminus, or side-chain amino group

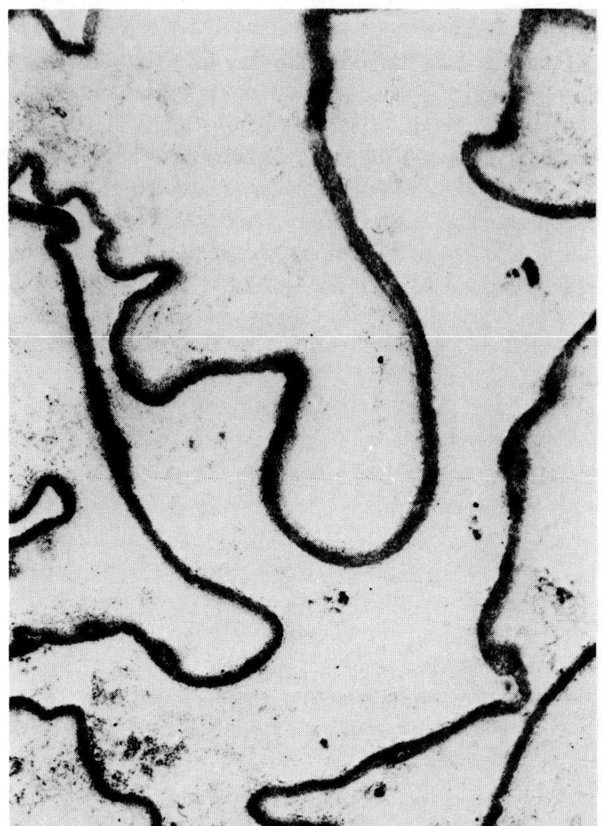

Figure 1. Electron micrograph of isolated and purified human GBM. The structure is free of cellular contamination.

of lysine, via a nucleophilic addition reaction, followed by the loss of a molecule of water. The first product formed is a labile chemical entity, named the Schiff base. With time, the Schiff base undergoes a slow Amadori-type chemical rearrangement which ends in the appearance of a more stable, although still reversible, sugar–protein adduct, the Amadori product (35). In structural long-lived proteins, such as collagen, myelin and crystallins, the Amadori adducts undergo a further series of dehydration, degradation and rearrangement reactions which results in the appearance of very stable, irreversible and highly reactive glycation end-products (20,36).

The importance of the non-enzymic glycation of body proteins has been highlighted by the large number of studies on human and animal tissues to investigate the origin of diabetic complications (15,16,22,37–39).

In vitro protein glycation is easily achieved by incubating the proteins with glucose. Our group has investigated the glycation of human albumin, fibrinogen and GBM at sugar molarities ranging from 5 to 100–500 mM (40,41). The high non-physiological concentrations of glucose used in these and other (42) studies were chosen for the specific purpose of maximizing its attachment rate to the proteins, at a physiological temperature and pH and in a relatively short reaction time. In vivo this process would occur over a much longer time-scale, as is demonstrated by the late appearance of complications in patients with insulin-dependent diabetes.

The degree of glycation can be quantified either colorimetrically, by means of the thiobarbituric reaction (5,43), or by adding radioactive D-glucose as tracer (44). The results of our experiments are shown in Figures 2 and 3. The data clearly confirm that the extent of the in vitro glycation of circulating and structural proteins is dependent on the concentration of sugar.

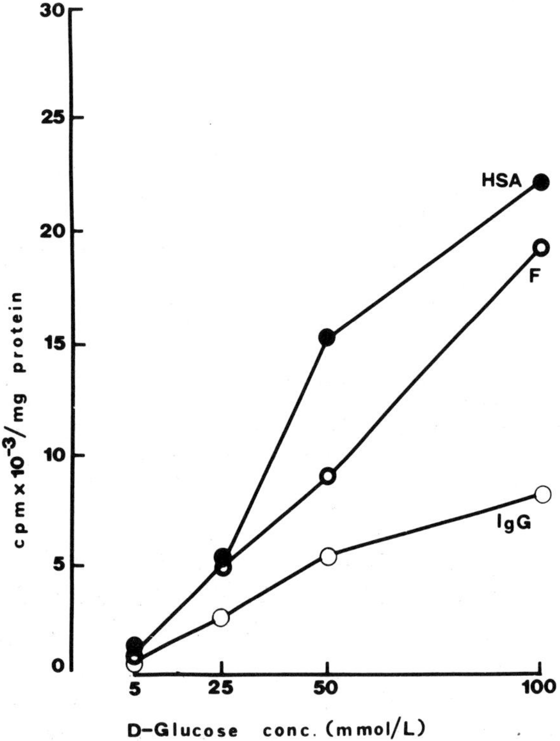


Figure 2. In vitro non-enzymic glycation of human albumin (HSA), fibrinogen (F) and immunoglobulin G (IgG). The amount of $^{14}$C-labelled glucose bound to each protein increases as the sugar concentration increases.

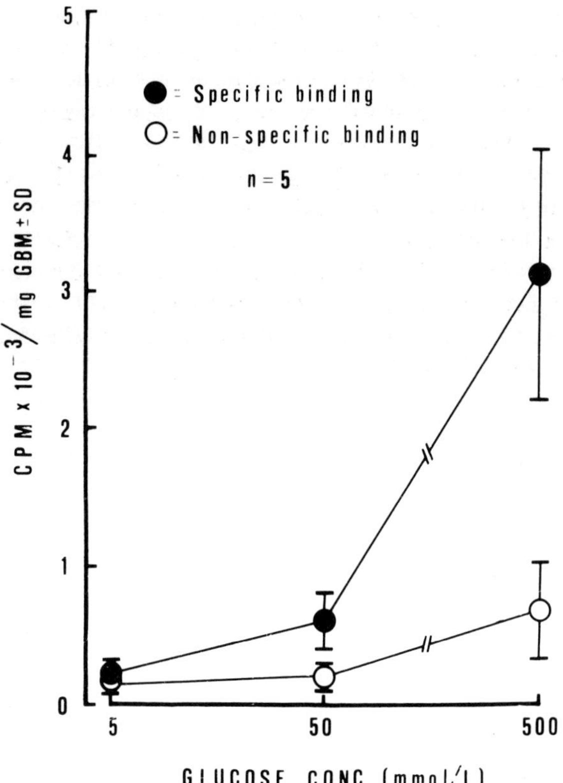


Figure 3. In vitro non-enzymic glycation of human GBM. As for circulating proteins, the amount of glucose bound to the GBM depends upon the sugar concentration in the medium. The non-specific binding was measured by a 30-min incubation of GBM in the sugar solution (as opposed to a 10-day incubation for the specific binding). At 5 mM there is little difference between specific and non-specific glucose binding.

## EFFECT OF NON-ENZYMIC GLYCATION ON STRUCTURAL AND FUNCTIONAL CHARACTERISTICS OF PROTEINS WITH REFERENCE TO DIABETIC NEPHROPATHY

### Circulating Proteins

Although glycation can alter the function of several circulating proteins, including hormones and enzymes (37,45), only albumin, the principal protein involved in diabetic nephropathy, will be discussed.

One of the main pathological signs of developing diabetic nephropathy is the slow but continuous increase of hyperfiltration of albumin (46). Many factors have been advocated to explain this phenomenon, including the non-enzymic glycation of the GBM itself (44). It is now accepted that hyperfiltration of albumin and other negatively charged proteins is electrostatically prevented by the negatively charged GBM pores (47). One of the theories to explain the appearance of microalbuminuria was based on the altered permeability selectivity of the GBM, due to the loss of anionic charges caused by non-enzymic glycation (44). Now the theory has been slightly modified, since, as will be mentioned later, the loss of fixed GBM negative charges is probably not dependent on glycation alone. Furthermore, the apparently altered permeability selectivity of the GBM could be the result of a modified albumin molecule. It has thus been shown that the urinary concentration of glyclated albumin is 5–10 times greater than its plasma concentration (48). Like albumin, other glycated proteins can be found in larger amounts in the urine than in the circulation (49). Although there is still controversy on the exact effect exerted by non-enzymic glycation on the overall electric charge of albumin, it is suggested that the conformational and spatial arrangement of the molecule is altered by the introduction of the large glucose molecule, causing the rearrangement and surfacing of normally hidden, positively charged, chemical groups (50,51). These could reduce the overall surface electrostatic repulsion at the level of the negatively charged GBM pores.

### Structural Proteins

Non-enzymic glycation of long-lived structural proteins, such as those constituting basement membranes and collagen, could induce electrical, biochemical and possibly immunological alterations. Similarly to circulating proteins, only the effect of glycation on a structure directly involved in diabetic nephropathy, such as the GBM, will be described here.

It was originally suggested that the introduction of glucose groups within the molecular structure of the filtering surface of the GBM could lead to a rearrangement or reduction of negatively charged ions, thus facilitating the passage of macromolecules which normally do not escape the circulating bed (44). It now appears more likely that the reduction of fixed *electric* negative charges on the GBM is mainly due to a reduced synthesis of two negatively charged non-proteinaceous components of the GBM, sialic acid (52) and heparan sulphate (53), both of which are negatively charged.

More interesting and possibly more relevant to the later stages of diabetic nephropathy are the *biochemical alterations* induced within the over-glycated GBM. It has already been mentioned that in longer-lived structural proteins non-enzymic glycation proceeds to the stage of formation of advanced glycation end-products. These groups are highly reactive for the presence of free carbonyls which can react with free amino groups and thus cross-link with other proteins (54,55). We have found that human insulin, albumin, IgG, and fibrinogen show an increased binding over isolated GBM following its glycation in vitro (41) (Figure 4). This result is consistent with the findings obtained with glycated animal skin collagen (42) and confirms the presence of some reactive chemical groups along the non-enzymically glycated GBM.

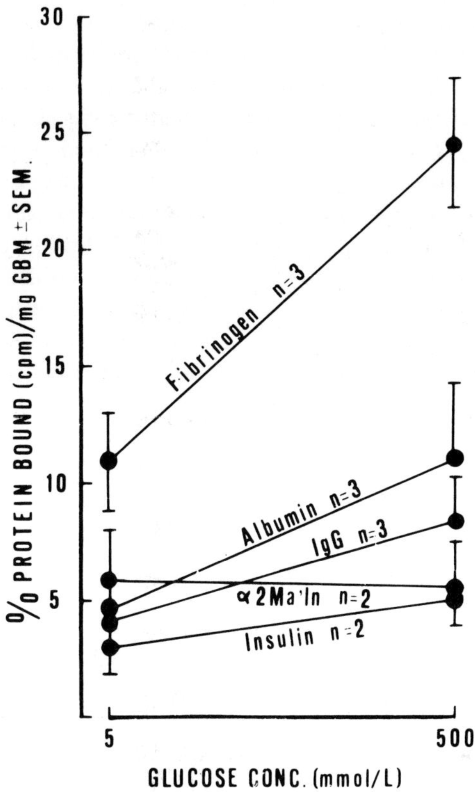


Figure 4. Binding of circulating proteins on human GBM non-enzymically glycated in vitro. Four out of the five proteins investigated show an increased binding over GBM pre-incubated in 500 mM D-glucose.

The phenomenon of the enhanced reactivity of glycated GBM is probably a reflection of what occurs—obviously on a different time-scale—in patients with long-standing diabetes mellitus.

The mechanism of the linear deposition of albumin, IgG, fibrin and other proteins over the GBM of many of these patients could be explained in terms of increased cross-linkage between these proteins and the reactive glycation end-products formed over the GBM. Deposition of these proteins over the glomerular membrane could also initiate an *immunological reaction*, leading to the formation of tissue-damaging immune complexes (56). The increased thickening of the GBM in diabetic patients (26) might also be the result of the pathological deposition of extraneous proteinaceous materials over glycated GBM (44). It is probable, however, that other factors are principally involved in the thickening phenomenon: firstly, a reduced turnover of the diabetic GBM due to a combination of two events, such as the inhibition of collagenase by increased plasma levels of alpha-2-macroglobulin, along with a reduced susceptibility of glycated GBM to proteolysis (57); secondly, the reduced synthesis of heparan sulphate proteoglycans in the course of diabetes could stimulate a hypersecretion of type IV collagen and laminin (58).

Very few data are available in the literature on the antigenic properties of glycated proteins. Bassiouny et al. (59) reported the production in the rat of antibodies directed against glycated, but not against unmodified, collagen. Other authors have claimed that only advanced glycation end-products are capable of eliciting an immunological response in the host, while the early Amadori products have scarce or no immunogenic activity (60). Thus, attempts to produce antibodies directed towards glycated plasma proteins, with the aim of measuring them radioimmunologically in the plasma of diabetic patients, have met with little success. However, antibodies could be produced against reductively glycated, low density lipoproteins (61) and albumin (62). Although this is clearly useful from a radioimmunoassay point of view, the fact that only the sodium borohydride reduced form, and thus the artificial and non-physiological form, of a glycated protein has antigenic properties is not helpful in the search for early markers of protein glycation.

## THERAPEUTIC INTERVENTION

Based on the present evidence, non-enzymic glycation could play a role in the development of diabetic nephropathy and obviously of any other late diabetic complication. The next step is therefore to find the means to inhibit, or at least to reduce, this reaction. Ideally, the main approach to reach this goal is the optimization of glycemic control. Since, however, this is not yet easy to obtain, a second possible approach is pharmaceutical intervention.

An important step in this direction has been the observation that aspirin, like glucose, can react with the same free amino group of the lysine residue to form an acetyl derivative (63). This property has been studied by Day et al. (5), Kennedy et al. (38) and Rendall et al. (64), who showed that aspirin could indeed reduce the in vitro non-enzymic glycation of human serum albumin, hemoglobin and other plasma proteins. Our group has also confirmed these findings not only in the case of human albumin and fibrinogen (Table 1), but also in human GBM (49) (Figure 5). The mechanism with which aspirin inhibits glycation is by rapidly acetylating the same amino group that reacts with glucose (64), thus preventing the initial formation of the Schiff base. Although interesting, the use of aspirin as a glycation inhibitor must be approached with caution in the light of its side-effects, especially at the doses that would be required to obtain a clinically significant inhibition. In addition, it would be necessary to make a very thorough study of the chemical characteristics of the

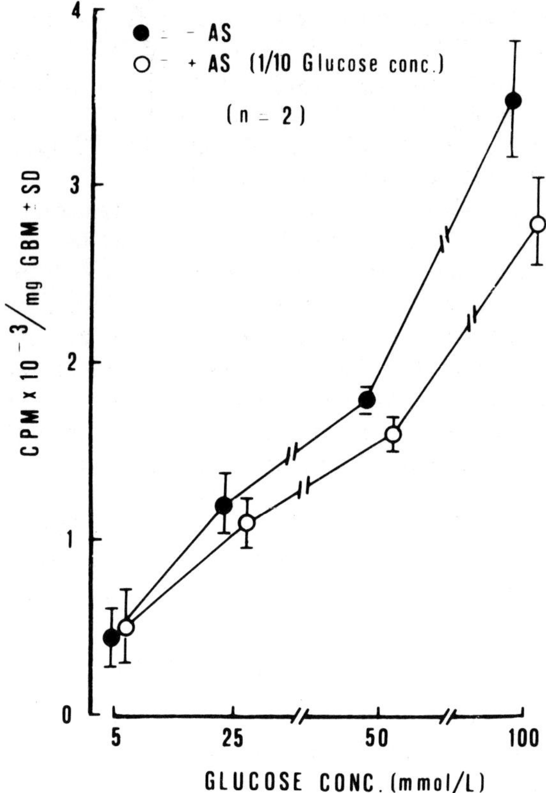


Figure 5. Effect of aspirin (AS) on the in vitro glycation of human GBM. The aspirin concentration was one-tenth that of glucose. Although the maximum inhibition occurs at the highest glucose levels, significant inhibition is present also with 25 mM D-glucose.

acetyl–protein adducts, since they could turn out to be more damaging than the chemical structure whose formation they prevent. At present, other related, less toxic, compounds to inhibit protein glycation are being investigated.

An alternative method to prevent the formation of damaging late glycation end-products entails the use of aminoguanidine. This nucleophilic hydrazine compound has been shown to prevent the formation of late glycation end-products and thus the formation of protein–protein cross-links (65). The inhibitory mechanism is different from that of aspirin and other acetylating compounds: whereas the latter inhibit the initial reaction between glucose and the protein amino groups, aminoguanidine reacts irreversibly with the carbonyl group of the early glycation products (65).

A third method to reduce the extent of non-enzymic protein glycation is the use of lysine. In principle, this amino acid and glucose should react very readily in

Table 1. The effect of aspirin on the in vitro non-enzymic glycation of human albumin and human fibrinogen

| | Albumin ($n$ = 3) | | Fibrinogen ($n$ = 2) | |
|---|---|---|---|---|
| | −AS | +AS | −AS | +AS |
| Glucose conc. (mmol/l) | | | | |
| 5 | 1 070±95 | 956±54 | 1 019±46 | 1045±125 |
| 25 | 4 963±535 | 3709±385 | 4 715±482 | 3678±491 |
| 50 | 11 630±3096 | 6717±642 | 7 898±1184 | 6136±1338 |
| 100 | 18 040±4244 | 9285±501 | 13 936±3808 | 9591±1646 |
| ANOVA | | | | |
| Glucose effect | $F$ (df 3,16) = 356 $p<0.001$ | | $F$ (df 3,8) = 129 $p<0.01$ | |
| Aspirin effect | $F$ (df 1,16) = 44.20 $p<0.001$ | | $F$ (df 1,8) = 5.41 $p<0.05$ | |

The data are expressed as cpm D-[$^{14}$C] glucose per mg protein. The ratio between radioactive and unlabelled sugar was kept constant. The concentration of aspirin used was one-tenth that of glucose.

solution, given the steric accessibility of both molecules. High blood levels of lysine could therefore prevent a substantial amount of glucose from reacting with less accessible amino groups in circulating and structural proteins. This problem has been investigated with D-lysine, which has the fundamental property of not being utilized in vivo for the synthesis of proteins. The preliminary results are encouraging (Sensi et al. unpublished data) and confirm that D-lysine possesses a considerable in vitro inhibitory capacity (Table 2).

Table 2. The effect of D-lysine on the in vitro non-enzymic glycation of human albumin, fibrinogen and GBM

| Glucose conc. (mmol/l) | Albumin | Fibrinogen | GBM |
|---|---|---|---|
| 5 | 0.85 (0.89) | 0.95 (1.02) | 0.79 (1.03) |
| 25 | 0.85 (0.74) | 0.50 (0.78) | 0.66 (0.90) |
| 50 | 0.46 (0.58) | 0.45 (0.77) | 0.78 (0.89) |
| 100 | 0.40 (0.51) | 0.49 (0.69) | 0.72 (0.79) |

The data are expressed as:

$$\frac{\text{cpm D-[}^{14}\text{C]glucose per mg protein in the presence of D-lysine}}{\text{cpm D-[}^{14}\text{C]glucose per mg protein in the absence of D-lysine}}$$

Similarly to aspirin, the concentration of D-lysine employed was one-tenth that of glucose. The values in parentheses are ratios calculated in the experiments with aspirin as inhibitor of glycation.

## FINAL COMMENTS

Evidence is accumulating that the non-enzymic glycation of proteins plays a role, if not the major one, in the pathogenesis of diabetic nephropathy. Glycation of albumin might lead to its loss via an increased permeability selectivity across an electrically and biochemically altered GBM. In addition, glycation of the GBM might enhance trapping and deposition of plasma proteins and immune complexes by increased protein–protein cross-links, ultimately leading to a gross dysfunction of the glomerular filtration barrier and thus to the final stages of diabetic renal failure.

Optimization of metabolic control together with early pharmaceutical/chemical inhibition of non-enzymic glycation might reduce the incidence of diabetic nephropathy.

## REFERENCES


1. Deckert T, Poulsen JE, Larsen M (1978) Prognosis of diabetics with diabetes onset before the age of thirty-one. Diabetologia 14: 363–370
2. Bunn HF, Gabbay KH, Gallop PM (1978) The glycosylation of hemoglobin: relevance to diabetes mellitus. Science 100: 21–27
3. Graham JJ, Ryall RG, Wise PM (1980) Glycosylated hemoglobin and relative polycythaemia in diabetes mellitus. Diabetologia 18: 205–207
4. Cerriello A, Dello Russo P, Sgambato S, Giugliano D (1982) Glycosylated hemoglobin and reticulocyte count in diabetes mellitus. Diabetologia 22: 223
5. Day JF, Thorpe SR, Baynes JW (1979) Nonenzymatically glycosylated albumin. J Biol Chem 254: 595–597
6. Guthrow CE, Morris MA, Day JF, Thorpe SR, Baynes JW (1979) Enhanced nonenzymatic glycosylation of human serum albumin in diabetes mellitus. Proc Natl Acad Sci USA 76: 4258–4261
7. Dolhofer R, Wieland OH (1979) Glycosylation of serum albumin. Elevated glycosyl–albumin in diabetic patients. FEBS Lett 103: 282–286
8. Dolhofer R, Wieland OH (1980) Increased glycosylation of serum albumin in diabetes mellitus. Diabetes 29: 417–422
9. Williams SK, Devenny JJ, Bitensky (1981) Micropinocytotic ingestion of glycosylated albumin by isolated microvessels: possible role in pathogenesis of diabetic microangiopathy. Proc Natl Acad Sci USA 78: 2393–2397
10. Schleicker E, Deufel T, Wieland OH (1981) Non-enzymatic glycosylation of human serum lipoproteins: elevated epsilon-lysine glycosylated low density lipoproteins in diabetes patients. FEBS Lett 129: 1–4
11. Gonen B, Baezinger J, Schonfeld G, Jacobson D, Farrar P (1981) Nonenzymatic glycation of low-density lipoproteins in vitro. Effect on cell-interactive properties. Diabetes 30: 875–878
12. Witztum SL, Mahoney EM, Branks MJ, Fisher M, Elam R, Steinberg D (1982) Nonenzymatic glycosylation of low density lipoprotein alter its biological activity. Diabetes 31: 283–291
13. Lorenzi M, Cagliero E, Markey B, Henriksen T, Wiztzum JL, Sanpietro T (1984) Interaction of human endothelial cells with elevated glucose concentrations and native and glycosylated low density lipoproteins. Diabetologia 26: 218–222
14. Stevens VS, Rouzer CA, Monnier VM, Cerami A (1978) Diabetic cataract formation: role of glycosylation of lens crystallins. Proc Natl Acad Sci USA 75: 2918–2922

15. Monnier UM, Cerami A (1982) Non enzymatic glycosylation and browning in diabetes and aging: studies on lens proteins. Diabetes 31: 57–63
16. Liang JN, Hershorin LL, Chylack LT Jr (1986) Non enzymatic glycosylation in human diabetic lens crystallins. Diabetologia 29: 225–228
17. Schnider SL, Kohn RR (1980) Glycosylation of human collagen in aging and diabetes mellitus. J Clin Invest 66: 1179–1181
18. Schnider SL, Kohn RR (1981) Effect of age and diabetes mellitus on the solubility and nonenzymatic glycosylation of human skin collagen. J Clin Invest 67: 1630–1635
19. Buckingham BA, Uitto J, Sandborg C, Keens T, Kaufmann F, Landing B (1981) Scleroderma-like syndrome and non-enzymatic glucosylation of collagen in children with poorly controlled insulin dependent diabetes (IDDM). Pediatr Res 15 (part 2): 626 (Abstract)
20. Monnier UM, Kohn RR, Cerami A (1984) Accelerated age-related browning of human collagen in diabetes mellitus. Proc Natl Acad Sci USA 81: 583–587
21. Yue DK, McLennan S, Delbridge L, Handelsman DJ, Reeve T, Turtle JR (1983) The thermal stability of collagen in diabetic rats: correlation with severity of diabetes and non-enzymatic glycosylation. Diabetologia 24: 282–285
22. Vlassara H, Brownlee M, Cerami A (1981) Non enzymatic glycosylation of peripheral nerve proteins in diabetes mellitus. Proc Natl Acad Sci USA 78: 5190–5192
23. Vlassara H, Brownless M, Cerami A (1983) Excessive non-enzymatic glycosylation of peripheral and central nervous system myelin components in diabetic rats. Diabetes 32: 670–674
24. Cohen MP, Urdanivia E, Surma M, Wu VY (1980) Increased glycosylation of glomerular basement membrane collagen in diabetes. Biochem Biophys Res Commun 95: 765–769
25. Uitto J, Grant CA, Perejda AJ, Rowald E, Williamson JR (1980) Glycosylation of human glomerular basement membrane collagen (GBMC): increased non-enzymatic glycosylation in diabetes. Fed Proc 39: 1972–1975
26. Osterby R (1972) Morphometric studies on the peripheral glomerular basement membrane in early juvenile diabetes. I. Development of initial basement membrane thickening. Diabetologia 8: 84–92
27. Brown DM, Steffes MW, Thibert P, Mauer SM (1983) Glomerular manifestations of diabetes in the BB rat. Metabolism 81: 131–135
28. Westberg G (1980) Diabetic nephropathy. Pathogenesis and prevention. Acta Endocrinol 94 (Suppl 238): 85–101
29. Michael AF, Brown DM (1981) Increased concentration of albumin in kidney basement membrane in diabetes mellitus. Diabetes 30: 843–846
30. Westberg G, Michael AF (1972) Immunohistopathology of diabetic glomerular sclerosis. Diabetes 21: 163–174
31. Greenspon SA, Krakower CA (1950) Direct evidence for the antigenicity of the glomeruli in the production of nephrotoxic serum. Arch Pathol 49: 291–297
32. Spiro GR (1967) Studies on the renal glomerular basement membrane. Preparation and chemical composition. J Biol Chem 242: 1915–1922
33. Carlson EC, Brendel K, Hjelle JT, Meezan E (1978) Ultrastructural and biochemical analyses of isolated basement membranes from kidney glomeruli and tubules and brain and retinal microvessels. J Ultrastruct Res 62: 26–53
34. Sensi M, Tanzi P, Bruno MR, Pozzilli P, Mancuso M, Gambardella S, Di Mario U, Andreani D (1987) Binding of plasma proteins on normal human glomerular basement membrane non-enzymatically glycosylated in vitro (submitted for publication)
35. Higgins PJ, Bunn HF (1981) Kinetic analysis of the nonenzymatic glycosylation of hemoglobin. J Biol Chem 256: 5204–5028

36. Monnier VM, Cerami A (1983) Nonenzymatic glycosylation and browning of proteins in vivo. In: Waller GR, Flather MS (eds) The Maillard reaction in foods and nutrition. American Chemical Society Symposium Series, No 215, Washington DC, pp 431–439
37. Brownlee M, Vlassara H, Cerami A (1984) Nonenzymatic glycosylation and the pathogenesis of diabetic complications. Ann Intern Med 101: 527–537
38. Kennedy A, Mehe TD, Elder E, Varghese M, Merimee TJ (1982) Nonenzymatic glycosylation of serum and plasma proteins. Diabetes 31 (Suppl): 52–56
39. Kohn RR, Schnider SL (1982) Glycosylation of human collagen. Diabetes 31 (Suppl): 47–51
40. Sensi M, Bruno MR, Pozzilli P (1987) In vitro inhibition of non-enzymatic glycosylation induced by aspirin. Med Sci Res 15: 99–100
41. Sensi M, Tanzi P, Bruno MR, Mancuso M, Andreani D (1987) Human glomerular basement membrane: altered binding characteristics following in vitro non-enzymatic glycosylation. Ann NY Acad Sci (in press)
42. Brownlee M, Pongor A, Cerami A (1983) Covalent attachment of soluble proteins by nonenzymatically glycosylated collagen. J Exp Med 158: 1739–1744
43. Fluckiger R, Winterhalter KH (1976) In vitro synthesis of $HbA_1c$. FEBS Lett 71: 356–360
44. Cohen MP, Urdanivia E, Surma M, Ciborowski CJ (1981) Nonenzymatic glycosylation of basement membranes. In vitro studies. Diabetes 30: 367–371
45. Means GE, Min Kun Chang (1982) Nonenzymatic glycosylation of proteins. Structure and function change. Diabetes 31 (Suppl): 1–4
46. Viberti G, Keen H (1983) The patterns of proteinuria in diabetes mellitus. Diabetes 33: 686–692
47. Brenner BM, Hostetter TH, Humes HD (1978) The molecular basis of proteinuria of glomerular origin. N Engl J Med 298: 826
48. Ghiggieri GM, Candiano G, Delfino G, Bianchini F, Queirolo C (1984) Glycosyl albumin and diabetic microalbuminuria: demonstration of an altered renal handling. Kidney Int 25: 565–570
49. Williams SK, Siegal RK (1985) Preferential transport of non-enzymatically glycosylated ferritin across the kidney glomerular. Kidney Int 29: 146–157
50. Jovanovic L, Peterson CM (1981) The clinical utility of glycosylated hemoglobin. Am J Med 70: 331–338
51. Shaklai N, Garlich RL, Bunn HF (1984) Non-enzymatic glycosylation of human serum albumin alters its conformation and function. J Biol Chem 259: 3812–3817
52. Carnivet J, Cruz A, Moreau-Lelande H (1979) Biochemical abnormalities of human diabetic glomerular basement membrane. Metabolism 28: 1206–1210
53. Williamson JR, Kilo C (1983) Extracellular matrix changes in diabetes mellitus. In: Wiliam JR, Kilo C (eds) Proceedings of the comparative pathobiology of age-related diseases. Alan R Liss, New York
54. Reynolds TM (1963) Chemistry of nonenzymatic browning. I. Adv Food Res 12: 1–52
55. Reynolds TM (1965) Chemistry of nonenzymatic browning. II. Adv Food Res 14: 167–183
56. Couser WG, Salant DJ (1980) In situ immune complex formation and glomerular injury. Kidney Int 17: 1
57. Williamson JR, Kilo C (1984) Pathogenetic mechanisms of diabetic microvascular disease. In: Andreani D, Di Mario U, Federlin KF, Heding LG (eds) Immunology in diabetes. Kimpton Medical Publications, London and Edinburgh, pp 245–254
58. Rohrbach DH, Hanel JR, Kleinman HK, Martin GR (1982) Alterations in basement membrane (heparan sulphate) proteoglycans in diabetic mice. Diabetes 31: 185–188
59. Bassiouny AR, Rosenberg H, McDonald TL (1983) Glycosylated collagen is antigenic.

Diabetes 32: 1182–1184

60. Kato Y Matsuda, Watanabe K, Nakamura R (1985) Alteration of ovalbumin immunogenic activity by glycosylation through the Maillard reaction. Agric Biol Chem 49: 423–427
61. Curtiss LK, Witztum JL (1983) A novel method for generating region-specific monoclonal antibodies to modified protein: application to the identification of human glucosylated low density lipoproteins. J Clin Invest 72: 1427–1438
62. Nakayama H, Taneda S, Manda N, Aoki S, Komori K, Kuroda Y, Misawa K, Tsushima S, Nakagawa S (1986) Radioimmunoassay for nonenzymatically glycated protein in human serum. Clin Chim Acta 158: 293–299
63. Hawkins D, Pinckard RN, Crawford IP, Farr RS (1969) Structural changes in human serum albumin induced by ingestion of acetylsalicylic acid. J Clin Invest 48: 536–542
64. Rendell M, Nierenberg J, Brannan C, Velentine JL, Stephen PM, Dodds S, Mercer P, Smith PK, Walder J (1986) Inhibition of glycation of albumin and hemoglobin by acetylation in vitro and in vivo. J Lab Clin Med 108: 286–293
65. Brownlee M, Vlassara H, Kooney A, Ulrich P, Cerami A (1986) Aminoguanidine prevents diabetes-induced arterial wall protein cross-linking. Science 232: 1629–1632

Diabetic Complications: Early Diagnosis and Treatment
Edited by D. Andreani, G. Crepaldi, U. Di Mario and G. Pozza


CHAPTER 23

# *Influence of Metabolic Control on the Development of Diabetic Nephropathy*

S. Gambardella, G. Pugliese and D. Andreani
*Cattedra di Endocrinologia 1, Clinica Medica 2, University of Rome 'La Sapienza', Italy*

The question of whether diabetic complications are correlated to metabolic control has been a subject of controversy for many years. The lack of overt microvascular lesions in some poorly controlled diabetic patients and the presence of advanced renal and/or retinal abnormalities in a few patients, both at onset and in others without known diabetes, have raised the possibility that microangiopathy may develop independently of metabolic derangement in a number of patients (1,2).

Furthermore, reports of the increased width of the capillary basement membrane in quadriceps muscle of euglycemic glucose-tolerant offspring of diabetic patients and in non-diabetic HLA-DR4 parents of Type 1 diabetic subjects (3,4) have suggested that microangiopathy and diabetes may be inherited together due to a common genetic background, although they may subsequently be expressed independently.

This view was confuted on the basis of several observations which demonstrated that hyperglycemia and microangiopathic changes are closely linked. The cited reports of complications in the absence of diabetes are still scarce; on the other hand, populations with a high incidence of hyperglycemia, like the Pima Indians (5), show increased risks of developing glomerulosclerosis and retinopathy in correlation to the oral glucose tolerance test (OGTT) (6). Nevertheless, a wide variation can be observed in the individual patient regarding the relationship between the degree of metabolic control and the appearance and development of microangiopathic complications. Some cases of rapid onset and development have been defined as 'malignant' microangiopathy (7) and a correlation with poor control has been surmised. Both clinical and experimental studies have been performed in order to clarify the influence of chronic hyperglycemia on the development of diabetic nephropathy and to investigate the mechanisms through which metabolic factors can induce small vessel damage.

Unfortunately, all the approaches that have been used possess varying degrees of limitation. Human studies are extremely difficult to perform because of the long latency period which precedes the appearance of proteinuria, that follows structural abnormalities after many years. In animal models, on the other hand, it is not possible to observe advanced lesions which are identical to those in man, and in vitro models are not capable of reproducing exact in vivo conditions.

## CLINICAL STUDIES

The role of metabolic control in the development of diabetic nephropathy has been investigated in man by means of both retrospective and prospective studies.

### Retrospective Studies

These studies have allowed the evaluation of large populations over long periods of time, but have at the same time revealed several shortcomings: the non-random distribution of patients in different groups according to the degree of control, and the lack of a reliable long-term control index, such as $HbA_{1c}$, which has only recently been introduced into clinical practice. In spite of these limitations, the studies have shown interesting results which suggest a correlation between metabolic control and kidney damage.

In the study performed by Johnson (8), patients treated with one daily injection of intermediate-acting insulin (poorly controlled) showed a higher frequency of nephropathy and other complications than patients treated with multiple injections of regular insulin (better controlled), despite the shorter duration of diabetes.

The extensive study carried out by Pirart (9) yielded three main findings: (1) the complications were inversely correlated with the degree of metabolic control; (2) the complications increased with the duration of the disease; (3) the three major complications (nephropathy, retinopathy and neuropathy) tended to occur in the same patients.

The study performed at the Joslin Clinic (10) obtained the same results. In addition, it showed that complications developed even in the group with good metabolic control, albeit at a low frequency (10–15%) and, conversely, in the poorly controlled group there were patients who were free from microangiopathic abnormalities after 20 years of the disease.

These findings underline the importance of other factors, in addition to metabolic derangements, in the development of diabetic complications. Unfortunately, all attempts to identify these factors have failed so far, and, in particular, the hypothesis of genetic susceptibility has not been verified; in fact, the reported link between HLA-DR4 (11) and retinopathy has been disproved.

### Prospective Studies

These are more controlled than retrospective studies and are usually based on continuous subcutaneous insulin infusion (CSII) which allows near normoglycemia to be attained in contrast to conventional therapy.

Strict glycemic control with CSII for up to 24 months in 6 patients with overt diabetic nephropathy (dip-stick positive) had no effect on the rate of decline of glomerular filtration rate (GFR) or on the fractional clearance of albumin and IgG compared with the run-in period before the start of strict control or with 6 conventionally-treated control subjects (12,13). An earlier uncontrolled study also confirmed the lack of effect of strict glycemic control on diabetic nephropathy (14). Even at the earlier stage of intermittent proteinuria, strict glycemic control had no effect (15), thus suggesting that the destructive process in the kidney becomes self-perpetuating and independent of the underlying diabetic abnormalities that initiate it. However, Hasslacher et al. (16) found a negative correlation in 52 sequentially recruited Type 1 diabetic patients between median postprandial blood glucose levels and median duration of diabetes until the onset of persistent proteinuria. The delay between the onset of proteinuria and the increase in serum creatinine concentrations was also negatively correlated with blood glucose levels. Once serum creatinine levels were elevated, metabolic control was demonstrated to have no effect at this stage of nephropathy.

Several longitudinal studies have recently suggested that the increased excretion of urinary albumin, so-called microalbuminuria which does not reach the level of clinical albuminuria, seems to be the most powerful indicator of the later stages of renal disease. Strict control using CSII or multiple insulin injections can reduce and in many cases normalize microalbuminuria (17–20). However, the preliminary results of a prospective randomized study of patients with persistent microalbuminuria (20–200 μg/min) have failed to show that metabolic control is able to lower albuminuria (21), thus suggesting that this stage (also termed 'incipient' nephropathy) may reflect the earlier phase of progressive diabetic nephropathy.

In conclusion, there is a need for prospective studies of diabetic patients prior to the onset of complications whose duration of the disease is long enough to cover the latency period that precedes the appearance of proteinuria. These studies are very difficult to perform but seem to be the only means of evaluating the importance of metabolic control on the development of diabetic nephropathy.

## EXPERIMENTAL STUDIES

Experimental evidence strongly suggests that metabolic control plays a major role in the genesis of diabetic nephropathy. The Minnesota group have shown that diabetic glomerulopathy develops in normal kidneys transplanted into diabetic rats (22). Islet-cell transplantation in highly inbred diabetic Lewis rats results in a marked reduction of immunofluorescence staining and mesangial volume (23). Moreover, meticulous glycemic control with insulin in rats with streptozotocin-induced diabetes early in the course of the disease prevents the development of glomerular lesions and the increase in urinary albumin excretion (24).

These findings are confirmed by the few experimental studies performed in vivo in man. Normal kidneys transplanted into human diabetic recipients develop hyaline arteriolar lesions in all renal biopsies in under 4 years (25). The report of the transplantation into non-diabetic recipients of kidneys taken from patients showing clinical signs of diabetic nephropathy caused much controversy. However, renal biopsies performed 7 months after the transplants indicated that mesangial expansion and glomerular basement membrane (GBM) thickness were almost completely reversed (26).

## POSSIBLE MECHANISMS

The widely accepted notion that metabolic control is a major factor in the development of the microangiopathic complications of diabetes has prompted research into the mechanism(s) through which chronic hyperglycemia triggers the pathogenetic sequence leading to small vessel lesions. Among other possible factors, the metabolic pathways followed by excessive glucose in tissues seem to be of major importance.

The first metabolic pathway is the non-enzymatic glycosylation of proteins (27,28), which is the subject of the chapter by Di Mario et al. In this context, it is worthwhile underlining that glycosylated GBM shows increased trapping of plasma proteins and that glycosylated collagen exhibits increased resistance to digestion because of the extensive intramolecular cross-linking, together with enhanced immunogenicity (29). Furthermore, glycosylated circulating macromolecules can only be cleared from tissues with difficulty.

The second metabolic pathway is the degradation of glucose into sorbitol by aldose reductase, whose activity is enhanced by increased substrate availability; sorbitol then accumulates in tissues due to the slow rate of conversion to fructose by sorbitol dehydrogenase. This mechanism has been shown to be of pathogenetic importance in peripheral neuropathy (30) and cataract (31) through the decrease in myoinositol content and/or the reduction of ATPase activity. Recently, convincing evidence has been reported on the role of polyol accumulation in the retina (32), as well as in the kidney (32,33). An aldose reductase activity has been demonstrated at the glomerular level (34) and has been found to be increased in isolated glomeruli from diabetic rats, together with a high polyol content and reduced ATPase activity (35). Furthermore, the use of aldose reductase inhibitors was able to prevent hyperfiltration (36) and proteinuria (37) in diabetic rats. To date no results of human studies are available.

In addition to the importance of the derangement of glucose metabolism, hemodynamic changes have been reported to characterize the early stage of Type 1 diabetes. Moreover, a few days of strict insulin control are able to normalize GFR and renal plasma flow (RPF) (38), as well as proteinuria (39), which seem dependent on hemodynamic factors. Hemodynamic changes have been postulated to play an important part in the initiation and progress of diabetic nephropathy (40) following the reports of several clinical and experimental studies that have stressed the role of increased intraglomerular pressure in glomerulosclerosis (41). These functional alterations may probably be followed by histological changes brought about by several factors, including protein and immunocomplex deposition, and clotting factors.

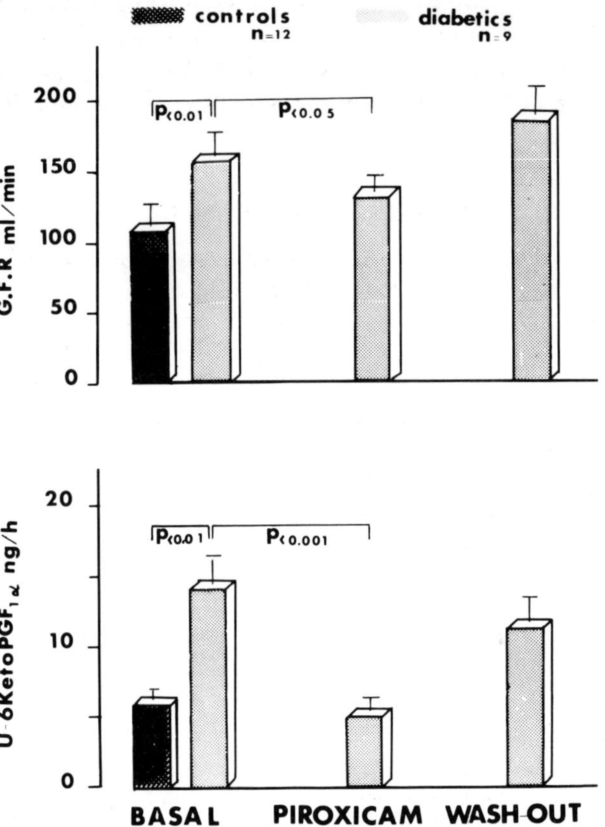


Figure 1. Basal values of 6-keto $PGF_{1\alpha}$ (the stable metabolite of prostacyclin) and GFR (measured as clearance of $^{99m}$Tc-DTPA) were significantly higher in untreated newly diagnosed Type 1 diabetic patients than in control subjects. After 1 week of piroxicam treatment (an inhibitor of cyclo-oxygenase activity) both GFR and 6-keto $PGF_{1\alpha}$ were significantly reduced.

Renal hyperfiltration has been attributed both to increased levels of growth hormone (42–44) and glucagon (45,46), and to hyperglycemia per se (47). Recent evidence seems also to involve other factors which normally modulate renal microcirculation, such as catecholamines, angiotensin and prostaglandins (PG). In particular, increased renal synthesis of vasodilating $PGE_2$ and $PGI_2$ has been shown in rats (48,49) and humans (50) respectively, whereas inhibition induced a decrease in GFR (51,52) (Figure 1). In addition, indomethacin prevented the glucose-induced increase of RPF in the isolated perfused rat kidney (53), adding further evidence to the relationship between high glucose levels, prostaglandins and hemodynamic changes.

In conclusion, if the hypothesis regarding the involvement of hemodynamic factors in the genesis of nephropathy were to be satisfactorily demonstrated, the influence of metabolic control on hyperfiltration would represent one of the principal starting mechanisms through which hyperglycemia induces kidney damage. Nevertheless, non-enzymatic glycosylation and polyol accumulation may play a role in the pathogenetic sequence leading to nephropathy and new evidence on this aspect is expected in the future.

## REFERENCES


1. Harrington AR, Hare HG, Chambers WN, Vattin H (1966) Nodular glomerulosclerosis suspected during life in a patient without demonstrable diabetes mellitus. N Engl J Med 275: 206–208
2. Strauss FG, Argy WG, Screiner GE (1971) Diabetic glomerulosclerosis in the absence of glucose intolerance. Ann Intern Med 75: 239–242
3. Siperstein MD, Unger RH, Madison LL (1968) Studies of muscle capillary basement membranes in normal subjects, diabetic and prediabetic patients. J Clin Invest 47: 1973–1999
4. Marks JF, Raskin P, Stastny P (1981) Increased capillary basement membrane width in parents of children with Type 1 diabetes mellitus. Association with HLA-DR4. Diabetes 30: 475–480
5. Kamenetzky SA, Bennett PH, Dippe SE, Miller M, LeCompte PM (1974) A clinical and histologic study of diabetic nephropathy in the Pima Indians. Diabetes 23: 61–68
6. Pettitt DJ, Knowler WC, Lisse JR, Bennet PH (1980) Development of retinopathy and proteinuria in relation to plasma glucose concentrations in Pima Indians. Lancet ii: 1050–1052
7. Andreani D (1980) Malignant microangiopathy. Diabetologia 18: 255
8. Johnson S (1960) Retinopathy and nephropathy in diabetes mellitus: comparison of the effects of two forms of treatment. Diabetes 9: 1
9. Pirart J (1978) Diabetes and its degenerative complications, a prospective study of 4400 patients observed between 1947 and 1973. Diabetes Care 1: 168
10. Keiding NR, Root HF, Marble A (1952) Importance of control of diabetes in prevention of vascular complications. J Am Med Assoc 150: 964
11. Dornan TL, Ting A, McPherson CK, Mann JI, Turner RC, Morris PJ (1982) Genetic susceptibility to the development of retinopathy in insulin-dependent diabetics. Diabetes 31: 226
12. Bending JJ, Pickup JC, Viberti GC, Keen H (1984) Glycemic control in diabetic nephropathy. Br Med J 288: 1187–1191
13. Viberti GC, Bilous RW, Mackintosh D, Bending JJ, Keen H (1983) Long term correction of hyperglycemia and progression of renal failure in insulin-dependent diabetes. Br Med J 286: 598–621
14. Tamborlane MV, Puklen JE, Bergamen M, Verdon KL, Rudolf MC, Felig P, Genel M, Sherwin R (1982) Long term improvement of metabolic control with insulin pump does

not reverse diabetic microangiopathy. Diabetes Care 5 (Suppl 1): 58–64

15. Bending JJ, Viberti GC, Watkins PJ, Keen H (1986) Intermittent clinical proteinuria and renal function in diabetes: evolution and the effect of glycemic control. Br Med J 292: 83–86
16. Hasslacher CH, Stech W, Wahl P, Ritz E (1985) Blood pressure and metabolic control as risk factors for nephropathy in Type 1 (insulin-dependent) diabetes. Diabetologia 28: 6
17. Steno Study Group (1982) Effect of 6 months of strict metabolic control in eye and kidney function in insulin dependent diabetics with background retinopathy. Lancet: 121–123
18. Beck-Nielsen H, Richelsen B, Mogensen CE, Olsen T, Ehlers N, Nielsen CB, Charles P (1985) Effect of insulin pump treatment for one year on renal function and retinal morphology in patients with IDDM. Diabetes Care 8: 585–589
19. The Kroc Collaborative Study Group (1984) Blood glucose control and the evolution of diabetic retinopathy and albuminuria. A preliminary multicenter trial. N Engl J Med 311: 365–372
20. Wiseman MJ, Saunders AJ, Keen H, Viberti GC (1985) Effect of blood glucose control on increased glomerular filtration rate and kidney size in insulin-dependent diabetes. N Engl J Med 312: 617–621
21. Feldt-Rasmussen B, Mathiesen ER, Hegedus L, Deckert T (1986) Kidney function during 12 months of strict metabolic control in insulin-dependent diabetic patients with incipient nephropathy. N Engl J Med 314: 665–670
22. Lee CS, Mauer SM, Brown DH, Sutherland ER, Michael AF, Najarian JS (1974) Renal transplantation in diabetes mellitus in rats. J Exp Med 139: 793–800
23. Steffes MW, Brown DM, Basgen JM, Mauer SM (1980) Amelioration of mesangial volume and surface alterations following islet transplantation in diabetic rats. Diabetes 29: 509–515
24. Mauer SM, Brown DM, Matas AJ, Steffes MW (1978) Effects of pancreatic islet transplantation on the increased urinary albumin excretion rates in intact and unnephrectomized rats with diabetes mellitus. Diabetes 27: 959–964
25. Mauer SM, Barbosa J, Vernier RL, Kjellsatrand CM, Buselmeier TJ, Simmons RL, Najaran JD, Goetz FC (1976) Development of diabetic vascular lesions in normal kidney transplanted into patients with diabetes mellitus. N Engl J Med 295: 916–920
26. Abouna GM, Kremer GD, Daddah SK, Al-Adnani MS, Kunar SA, Kusmag G (1983) Reversal of diabetic nephropathy in human cadaveric kidneys after transplantation into non-diabetic recipients. Lancet ii: 1274–1276
27. Brownleee M, Vlassara H, Cerami A (1984) Non-enzymatic glycosylation and the pathogenesis of diabetic complications. Ann Intern Med 101: 527–537
28. Sensi M, Tanzi P, Bruno MR, Pozzilli P, Di Mario U, Andreani D (1985) Binding properties of glycosylated human glomerular basement membrane. Diabetes Res Clin Pract Suppl 1: 810
29. Bassiouny AR, Rosenberg H, McDonald TL (1983) Glycosylated collagen is antigenic. Diabetes 32: 482–484
30. Finegold D, Lattimer SA, Nolle S, Bernstein M, Greene DA (1983) Polyol pathway activity and myoinositol metabolism. A suggested relationship in the pathogenesis of diabetic neuropathy. Diabetes 32: 988–992
31. Kinoshita JH, Fukushi S, Kodor P, Merola LO (1979) Aldose reductase in diabetic complications of the eye. Metabolism 28: 462–469
32. Beyer-Mears A, Ku L, Cohen MP (1984) Glomerular polyol accumulation in diabetes and its prevention by oral sorbinil. Diabetes 33: 604–607
33. Chandler HL, Shannon WA, De Santis L (1984) Prevention of retinal capillary basement

membrane thickening in diabetic rats by aldose reductase inhibitors. Invest Ophthalmol Vis Sci 25 (Suppl): 159
34. Ludvigson HA, Sorensen RL (1980) Immunohistochemical localization of aldose reductase. Diabetes 29: 450–459
35. Cohen HP, Dasmahapatra A, Shapiro E (1985) Reduced glomerular sodium/potassium adenosin triphosphatase activity in acute streptozotocin diabetes and its prevention by oral sorbinil. Diabetes 34: 1071–1074
36. Goldfarb S, Simmons DA, Kern E (1986) Amelioration of glomerular hyperfiltration in acute experimental diabetes by dietary myoinsoitol and by an aldose reductase inhibitor. Clin Res 34: 725A
37. Beyer-Mears A, Varagiannis E, Cruz E (1985) Effect of sorbinil on reversal of proteinuira. Diabetes 34 (Suppl 1): 101A
38. Christiansen JS, Gammelgaard T, Tronier B, Svendsen PA, Parving HH (1982) Kidney function and size in diabetics before and during initial insulin treatment. Kidney Int 21: 683–688
39. Viberti GC, Pickup JC, Jarret RJ, Keen H (1979) Effect of control of blood glucose on urinary excretion of albumin and beta 2-microglobulin in insulin-dependent diabetes. N Engl J Med 300: 638–641
40. Thomas H, Rennke HG, Brenner BM (1982) The case for intrarenal hypertension in the intial and progression of diabetic and other glomerulopathies. Am J Med 72: 375–380
41. Parving HH, Viberti GC, Kenn H, Christiansen JS, Lesser NA (1983) Hemodynamic factors in the genesis of diabetic microangiopathy. Metabolism 32: 943
42. Ikkos D, Luft R, Gemzell CA (1954) The effect of human growth hormone in man. Acta Endocrinol 32: 341–361
43. Christiansen JS, Gammelgaard J, Frandsen M, Orskov H, Parving HH (1982) Kidney function and size in Type 1 diabetic patients before and during growth hormone administration for one week. Diabetologia 22: 333–337
44. Christiansen JS, Gammelgaard J, Orskov H, Andersen AR, Telmer S, Parving HH (1981) Kidney function and size in normal subjects before and during growth hormone administration for one week. Eur J Clin Invest 11: 487–490
45. Parving HH, Noer I, Kehlet H, Mogensen CE, Svendsen PA, Heding LG (1977) The effect of short-term glucagon infusion on kidney function in normal man. Diabetologia 13: 323–325
46. Parving HH, Christiansen JS, Noer I, Tronier B, Mogensen CE (1980) The effect of glucagon infusion on kidney function in short-term insulin-dependent juvenile diabetics. Diabetolgia 19: 350–354
47. Christiansen JS, Frandsen M, Parving HH (1981) Effect of intravenous glucose infusion on renal function in normal man and in insulin-dependent diabetes. Diabetologia 21: 368
48. Schambelan M, Blake J, Sraer S, Bens M, Niver MP, Wahbe F (1985) Increased prostaglandin production by glomeruli isolated from rats with streptozoctocin-induced diabetes. J Clin Invest 75: 404
49. Rogers SP, Larkins RG (1982) Production of 6-oxo-prostaglandin F1 and E2 by isolated glomeruli from normal and diabetic rats. Br Med J 284: 1215–1217
50. Gambardella S, Puliese G, Napoli A, Morano S, Pietravalle P, Pugliese F, Stirati G, Andreani D (1986) Urinary excretion of prostaglandins and renal hemodynamics in Type 1 (insulin-dependent) diabetes at onset: effect of piroxicam. Diabetologia 29: 539A
51. Kich-Jensen P (1985) Modulating factors of renal hemodynamics in experimental diabetes. Diabetic Nephropathy 4: 17
52. Craven PA, De Robertis FR (1985) Glomerular Prostaglandins (PG) in the hyper-

filtration (H) of early diabetes. Kidney Int 28: 332A
53. Kasike BL, O'Donnel MP, Keane WF (1985) Glucose induced increases in renal hemodynamic function. Possible modulation by renal prostaglandins. Diabetes 34: 360–364

Diabetic Complications: Early Diagnosis and Treatment
Edited by D. Andreani, G. Crepaldi, U. Di Mario and G. Pozza


# CHAPTER 24

# *Proteinuria, an Indicator of Malignant Angiopathy*

T. Deckert, B. Feldt-Rasmussen, K. Borch-Johnsen, T. Jensen,
L. Bent-Hansen and A. Kofoed-Enevoldsen
*Steno Memorial Hospital, Gentofte, Denmark*

The prognosis of Type 1 (insulin-dependent) diabetes mellitus has improved considerably during the last 20 years. Thus, a study performed at the Steno Memorial Hospital, which included about 20% of insulin-dependent diabetic patients of juvenile onset in Denmark, demonstrated that the relative mortality among patients with diabetes onset after 1952 was 30–40% lower compared to patients who had developed the disease between 1933 and 1942 (1). The improved survival was due to a lower incidence of clinical nephropathy (2). The mortality rate of diabetic patients aged about 25 years is, however, still about 10 times higher compared with that of the background population (1). It may be demonstrated that the severity of these figures is mainly due to the excessively high mortality among patients with proteinuria. Patients not developing proteinuria have a near normal survival rate (3).

## Malignant Angiopathy

Proteinuria is associated not only with high mortality but also with severely invaliding non-renal complications. Not only do serum creatinine and blood pressure increase slowly in these patients, but also higher levels of fibrinogen and blood lipids are found in patients with clinical nephropathy (4). Patients with persistent proteinuria are also characterized by a ten-fold increase in cardiovascular mortality, an eight-fold increase in the cumulative incidence of coronary heart disease and a ten-fold increase in the incidence of proliferative retinopathy (5,6). Micro- and macrovascular complications develop simultaneously. However, hypertension, lipids, fibrinogen, free plasma insulin and smoking habits cannot explain the ten-fold increase in cardiovascular mortality in patients with proteinuria. Therefore another pathogenetic link between micro- and macroangiopathy may be surmised. This link is probably associated with increased endothelial permeability (7). Since micro- and macroangiopathic complications develop simultaneously, since there seems to be a non-renal pathogenetic link between these complications, and since these patients suffer not only from impaired renal function but also from widespread non-renal lesions, it is preferable to speak of malignant angiopathy instead of clinical nephropathy in patients with persistent proteinuria. Thus, persistent proteinuria indicates malignant angiopathy.

## Benign Angiopathy

In addition, those patients who escape the development of persistent proteinuria will after some years reveal morphological signs of angiopathy, such as increased basement membrane thickness, retinal microaneurysms, increased mesangium volume density, and media calcification of larger vessels. As long as these alterations do not progress to malignant angiopathy, they seem to be of no clinical importance, since patients can live with these alterations for more than 40 years without becoming invalided (8). Therefore, it is preferable to speak of benign angiopathy in these patients.

## The Onset of Persistent Proteinuria

The onset of proteinuria (>0.5 g protein per 24 h) is a late stage in the development of malignant angiopathy, and in fact is the last stage of a long-term process. From studies of the incidence of proteinuria and from prospective studies of microalbuminuric patients it has been calculated that the process of increased glomerular leakage of albumin starts at the onset of diabetes in those patients (45%) who later develop persistent proteinuria (9). Since the increase in urinary albumin excretion (UAE) is exponential, 15–25%/year, these patients will enter the range of microalbuminuria (30–300 mg albumin per 24 h) about 6 years after the onset of diabetes. During the next 10 years these patients can be identified by repeated measurements of UAE, and over this period—many years prior to the onset of persistent proteinuria—lipids, fibrinogen and blood pressure will gradually increase, plasma albumin will decrease, and the transcapillary escape rate of albumin and fibrinogen will gradually rise (10), possibly leading to increased extravascular coagulation (11). The incidence of retinopathy also increases during this period to a level ten times higher than in patients of similar age, blood pressure and diabetes duration (6).

## Identification and Therapy

The identification of patients with persistent microalbuminuria appears to be important for the following reasons. Firstly, the retina should be examined much more frequently in these patients than in patients with normo-albuminuria. Indeed, since blindness can be prevented by photocoagulation and since the incidence of proliferative retinopathy is much higher in this group of patients compared to any other group of diabetic patients, candidates for laser treatment can be identified early. Secondly, blood pressure should be measured much more frequently since hypertension is much more commonplace in this group of young patients (5,6). Finally patients with persistent microalbuminuria should be identified because progression to persistent proteinuria can be prevented by strict metabolic control.

Table 1. Clinical data of 51 patients with IDDM and persistent microalbuminuria included in the prospective Steno studies I + II (mean or median and range)

| | CSII | CIT |
|---|---|---|
| Number of patients | 26 (15 M) | 25 (13 M) |
| Age (years) | 31.7 (17–48) | 30.4 (18–47) |
| Duration (years) | 15.9 (10–26) | 16.3 (5–27) |
| $HbA_{1c}$ | 9.6 (6.6–13.6) | 9.2 (7.0–11.7) |
| GFR (ml/min/1.73 $m^2$) | 116 (81–169) | 116 (75–170) |
| Blood pressure (mmHg) | 130 (102–160) | 130 (110–153) |
| | 83 (73–90) | 84 (65–110) |
| Urinary albumin (median mg/24 h) | 126 (30–300) | 124 (30–300) |

CSII = continuous subcutaneous insulin infusion, CIT = conventional insulin treatment, GFR = glomerular filtration rate.

A recently published prospective randomized study of patients with persistent microalbuminuria demonstrated that strict metabolic control given by continuous subcutaneous insulin infusion (CSII) stopped the increase in UAE (12), thus confirming our earlier results (13). In both these studies, which were performed at the Steno Memorial Hospital, 51 patients with persistent microalbuminuria were recruited. After allocating them either to CSII or conventional insulin treatment, the two groups were well matched for age, diabetes duration, hemoglobin $A_{1c}$ at the onset of the study, glomerular filtration rate (GFR) and blood pressure (Table 1). The levels of UAE at the onset of the study were nearly identical. After 2 years of treatment only 1 out of 26 patients in the CSII group developed persistent proteinuria, whereas 10 patients out of 25 in the control group treated with conventional therapy progressed to persistent proteinuria ($2p<0.004$). Blood pressure increased significantly in the conventionally treated group, but was unchanged in the CSII group (Table 2). UalbV decreased significantly from 126 to 106 in the CSII group and more than doubled in the conventionally treated group. Fractional IgG clearance, which was only studied in the second Steno study, increased significantly in the pump-treated patients (Table 3). Since the mean level of $HbA_{1c}$ during the experimental period was the only factor which differed significantly between the two groups (7.28 ± 0.80% and 8.95 ± 1.34%, $p<0.00001$ for CSII and conventionally treated patients, respectively) near normalization of blood glucose in microalbuminuric patients is held to be important for the prevention of malignant angiopathy. Whether near normalization of blood glucose in these patients will also reduce the incidence of proliferative retinopathy and of coronary heart disease awaits further clarification.

Table 2. Incipient nephropathy, Steno I + II: blood pressure (mmHg)

| | Before | After 24 months | |
|---|---|---|---|
| CSII ($n$ = 26) | 130/83 | 132/84 | n.s. |
| CIT ($n$ = 25) | 130/84 | 135/89 | $p < 0.05$ |

Table 3. Incipient nephropathy, Steno II: fractional IgG clearance × $10^{-6}$ median (mean)

| | Before | After 24 months | |
|---|---|---|---|
| CSII ($n$ = 18) | 2.65 (5.57) | 2.30 (2.71) | 2 < 0.05 |
| CIT ($n$ = 17) | 2.30 (4.11) | 3.10 (7.78) | 2 < 0.02 |

## REFERENCES


1. Borch-Johnsen K, Kreiner S, Deckert T (1986) Mortality of Type 1 (insulin-dependent) diabetes mellitus in Denmark: a study of relative mortality in 2930 Danish Type 1 diabetic patients diagnosed from 1933 to 1972. Diabetologia 29: 767–772
2. Kofoed-Enevoldsen A, Borch-Johnsen K, Kreiner S, Nerup J, Deckert T (1987) Declining incidence of persistent proteinuria in Type 1 (insulin-dependent) diabetic patients in Denmark. Diabetes (in press)
3. Borch-Johnsen K, Andersen PK, Deckert T (1985) The effect of protcinuria on relative mortality in Type 1 (insulin-dependent) diabetes mellitus. Diabetologia 28: 590–596
4. Valdorf-Hansen F, Jensen T, Borch-Johnsen K, Deckert T (1987) Cardiovascular risk factors in Type 1 (insulin-dependent) diabetic patients with and without proteinuria (submitted for publication)
5. Jensen T, Borch-Johnsen K, Kofoed-Enevoldsen A, Deckert T (1987) Coronary heart disease in young Type 1 (insulin-dependent) diabetic patients with and without diabetic nephropathy: incidence and risk factors. Diabetologia (in press)
6. Kofoed-Enevoldsen A, Jensen T, Borch-Johnsen K, Deckert T (1987) Incidence of retinopathy in Type 1 (insulin-dependent) diabetes association with clinical nephropathy. Diabetic Complications (in press)
7. Feldt-Rasmussen B (1986) Increased transcapillary escape rate of albumin in Type 1 (insulin-dependent) diabetic patients with microalbuminuria. Diabetologia 29: 282–286
8. Borch-Johnsen K, Nissen H, Henriksen E, Kreiner S, Salling N, Deckert T, Nerup J (1987) The natural history of insulin-dependent diabetes mellitus in Denmark: long-term survival with and without late diabetic complications. Diabetic Med (in press)
9. Deckert T, Feldt-Rasmussen B, Borch-Johnsen K, Kverneland A, Frokjaer Thomsen O (1986) Clinical assessment and prognosis of complications of diabetes. Transplant Proc 18: 1636–1638
10. Bent-Hansen L, Deckert T (1987) Metabolism of albumin and fibrinogen in Type 1 (insulin-dependent) diabetes mellitus (to be published)

11. Dvorak H, Senger DR, Dvorak AM, Harvery VS, McDonah J (1985) Regulation of extravascular coagulation by microvascular permeability. Science 27: 1059–1061
12. Feldt-Rasmussen B, Mathieson ER, Deckert T (1986) Effect of two years of strict metabolic control on progression of incipient nephropathy in insulin-dependent diabetes. Lancet ii: 1300–1304
13. Deckert T, Lauritzen T, Parving H-H, Sandahl Christiansen J, Steno Study Group (1983) Effect of two years of strict metabolic control on kidney function in long-term insulin-dependent diabetics. Diabetic Nephropathy 2: 6–10

Diabetic Complications: Early Diagnosis and Treatment
Edited by D. Andreani, G. Crepaldi, U. Di Mario and G. Pozza


# CHAPTER 25

# *Hypertension and Diabetic Nephropathy. Notes on Screening, Diagnosis and Treatment, with Emphasis on Insulin-dependent Patients*

C. E. MOGENSEN
*Second University Clinic of Internal Medicine, Kommunehospitalet, Aarhus, Denmark*

When treating patients with various kinds of nephropathies it is an important clinical observation that reduced kidney function is associated with an elevation in blood pressure. This is so whatever the genesis of the renal disease—including diabetic nephropathy (1,2). It is generally assumed that treatment of elevated blood pressure will have a beneficial long-term effect on the rate of deterioration of renal function in all kinds of renal diseases (1,3). However, long-term studies have only been carried out in diabetic nephropathy in *insulin-dependent patients*, where there is evidence to suggest a long-term beneficial effect of antihypertensive treatment on renal function. In proteinuric diabetic patients not under going treatment, the rate of fall in glomerular filtration rate (GFR) is around 1 ml/min/month, with an almost linear deterioration in renal function. With effective antihypertensive treatment, the rate of fall may be reduced by about 60% according to available studies. Thus uremia can be considerably postponed in these patients (4,5).

Recent evidence suggests that hypertension is frequently present in *non-insulin-dependent diabetic patients* and antihypertension here may be related to obesity, or hyperinsulinism, which is commonly found in non-insulin-dependent patients (8,9). According to recent epidemiological studies, nephropathy is an important feature also in elderly diabetic subjects (10). A fairly close association exists between urinary albumin excretion rate or clinical proteinuria and blood pressure elevation in known non-insulin-dependent diabetic patients (11).

The issue of increased blood pressure in diabetes has, however, been analysed most fully in insulin-dependent patients. Over the last decade, intensive research into the renal changes in diabetes aroused increasing interest in the mechanisms of hypertension and the majority of these studies investigated insulin-dependent patients (12–19). In this category of patient, elevated blood pressure is closely associated with the degree of nephropathy.

Early elevation of blood pressure as well as early renal changes in diabetes are without any subjective complaints whatsoever. When clinical signs appear, the first sign usually being edema, the disease process is far advanced and may be difficult to treat. Therefore, early detection programmes are required in diabetic patients. Since the long-term vascular and neurological complications are closely associated, such programmes should include attempts to detect a number of other long-term diabetic complications early in the course of the disease, in addition to early nephropathy and elevated blood pressure.

This chapter will describe a framework for (1) the clinical understanding of renal disease in diabetes, (2) an early detection programme for diabetic complications, including hypertension, and (3) give guidelines and suggestions or antihypertensive treatment and additional measures in diabetic nephropathy.

Table 1. Classification of diabetes

| |
|---|
| Type 1 diabetes |
| Hypertension associated with diabetic nephropathy |
| Essential hypertension (occurring by chance) |
| Secondary hypertension |
| Type 2 diabetes |
| Hypertension associated with obesity |
| Hypertension associated with diabetic nephropathy |
| Essential hypertension (occurring by chance) |
| Secondary hypertension |
| Endocrine causes of both abnormalities |
| Pheochromocytoma |
| Cushing's syndrome |
| Acromegaly |
| Steroid administration |

## CLASSIFICATION OF HYPERTENSION AND RENAL INVOLVEMENT IN DIABETES

Since nephropathy is an important factor in hypertension, it is necessary to classify diabetic patients according to the extent of renal involvement and according to the type of diabetes (Table 1) (14,20,21). The main measure of renal involvement in the diabetic patient is the urinary albumin excretion rate (UAE). Figure 1 shows a correlation between UAE and blood pressure in all phases of the disease. Sensitive assays such as radioimmunoassay or immunochemical assay (e.g. ELISA or nephelometric methods) are required in the early phases of renal involvement (20,22–24). When the disease becomes overt, standard clinical protein assays are sufficient.

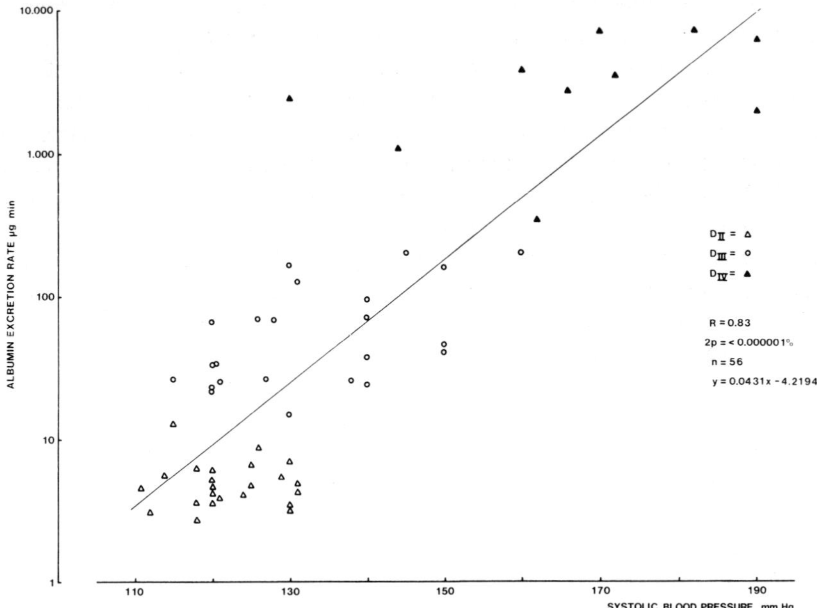


Figure 1. Urinary albumin excretion (UAE) rate plotted against systolic blood pressure in diabetic patients with normal albumin excretion rate ($D_{II}$), diabetic patients with incipient diabetic nephropathy (persistently elevated UAE rate) ($D_{III}$), and overt diabetic nephropathy ($D_{IV}$).

A number of stages in the development of renal disease have been described. Since UAE is a key parameter in the evaluation of renal function, definitions on the basis of this parameter are required.

## EXACT DEFINITIONS OF MICROALBUMINURIA AND INCIPIENT DIABETIC NEPHROPATHY

New exact definitions in assessing insulin-dependent patients with early diabetic nephropathy have recently been proposed (25).

*Microalbuminuria* is considered present when the urinary albumin excretion rate (UAE) is greater than 20 $\mu$g/min and less than or equal to 200 $\mu$g/min. This level of UAE corresponds to approximately 30 to 300 mg per 24 hours.

*Incipient diabetic nephropathy (Stage III)* is considered present when microalbuminuria is found in two out of three urine samples collected consecutively, preferably within no more than 6 months and no less than 1 month. If more than three samples are available mean values should correspond to a microalbuminuria level of 20–200 μg/min. Urine should be sterile and obtained in the non-ketotic state. It is recommended that the best possible conventional control of diabetes should be achieved prior to determining UAE. Other causes of increased UAE should be excluded, especially if diabetes has been present less than 6 years.

Finally, *overt diabetic nephropathy (Stage IV)* is considered present when the UAE is greater than 200 μg/min in at least two out of three urine samples, preferably collected within no more than 6 months, and no less than 1 month, or when the mean value of the UAE of multiple collections exceeds 200 μg/min. As in the case of incipient diabetic nephropathy, urine samples should be sterile and obtained in the non-ketotic state; other causes of increased UAE should be excluded. According to these definitions, the dip-stick tests for urinary protein should not be applied when classifying diabetic renal disease.

## NORMAL VALUES OF UAE

Since UAE is an important parameter of renal involvement in diabetes, now introduced into clinical medicine (20), the definition of normal excretion rates is essential.

*Normal values (non-diabetic subjects)*: UAE measured in 24-hour samples in 20 normal women and 23 normal men (aged 22–40 years) averaged 4.3 ± 4.8 (SD) (range 1.1–21.9) and 4.7 ± 4.7 μg/min (range 2.6–12.6), respectively. The day-to-day variation of 24 normal subjects estimated as the coefficient of variation of three 24-hour samples was 31.3. Mean values in excretion rate at rest (short-term collections over few hours) was at the same level: 4.8 ± 1.4 (SD) but with a narrower range (range 2.3–8.3, $n$ = 18, all males). In elderly non-diabetic individuals higher values may be seen (10).

Because UAE varies with posture (26) and with exercise (27), urine should be collected under standardized conditions. The following procedures are considered acceptable: (1) short-term collection over several hours in the laboratory or clinic; (2) overnight (about 8-hour) urine collection; (3) a 24-hour collection; (4) an early morning urine sample corrected for urine flow by creatinine measurements (26,28). Because of coefficients of variance in UAE of approximately 30–45%, at least three urine collections are recommended (26,29).

## STAGES OF RENAL INVOLVEMENT

Figure 2 summarizes the course of UAE in insulin-dependent diabetes. Table 2 provides more detailed information on renal and blood pressure involvement in the stages of renal change in diabetes.

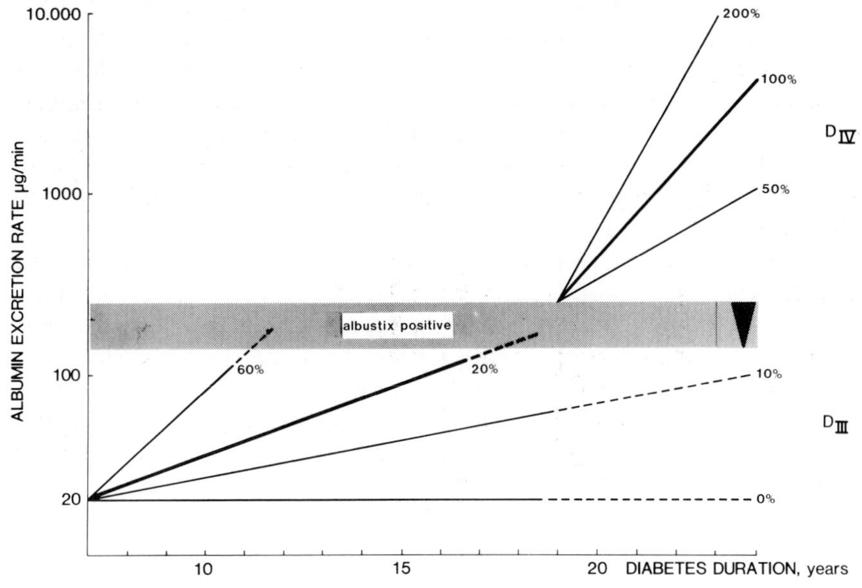


Figure 2. Outline of renal function changes (UAE) in the course of diabetes. $D_{III}$ and $D_{IV}$ refer to the stages shown in Table 2.

*Stage I* is the early hyperfunction–hypertrophy stage found at diagnosis. Increase in glomerular and kidney size is a prominent finding (30–33). Microalbuminuria may be present at diagnosis but is readily reversible by insulin treatment. Glomerular filtration rate (GFR) is high in these patients; this abnormality is also reversible, but in most cases only partially.

*Stage II* is the stage of renal lesion without clinical signs (the 'silent stage'). The hallmark of diabetic glomerulopathy, the thickening of the basement membrane, is detectable after about 2–3 years of diabetes (34). Some years later, the relative expansion of mesangial regions (mesangium as percentage of tuft) becomes evident. By definition UAE is normal. A number of patients continue in this stage throughout their lifetime.

*Stage III* is the stage of incipient diabetic nephropathy, typically found after 10–15 years. Microalbuminuria increases steadily over the years (20–200 $\mu$g/min). However, GFR is still high or normal. Blood pressure starts to increase at this stage. Structural lesions are more advanced and glomerular closure probably starts at this stage (35).

*Stage IV* is the well-known stage with clinical nephropathy and is eventually found in 30–40% of patients, often after 15–25 years of diabetes. It is characterized by the classical morphological lesions (36), but the diagnosis is most often made on clinical manifestations. Microalbuminuria has now developed into clinical proteinuria and

Table 2. Microalbuminuria and diabetic nephropathy stages in diabetic renal involvement and nephropathy (DN)

| Stage | Designation | Main characteristics | Main structural changes | GFR (ml/min) | Albumin exretion (UAE) | Blood pressure | Suggested main pathophysiologic change |
|---|---|---|---|---|---|---|---|
| *Stage I* | Hyperfunction and hypertrophy stage* | Large kidneys and glomerular hyperfiltration | Glomerular hypertrophy; normal | ~150 | May be increased | Normal (may initially increase during insulin treatment) | Glomerular volume expansion and increased intraglomerular pressure |
| *Stage II* | | | | | | | |
| In short-term diabetes (7–15 years) | 'Silent' stage with normal UAE | Normal UAE | Increasing basal membrane thickness and mesangial expansion | With or without hyperfiltration* | Normal (often increased in stress situations) | Normal | Changes as indicated above but quite variable (dependent on metabolic control?) |
| In long-term diabetes | Structural lesion present | | No or few studies | With or without hyperfiltration** | Normal (often in stress situations) | Normal or slightly elevated | In addition increased accumulation of basement membrane and basement-membrane-like material |

| | | | | | | | |
|---|---|---|---|---|---|---|---|
| *Stage III* Early | Incipient DN (or 'at-risk patient') | Persistently elevated UAE (20–200 μg/min) | Severity probably between Stages II and IV | ~160 | 20–70 μg/min | Often elevated compared to healthy subjects; | Glomerular closure probably starts in this stage. |
| Late | | | | ~130 (considerable range) | 70–200 μg/min | also blood pressure elevated during exercise. Increase by 3.5% per year | In some patients high intraglomerular pressure |
| *Stage IV* | | | | | | | |
| Early | | Clinical proteinuria or UAE >200 μg/min | Further increase in basement membrane thickening and mesangial expansion. Increasing rate of glomerular closure | ~130–70 | >200 μg/min | Often frank hypertension. Hypertension almost ubiquitous. Increase by 8% per year | High rate of glomerular closure and advancing mesangial expansion. Hyperfiltration in remaining glomeruli (deleterious) |
| Intermediate | Overt DN | | Hypertrophy of remaining glomeruli | ~70–30 | | | |
| Advanced | | | | ~30–10 | | | |
| *Stage IV* | Uremia | End-stage renal failure | Generalized glomerular closure | 0–10 | Decreasing (due to nephron) | High but often controlled by dialysis treatment | Advanced lesions and glomerular closure |

* Changes present probably in all stages when control imperfect.
** Marker of future nephropathy (if GFR > 150 ml/min).

GFR is declining. The fall in GFR can often be reduced by effective antihypertensive treatment (4,5).

*Stage V* is end-stage renal failure (ESRF) occurring after many years of diabetes and characterized by generalized glomerular closure and very low GFR.

Renal involvement can thus be traced throughout the course of diabetes, either by renal function tests or by biopsy procedures. It is important to stress that control and evaluation of diabetic nephropathy has to start very early. If delayed until advanced overt nephropathy or ESRF appears the game is already lost, and treatment must be directed towards renal supportive measures with dialysis and transplantation.

Table 3. Characteristics of incipient diabetic nephropathy

| |
|---|
| Elevated urinary albumin excretion rate (20–200 μg/min)<br>Rate of albumin excretion increased by 20% per year<br>80% risk of diabetic nephropathy over the next 10 years |
| Early hyperfiltration |
| Considerably increased risk of proliferative diabetic retinopathy |
| Increase in blood pressure |
| Increase in transcapillary escape rate of albumin (60) |
| Insulin pump treatment reverses disease or arrests progression; new data suggest partial reversion by antihypertensive treatment |

## VASCULAR LESIONS IN INCIPIENT NEPHROPATHY

Generalized vascular damage is a prominent feature in overt nephropathy but a number of abnormalities can already be observed in patients with incipient diabetic nephropathy (Table 3) (25). The main characteristic is, of course, a persistently elevated UAE rate. According to three studies the blood pressure is slightly but significantly elevated in patients with a UAE rate exceeding 30 mg/min. Very similar elevations in blood pressure were observed in three studies: 134/87, 138/91, 136/87 mmHg as compared with 120/72 mmHg in control subjects (15,37,38). In one study the rate of progression of renal disease, expressed as an increase in UAE rate per year, was highest in patients with the highest blood pressure values (12). According to recent studies, blood pressure rises by around 4% per year in incipient nephropathy, and by 8% per year in overt nephropathy (5,39) in patients on conventional insulin treatment. Interestingly, blood pressure elevation was not found in incipient nephropathy if patients were treated with the insulin pump (39).

Glomerular hyperfiltration may be found in the early stages of incipient diabetic nephropathy. Later, when the UAE rate reaches over 70 mg/min, the GFR starts to decline. It has recently been reported that the rate of transcapillary escape is increased in incipient diabetic nephropathy. Diabetic retinopathy is more pronounced in these patients, and indeed microalbuminuria can be used as a predictor of both proliferative diabetic retinopathy (40) and of elevation of blood pressure (15,16) as seen in Table 4. An increased incident of retinopathy is seen in diabetic patients with elevated blood pressure (41,42).

Table 4. Risk for development of nephropathy, proliferative diabetic retinopathy, and high blood pressure based on early measurement of urinary albumin excretion rate in 10-year follow-up study

| Urinary albumin excretion ($\mu$g/min) | Age at diagnosis (years) | Diabetes duration (years) | Follow-up (years) | Diabetic nephropathy at follow-up (%) | Proliferative diabetic retinopathy at follow-up (%) | Blood pressure at follow-up (mmHg) |
|---|---|---|---|---|---|---|
| $<15$ $\mu$g/min | 12 | 13 | 11 | 0 | 3 | 123/84 |
| $\geqslant 15$ $\mu$g/min | 13 | 13 | 11 | 80 | 70 | 149/99 |

## PATHOGENESIS OF HYPERTENSION IN DIABETES

The development of hypertension in diabetic patients is incompletely understood, although renal involvement is a major determinant (43), at least in insulin-dependent patients. Which structural lesions in the glomeruli are responsible for the high blood pressure is not clear. However, mesangial expansion seems to be closely associated with elevated blood pressure (44) and it is also possible that structural lesions in both the afferent and efferent glomerular vessels play a role. Microscopic lesions in the glomerulus, of both diffuse and nodular nature, are also characteristic of hypertensive diabetes (36,45). Sodium retention seems to be important in the genesis of hypertension in diabetes, particularly in patients with proteinuria and severe urinary protein loss, but also in non-azotemic patients (46,47), and in patients with microalbuminuria (B. Feldt-Rasmussen, personal communication). Renal arterial stenosis seems not to be more frequent in diabetic subjects than in the non-diabetic population (48). Abnormal increases in blood pressure are seen during physical exercise (27,49).

## LONG-TERM BENEFICIAL EFFECT OF ANTIHYPERTENSIVE TREATMENT

Two long-term studies have now shown that the rate of decline in GFR in overt nephropathy can be considerably reduced by effective antihypertensive treatment (4,5). Data from these studies are shown in Table 5. In these studies pretreatment fall in GFR was used as an internal control. Antihypertensive treatment also seems

Table 5. Effect of antihypertensive treatment on blood pressure and renal function in diabetic nephropathy

| | Treatment | No. of subjects | Age (years) | Duration of diabetes (years) | Observation period (months) | Glomerular filtration rate before treatment (ml/min) | Blood pressure before and during treatment (mmHg) | Decrease in glomerular filtration rate (ml/min/month) | Albumin excretion (yearly increase) % |
|---|---|---|---|---|---|---|---|---|---|
| Mogensen (4) | Before treatment | 6 | 30 | 18 | 28 | 86 | 162/103 | 1.23 | 107 |
| | During treatment | | | | 73 | | 144/95 | 0.49 | 5 |
| Parving et al. (61) | Before treatment | 10 | 29 | 16 | 29 | 80 | 144/97 | 0.91 | Further increase |
| | During treatment | | | | 69 | | 129/85 | 0.25 | Reversed |

effective in incipient diabetic nephropathy (50). In these patients GFR is still well preserved and the increase in UAE is the main effect parameter. As seen in Figure 3, progression can be reversed by antihypertensive treatment (cardioselective beta-blockers and diuretics).

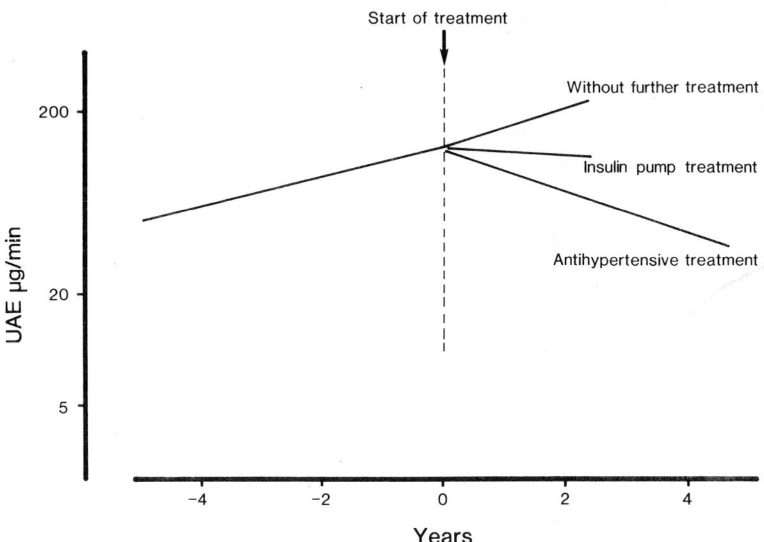


Figure 3. Outline of increase in urinary albumin excretion (UAE) rate before and during antihypertensive treatment in incipient diabetic nephropathy as compared to the effect of insulin pump treatment.

These results suggest that the elevation of blood pressure is an important modulating factor in the development of diabetic nephropathy.

Table 6. Blood pressure level during treatment and fall in GFR

| Author | Fall rate of GFR (ml/min/month) | Blood pressure (mmHg) |
|---|---|---|
| Mogensen (overt DN) | 0.49 | 144/95 (111) |
| Parving et al. (overt DN) | 0.39 | 128/85 (99) |
| Christensen (incipient DN) | No fall | 125/84 (97) |

## OPTIMAL BLOOD PRESSURE LEVEL DURING TREATMENT

The optimal blood pressure level during antihypertensive treatment in patients with diabetic nephropathy is not clearly defined. The rate of fall in GFR and blood pressure levels during antihypertensive treatment are shown in Table 6 (4,5,50). The lowest decline in blood pressure is found in patients with blood pressure levels around 130/85. As practical guidelines we therefore propose that during antihypertensive treatment in young patients below the age of 40 blood pressure should be below 130-40/85-90.

Table 7. A diabetic complication follow-up system

*Examinations*

- I. Measurements for micro- or macroalbuminuria
- II. Eye examination including ophthalmoscopy
- III. Screening for peripheral neuropathy
  - a. Vibration threshold examination (Biothesiometer)
  - b. Clinical examination
- IV. Resting blood pressure
- V. Clinical history and examinations regarding cardiovascular disease
- VI. Foot examination

*Metabolic control*

Multiple measurements of blood glucose and $HbA_{1c}$

*Time course*

- A. Without symptoms and/or signs and/or laboratory changes
  - a. At admission
  - b. Every third year during the first 9 years of diabetes (must include INFORMATION), blood pressure measurements more often (at least yearly)
  - c. Thereafter annually
- B. With symptoms and/or signs and/or laboratory changes
  Immediate examination
  Time course to be decided in the individual patient (examination every 3–6 months)

*Metabolic control*

Every 1–3 months

## CLINICAL MANAGEMENT OF EARLY PHASES OF DIABETIC NEPHROPATHY

It is proposed that UAE should be measured quite early in the course of diabetes, e.g. following metabolic stabilization after diagnosis, or when first admitted to hospital. Thereafter examinations should be carried out after 3, 6, and 9 years and then at yearly intervals, along with other examinations for diabetic complications, e.g. retinopathy and neuropathy (Table 7). Blood pressure should be taken more often. In the early examinations it is essential to give information to patients regarding the nature of diabetes and its complications (Table 7). Using these methods incipient diabetes can be diagnosed early in the course.

The management of patients with incipient diabetic nephropathy must be individualized. First of all, in the clinical situation, knowledge of the prognosis of a patient is clearly of importance in itself. Apart from its prognostic value, the identification of persisting microalbuminuria in a patient may have the following consequences:

1. Urinary albumin excretion should be monitored every 3–6 months, to follow the development of early renal damage.
2. If patient's diabetes is poorly or semipoorly controlled, the best possible control should be achieved either with conventional insulin treatment, including self-monitoring of blood glucose levels, or possibly with multiple injection therapy using new devices, such as the 'insulin-pen' (51) or the insulin-pump (39).
3. Baseline blood pressure should be closely monitored. If blood pressure should exceed 145/90-94 mmHg while the patient is receiving non-pharmacological therapy, most authors would agree that antihypertensive treatment is indicated in young diabetic subjects (17).
4. Since microalbuminuria to some extent also predicts proliferative retinal lesions, patients should undergo regular fundoscopic examinations (40).
5. Patients should be informed that the observed values of UAE indicate a certain risk of subsequent nephropathy and that closer control is required. Smoking is ill-advised. Patients who do not follow diabetic control should be warned of the potential consequences of their non-compliance.
6. Urinary tract infection should be treated.

Insulin pump treatment, resulting in improved metabolic control in the average controlled patient, has stopped or even reversed the progression of microalbuminuria (39). Insulin pumps are less effective in overt nephropathy (52). Therefore, there may be an indication for pump treatment in patients with incipient nephropathy. However, long-term studies over several years are required, and are currently being carried out.

## EVALUATION BEFORE PHARMACOLOGICAL TREATMENT

Table 8 outlines a diagnostic and treatment programme. I propose the following guidelines for the treatment of hypertension in diabetes. Before treatment, the following points are to be clarified: (a) what is the exact level of blood pressure at repeated measurements? (b) what is the underlying cause of hypertension? (secondary causes should be excluded); (c) are there contributory or modulating factors present, such as high salt intake, heavy smoking, poor control of diabetes? and (d) what is the extent

Table 8. Diabetes and hypertension

| | | |
|---|---|---|
| I. *Evaluation* | | |
| Elevated casual blood pressure (BP) (for patients aged less than 40 years): BP > 145/90−94 mmHg | Observation, measurement of UAE repeated measurements of BP and UAE under peaceful circumstances (possibly at hospital) | Consider screening for secondary hypertension. Evaluation of renal function |
| II. *Non-pharmacological intervention* | | |
| Still high BP. Information on the nature of elevated BP ('blood pressure school') | Relative normalization: BP < 140/90<br>Ensure modern dietary treatment of diabetes (low fat diet, high amount of complex carbohydrate). Low salt intake and good diabetes control | Relative normalization: BP < 140/90<br>Weight reduction<br>Reduced smoking<br>Alter stressful lifestyle<br>No heavy exercise |
| III. *Pharmacological intervention** | | |
| Diuretics | Relative normalization: BP < 140/90<br>+ Calcium antagonist or cardioselective beta-blockers | Relative normalization < 140/90<br>+ Vasodilators |
| or Calcium antagonist | | Angiotensin-converting enzyme inhibitors** (alone or with diuretics or other combinations) |
| or Cardioselective beta-blockers | + Diuretic (in case of impaired renal function, loop diuretics) | |
| IV. *No or insufficient effect* | | |
| Consider compliance (does the patient take the drugs) | Re-evaluation of genesis of hypertension | Try unusual combinations. If renal function stable accept some elevation of blood pressure |

* Always consider side-effects (Table 9).
** May also be used as first choice.

of damage to the kidneys, eyes, heart, and peripheral vessels? General measures are taken such as encouraging weight loss, modifying smoking habits, reducing salt intake, altering a stressful lifestyle, and encouraging the best possible control of diabetes, including modern dietary treatment, which seems to possess some antihypertensive effect (53).

## TREATMENT OF HYPERTENSION IN DIABETES

A conventional scheme of antihypertensive treatment, with some modification, can be used in diabetic patients, starting with beta-blockers, diuretics or calcium antagonists.

Table 9. Undesirable effects of antihypertensive drugs in diabetes

| Drug | Problem | Promoted by | Ameliorated by |
|---|---|---|---|
| Beta-blockers | Hypoglycemic-unaware and delayed recovery (sweating is enhanced) | Autonomic neuropathy | Use of cardio-selective blockers Information to the patient |
| Diuretics ($K_+$-losing) | Increase in blood glucose and hypokalemia | Loss in potassium | Potassium supplementation |
| Diuretic ($K_+$-sparing) | Hyperkalemia | Impaired renal function | Discontinuing or reducing the drug |
| Some diuretics and beta-blockers | Dyslipoproteinemia | ? | Discontinuing or reducing the drug |
| Especially sympatholytics and alpha-blockers and vasodilators | Orthostatic hypotension | Autonomic neuropathy | Discontinuing or reducing the drug |
| Sympatholytics, diuretics | Sexual dysfunction | Autonomic neuropathy | Discontinuing or reducing the drug |
| Most antihypertensive drugs | Claudication and dizziness | Arteriosclerosis | Discontinuing or reducing the drug |

Cardioselective beta-blockers, in contrast to non-selective blockers, should strongly be recommended, since problems with hypoglycemic unawareness only seldom occur with these agents when used in moderate doses. This is occasionally found in propranolol-treated patients. The relative safety of cardioselective beta-blockers in diabetic patients has recently been further established, at least when used in moderate doses (4,5,54). However, some patients experience problems with hypoglycemic unawareness, also with selective blockers. Information is important but it may be required to reduce the dose or discontinue the drug. When diuretics are used in the treatment of diabetic patients one should bear in mind the possible aggravation of the diabetic state in non-insulin-dependent patients (55). This may be related to potassium loss and therefore serum potassium should be monitored regularly along with the evaluation of kidney function and clinical status. Table 9 provides an outline of the side-effects of antihypertensive regimens. In diabetic nephropathy loop diuretics, often in high doses, are useful for eliminating edema, and for reducing blood pressure. Subsequently, vasodilators such as Apresoline (hydralazine) or prazosin are used, and with these programmes a fair reduction in blood pressure is obtained, although normalization is not always found.

ACE inhibitors (angiotensin-converting enzyme inhibitors) may also prove useful in the treatment of diabetic hypertension (56–59), even over years of therapy. ACE inhibitors may also be used as first drugs, often along with diuretics.

## REFERENCES

1. Pohl JEF, Thurston H, Swales JD (1974) Hypertension with renal impairment. Influence of intensive therapy. Q J Med 172: 569–581
2. Mogensen CE (1976) Progression of nephropathy in long-term diabetics with proteinuria and effect of initial antihypertensive treatment. Scand J Clin Lab Invest 36: 383–388
3. Shimamatsu K, Onoyama K, Harada A, Kumagai H, Hirakata H, Miishima C, Inenaga T, Fujimi S, Fujishima M, Omae T (1985) Effect of blood pressure on the progression rate of renal impairment in chronic glomerulonephritis. J Clin Hypertension 3: 239–244
4. Mogensen CE (1982) Long-term antihypertensive treatment inhibiting progression of diabetic nephropathy. Br Med J i: 2–7
5. Parving H-H, Andersen AR, Smidt UM, Svendsen PAA (1983) Early aggressive antihypertensive treatment reduces rate of delcine in kidney function in diabetic nephropathy. Lancet i: 1175–1179
6. Fabre J, Balant LP, Dayer PG, Fox HM, Vernet AT (1982) The kidney in maturity-onset diabetes mellitus: a clinical study of 510 patients. Kidney Int 21: 730–738
7. Prevalence of small vessel and large vessel disease in diabetic patients from 14 centres: The World Health Organization Multinational Study of Vascular Disease in Diabetics (1985) Diabetologia 28: 615–640
8. Lucas CP, Estigarribia JA, Darga LL, Reaven GM (1985) Insulin and blood pressure in obesity. Hypertension 7: 702–706
9. Christlieb AR, Krolewski AS, Warram JH, Soeldner JS (1985) Is insulin the link between hypertension and obesity? Hypertension 7 (Suppl II): II-54-II-57
10. Klein R, Klein BEK, Moss SE, Demets DL (1985) Blood pressure and hypertension in diabetes. Am J Epidemiol 122: 75–89
11. Damsgaard EM, Binder C, Dyerberg J, Faber OK, Frøland A, Mogensen CE (1985) Factors associated with increased urinary albumin excretionin occult and known IDDM. Diabetes Res Clin Pract Suppl 1: 119
12. Christensen CK, Mogensen CE (1985) The course of incipient diabetic nephropathy: Studies of albumin excretion and blood pressure. Diabetic Med 2: 97–102
13. Hostetter TH (1985) Diabetic nephropathy. N Engl J Med 312: 642–643
14. Mogensen CE, Christensen CK, Vittinghus E (1983) The stages in diabetic renal

disease. With emphasis on the stage of incipient diabetic nephropathy. Diabetes 32: 64–78
15. Mogensen CE, Christensen CK (1984) Predicting diabetic nephropathy in insulin-dependent patients. N Engl J Med 311: 89–93
16. Mogensen CE, Christensen CK (1985) Blood pressure changes and renal function changes in incipient and overt diabetic nephropathy. Hypertension 7 (Suppl II): 64–73
17. Weidman P, Mogensen CE, Ritz E (1985) Hypertension associated with diabetes mellitus. Hypertension 7 (Suppl II): 1–2
18. Parving H-H, Anderson AR, Oxenbøll B, Christiansen JS (1983) Blood pressure and diabetic nephropathy. Diabetologia 24: 10–12
19. Parving H-H, Smidt UM, Friisberg B, Bonnevie-Nielsen V, Anderson AR (1981) A prospective study of glomerular filtration rate and arterial blood pressure in insulin-dependent diabetics with diabetic nephropathy. Diabetologia 20: 457–461
20. Krolewski AS, Warram JH, Christlieb AR, Bustick EJ, Kahn ER (1985) The changing natural history of nephropathy in type 1 diabetes. Am J Med 78: 785–794
21. Hasslacher C, Ritz E (1985) Diagnose der diabetischen Nephropathie. Dtsch Med Wochenschr 110: 1662–1663
22. Christensen CK, Ørskov C (1984) Rapid screening PEG radioimmunoassay for quantification of pathological microalbuminuria. Diabetec Nephropathy 3: 92–94
23. Feldt-Rasmussen B, Dinesen B, Deckert M (1985) Enzyme immunoassay—an improved determination of urinary albumin in diabetics with incipient nephropathy. Scand J Clin Lab Invest 45: 539–544
24. Miles DW, Mogensen CE, Gundersen HJG (1970) Radioimmunoassay for urinary albumin using a single antibody. Scan J Clin Lab Invest 26: 5–11
25. Mogensen CE (1987) Microalbuminuria as a predictor of clinical diabetic nephropathy. Kidney Int 31: 673–689
26. Mogensen CE (1971) Urinary albumin excretion in early and long-term juvenile diabetes. Scand J Clin Lab Invest 28: 183–193
27. Christensen CK (1984) Abnormal albuminuria and blood pressure rise in incipient diabetic nephropathy induced by exercise. Kidney Int 25: 819–823
28. Gatling W, Knight C, Hill RD (1985) Screening for early diabetic nephropathy. Which sample to detect microalbuminuria. Diabetic Med 2: 451–455
29. Feldt-Rasmussen B, Mathiesen ER (1984) Variability of urinary albumin excretion in incipient diabetic nephropathy. Diabetic Nephropathy 3: 101–103
30. Mogensen CE, Andersen MJF (1975) Increased kidney size and glomerular filtration rate in untreated juvenile diabetics. Normalization by insulin treatment. Diabetologia 11: 221–224
31. Kroustrup JP, Gundersen HJG, Østerby R (1977) Glomerular size and structure in diabetes mellitus. III. Early enlargement of the capillary surface. Diabetologia 13: 207–210
32. Østerby R, Gundersen HJG, Hørlyck A, Kroustrup JP, Nyberg GG, Westberg GG (1983) Diabetic glomerulopathy: structural characteristics of the early and advanced stages. Diabetes 32 (Suppl 2): 79–82
33. Østerby R, Gundersen HJG (1975) Glomerular size and structure in diabetes mellitus. I. Early abnormalities. Diabetologia 11: 225–229
34. Østerby R (1975) Early phases in the development of diabetic glomerulopathy. A quantitative electron microscopic study. Acta Med Scand Suppl 574
35. Østerby R (1986) Structural changes in the diabetic kidney. Clin Endocrinol Metab 15: 733–751
36. Gellman DD, Pirani CL, Soothill JF, Muehrcke RC, Kark RM (1959) Diabetic nephropathy: a clinical and pathologic study based on renal biopsies. Medicine 38:

321–367

37. Wiseman M, Viberti GC, Mackintosh D, Jarrett RJ, Keen H (1984) Glycaemia, arterial pressure and micro-albuminuria in type 1 (insulin-dependent) diabetes mellitus. diabetologia 26: 401–405
38. Mathiesen ER, Oxenbøll B, Johansen K, Svendsen PAa, Deckert T (1984) Incipient nephropathy in type 1 (insulin-dependent) diabetes. Diabetologia 26: 406–410
39. Feldt-Rasmussen B, Mathiesen ER, Deckert T (1986) Effect of two years of strict metabolic control on progression of incipient nephropathy in insulin dependent diabetes. Lancet ii: 1300–1304
40. Vigstrup J, Mogensen CE (1985) Proliferative diabetic retinopathy: at risk patients identified by early detection of microalbuminuria. Acta Ophthalmol 63: 530–534
41. Knowler WC, Bennett PH, Ballintine EJ (1980) Increased incidence of retinopathy in diabetics with elevated blood pressure. A six year follow-up study in Pima Indians. N Engl J Med 302: 645–650
42. Chahal P, Inglesby DV, Sleightholm M, Kohner EM (1985) Blood pressure and the progression of mild background diabetic retinopathy. Hypertension 7 (Suppl II): II-79–II-83
43. Mogensen CE (1982) Hypertension in diabetes and the stages of diabetic nephropathy. Editorial review. Diabetic Nephropathy 1: 2–7
44. Mauer SM, Steffes MW, Ellis EN, Sutherland DER, Brown DM, Goetz FC (1984) Structural–functional relationship in diabetic nephropathy. J Clin Invest 74: 1143–1155
45. Kuhlmann H, Mehnert H (1969) Zur Beeinflussung des Blutdrucks durch eine Nephropathie bei Diabetikern. Klin Wochenschr 47: 276–277
46. Weidmann P (1980) Recent pathogenic aspects in essential hypertension and hypertension associated with diabetes mellitus. Klin Wochenschr 58: 1071–1089
47. Weidmann P, Trost BN (1985) Pathogenesis and treatment of hypertension associated with diabetes. Horm Metab Res Suppl 15: 51–58
48. Munichoodappa C, D'Elia JA, Libertino JA, Gleason RE, Christlieb AR (1979) Renal artery stenosis in hypertensive diabetics. J Urol (Baltimore) 121: 555–558
49. Karlefors T (1966) Exercise tests in male diabetics, II. Heart rate and systolic blood pressure. Acta Med Scand 180 (Suppl 449): 19
50. Christensen CK, Mogensen CE (1985) Effect of antihypertensive treatment on progression of disease in incipient diabetic nephropathy. Hypertension 7 (Suppl II): 109–114
51. Berger AS, Saurbrey N, Kühl C, Villumsen J (1985) Clinical experience with a new device that will simplify insulin injections. Diabetes Care 8: 73–76
52. Viberti GC, Bilous RW, Mackintosh D, Bending JJ, Keen H (1983) Long-term correction of hyperglycaemia and progression of renal failure in insulin dependent diabetes. Br Med J 286: 598–600
53. Dodson PM, Pacy PJ, Bal P, Kuniki AJ, Fletcher RF, Taylor KG (1984) A controlled trial of a high-fibre, low-fat and low-sodium diet for mild hypertension in Type 11 (non-insulin-dependent) diabetic patients. Diabetologia 27: 522–526
54. Kølendorf K, Bonnevie-Nielsen V, Broch-Møller B (1982) A trial of metoprolol in hypertensive insulin-dependent diabetic patients. Acta Med Scan 211: 175–178
55. Struthers AD, Murphy MB, Dollery CT (1985) Glucose tolerance during antihypertensive therapy in patients with diabetes mellitus. Hypertension 7 (Suppl II): II-95–II-101
56. Gambaro G, Morbiato F, Cicerello E, Del Turco M, Sartori L, D'Angelo A, Crepaldi G (1985) Captopril in the treatment of hypertension in Type 1 and Type 11 diabetic patients. J Hypertension 3 (Suppl 2): 149–151
57. Taguma Y, Kitamoto Y, Futake G, Ueda H, Monma H, Ishizaki M, Takahashi H, Sekino H, Sasaki Y (1985) Effect of captopril on heavy proteinuria in azotemic diabetics. N Engl J Med 313: 1617–1620

58. Björck S, Nyberg G, Mulec H, Granerus G, Herlitz H, Aurell M (1986) Beneficial effects of angiotensin converting enzyme inhibition on renal function in patients with diabetic nephropathy. Br Med J 293: 471–474
59. Hommel E, Parving H-H, Mathiesen E, Edsberg B, Nielsen MD, Giese J (1986) Effect of captopril on kidney function in insulin-dependent diabetic patients with nephropathy. Br Med J 293: 467–470
60. Feldt-Rasmussen B (1986) Increased transcapillary escape rate of albumin in type 1 (insulin-dependent) diabetic patients with microalbuminuria. Diabetologia 29: 282–286
61. Parving H-H, Anderson AR, Smidt UM (1986) The effect of long-term antihypertensive treatment on kidney function in diabetic nephropathy. Diabetic Nephropathy 5: 48

Diabetic Complications: Early Diagnosis and Treatment
Edited by D. Andreani, G. Crepaldi, U. Di Mario and G. Pozza


CHAPTER 26

# *Diabetic Nephropathy: Identification and Treatment of the Susceptibles*

G. Viberti and R. Mangili
*Unit for Metabolic Medicine, Guy's Hospital, London, UK; Ospedale San Raffaele, Divisione Medica I, Milan, Italy*

## CLINICAL DIABETIC NEPHROPATHY

The clinical diagnosis of diabetic nephropathy relies on the detection of persistent proteinuria (i.e. urinary total protein excretion rate greater than 0.5 g/24 h) after 10 years or more of diabetes mellitus in an insulin-dependent patient with concomitant diabetic retinopathy and rising arterial pressure, but no signs of other renal disease, urinary tract infection or heart failure. Diabetic glomerulosclerosis is found at renal biopsy in over 90% of the cases (1,2), confirming the diagnosis.

Long-term follow-up studies show that diabetic nephropathy develops in approximately 35% of insulin-dependent patients (1,3) and it is mostly in this kind of patient that the natural history of this disorder has been outlined. Non-insulin-dependent diabetic patients of European origin seem to develop nephropathy less frequently than insulin-dependent patients, but because of their larger number the actual number of patients developing end-stage renal failure is approximately the same (4).

Persistent proteinuria is the forerunner of progressive deterioration of renal function. Glomerular filtration rate (GFR) declines linearly with time at rates ranging between 0.6 and 2.4 ml/min/month (5). The reasons for the different rates of decline are largely unknown but varying degrees of blood pressure and control may play a role. Indeed, arterial pressure starts to climb at a very early stage of renal involvement in diabetes (6). With the fall in GFR, proteinuria and the clearances of major plasma proteins such as albumin and IgG increase. There is a change from proteinuria characterized by a high selectivity for albumin in the early stages, when the GFR is still normal or only moderately reduced, to a low selectivity proteinuria with proportionally more IgG being cleared when the GFR is markedly reduced (7). In 50% of affected patients end-stage renal failure occurs within 7 years of the onset of persistent proteinuria (1).

Three different lines of treatment have been employed in the attempt to arrest this apparently inexorable evolution to end-stage renal failure. An obvious approach was the optimization of glycaemic control. Controlled trials of intervention with continuous subcutaneous insulin infusion (CSII) have been disappointing, however, in that correction of hyperglycaemia failed to influence the downhill course of established nephropathy. Our own experience, spanning a time period of from 2 to 6 years in patients with either persistent (8) or intermittent proteinuria (9), shows that the average rate of decline of GFR and the increase in the fractional clearance of albumin and IgG are by and large unchanged by improved metabolic control (Table 1). In this series of studies systemic blood pressure was maintained stable throughout and diet was unchanged to prevent possible confounding effects of these two factors.

Table 1. Effect of blood glucose (BG) control on rate of decline of GFR in patients with intermittent and persistent clinical proteinuria

| | Rate of GFR decline* (ml/min/month) | | |
|---|---|---|---|
| | Conventional BG control | Strict BG control | Significance level |
| Intermittent proteinurics ($n$=6) | 0.9 ± 0.2 | 0.8 ± 0.3 | NS |
| Persistent proteinurics ($n$=6) | 0.9 ± 0.3 | 0.7 ± 0.1 | NS |

* Data are mean ±SEM.

Studies with hypotensive treatment, started early in the course of diabetic renal failure, have had some success in slowing the deterioration of renal function. In a small but carefully followed series the rate of decline of GFR was lowered from 0.9 ml/min/month before treatment to 0.24 ml/min/month during treatment (6). This lower rate of fall could be maintained for several years and concomitantly the albuminuria was significantly reduced, though not entirely normalized. These results were obtained in the absence of change of blood glucose control or dietary habits. The hypotensive regimens used in these early studies included selective beta-blockers, vasodilators and diuretics. More recently a number of studies, though uncontrolled and small in size, seem to suggest that the administration of angiotensin-converting enzyme inhibitors to diabetic patients with renal failure may have an additional specific beneficial effect on the progression of renal disease (10–12). Some workers have claimed that these effects are independent of systemic blood pressure reduction, and animal studies suggest that they may be related to the lowering of intraglomerular pressure (10,12,13). The third line of intervention in the treatment of progressive diabetic nephropathy consists in the reduction of dietary protein intake. Surprisingly this manoeuvre, which is known to retard progression in other renal disease, has been inadequately explored in diabetic renal failure. We have preliminary data in 21 persistently proteinuric insulin-dependent diabetic patients (14 M, 7 F) aged between 30 and 64 years (mean 42 years), with duration of diabetes ranging between 16 and 41 years (mean 24 years) studied over a period of at least 3 years, the last of which on restricted protein intake (14). The low protein diet reduced protein intake to 45 ± 7 g/day and this was accompanied by a significant fall in total protein excretion and in the rate of decline of GFR (Table 2). No significant changes occurred in levels of arterial pressure or glycosylated haemoglobin concentrations. Even though the response to low protein diet was heterogeneous, with some individuals slowing markedly their rate of progression and others showing little change, these findings support the view that, on average, low protein diet has a beneficial and independent effect on the evolution of diabetic renal failure.

Table 2. Effect of low protein intake on the rate of GFR decline and total urinary protein excretion in 21 clinically proteinuric insulin-dependent diabetic patients

| | Normal protein diet (77 ± 22 g/day) | Low protein diet (45 ± 7 g/day) | Significance level (*p* value) |
|---|---|---|---|
| Total urinary protein (g/24 h) | 2.9 ± 0.4 | 1.5 ± 0.4 | <0.01 |
| GFR fall (ml/min/month) | 0.7 ± 0.1 | 0.3 ± 0.2 | <0.02 |
| Glycosylated haemoglobin (%) | 9.2 ± 0.4 | 9.4 ± 0.6 | NS |
| Mean blood pressure (mmHg) | 94 ± 4 | 97 ± 7 | NS |

Data are mean ± SEM.

Further controlled studies are clearly needed to substantiate the promising results obtained with reduction of blood pressure and dietary protein intake. However, the overall impression is that present therapeutic means can at best delay the development of end-stage renal failure without arresting the progression of the disease in the overt clinical stage.

## EARLY MARKERS OF DIABETIC KIDNEY DISEASE

The progressive nature of diabetic nephropathy and our relative therapeutic impotence, together with the elevated mortality associated with this disorder (15), emphasize the need for early identification of patients prone to develop the clinical stage of the disease.

Renal abnormalities in early diabetes mellitus have been recently described, some of which may be relevant to the progression to overt nephropathy. Their prognostic significance and present options for their treatment will be examined in turn.

### Microalbuminuria

Until recently, it was thought that the increase in albumin excretion above the detection threshold of current clinical methods (e.g. the Albustix test) was a sudden event, that was preceded by years of normal protein excretion. In 1963 a sensitive and specific radioimmunoassay for measuring urinary albumin in low concentration was developed (16). Using this method, a number of authors consistently found that the urinary albumin excretion rate (AER) may be subclinically elevated in diabetes mellitus (17–19). Approximately 40% of insulin-dependent diabetic patients have albumin excretion rates above the upper limit of the normal range (2.0–25 mg/24 h), but still well below the excretion rates which are conventionally used to diagnose clinical albuminuria (i.e. AER greater than 250 mg/24 h) (20). This subclinical increase in AER was defined as microalbuminuria. The biological variability of AER may be as high as 40–50% (21). Therefore, the extremes of AER ranges, and especially the limit between normo- and microalbuminuria, are not to be considered as rigid cut-off values, and common sense should be applied in assigning a given AER value to one range or another. AER does not seem to be related to age, sex and duration of diabetes; higher values are found during the day, in the upright, ambulant position, than during the night in the recumbent position (17,18,20) and the day-to-day variation seems lower in the latter circumstance (21).

The importance of subclinical elevations of AER remained unknown until it was shown that some degrees of microalbuminuria could be predictive of later development of clinical proteinuria. Insulin-dependent diabetic patients with an overnight AER $>30$ μg/min were found to have a 20-fold higher risk of developing nephropathy compared to patients with an AER $<30$ μg/min after a 14-year follow up (22). These results were substantially confirmed in two other independent studies (21,23) (Table 3). The different AER levels that were shown to predict nephropathy may be explained by the different duration of follow up and method of urine collection.

Table 3. Albumin excretion rates (AER) predictive of clinical diabetic nephropathy in three studies

| Study group | AER (μg/min) | Urine collection | Follow-up (years) |
|---|---|---|---|
| Guy's Hospital | >30 | Overnight | 14 |
| Aarhus University | >15 | 1–2 hours | 10 |
| Steno Memorial Hospital | >70 | 24 hours | 6 |

The microalbuminuria of early diabetes appears to be glomerular in origin and increases with time at an average rate estimated to be around 25% per year. Recent findings indicate that levels of albumin excretion rates identifying at-risk patients are absent during the first 5 years of diabetes in conventionally treated insulin-dependent diabetic patients; this suggests that microalbuminuria is a sign of early disease rather than a marker of susceptibility (24).

Different studies have shown that microalbuminuria is associated with poorer glycaemic control and independently and more strongly with raised levels of arterial pressure (21,23,25). Blood pressure in patients with microalbuminuria, although within the so-called normal range, is significantly higher than that of a matched normoalbuminuric group (Table 4). The elevation of blood pressure in these patients is of great interest since it occurs in the absence of any renal hypofunction (the glomerular filtration rate may be either normal or elevated) and raises the question as to whether rises in arterial pressure should be considered a consequence of the renal disease, as generally thought, or rather a phenomenon that may play a causal role in the pathogenesis of diabetic renal failure.

Table 4. Mean arterial pressure (diastolic and 1/3 of pulse pressure) in age-, sex- and duration-matched insulin-dependent diabetic patients with albumin excretion rates (AER) above 30 μg/min (high risk group), below 12 μg/min (upper limit of normal range) and between 12 and 30 μg/min

| | Mean blood pressure (mmHg) |
|---|---|
| AER >30 μg/min ($n$=12) | 103 ± 12 |
| AER 12–30 μg/min ($n$=16) | 92 ± 8* |
| AER <12 μg/min ($n$=12) | 87 ± 7** |

* = $p<0.02$ versus AER >30 μg/min.
** = $p<$ 0.001 versus AER >30 μg/min.
Data are mean ± SEM.

Microalbuminuria can also be found in diabetic subjects with supranormal GFR (23).

## Increased Glomerular Filtration Rate and Kidney Size

Microalbuminuria and elevated arterial pressure may not be the earliest signs of kidney involvement in diabetes.

The occurrence of glomerular hyperfiltration in diabetes mellitus has long been known. GFR is elevated on average by 20–40%; only 25–30% of patients have a higher than normal GFR (26). Whether diabetic patients with normal GFR really have a higher GFR than prior to the onset of diabetes is at present uncertain. The determinants of glomerular hyperfunction have been directly investigated using micropuncture techniques in diabetic rats and have been shown to consist mainly of renal vasodilation, more accentuated at afferent than efferent glomerular arterioles, thus resulting in both increased glomerular plasma flow rate and mean trans-glomerular hydraulic pressure gradient. Glycaemic, metabolic and hormonal alterations at least partially mediate these changes in kidney haemodynamics (26).

The elevated GFR in humans is strongly associated with increased kidney volume. Interestingly, even though a large kidney can be associated with a normal GFR, a high GFR is extremely unlikely to occur in normal size kidneys. Large kidneys reflect hyperplasia and hypertrophy of renal tubules, but only hypertrophy of the glomeruli (27). The latter phenomenon would increase the surface area available to filtration, and a strong correlation has been demonstrated between GFR and glomerular filtering surface area in diabetic patients (26).

The exact description of the relationship between GFR and albumin excretion rate in non-clinically proteinuric diabetic patients remains unresolved. Cross-sectionally an elevated GFR can be associated with either normal or subclinically elevated levels of albumin excretion and, vice versa, microalbuminuria may be accompanied by high or normal GFR. Whether there is a chronological relationship between increases in GFR and in albumin excretion rates, with the former preceding the latter, remains to be established in man. In experimental diabetic animals the elevated GFR has been implicated in the initiation and progression of diabetic renal disease but this has not as yet been proven in humans. In one study (23) a small selected group of hyperfiltering diabetic patients (in whom, admittedly, the high GFR was coupled with microalbuminuria) progressed to persistent proteinuria and lost glomerular function, over a 10-year period, at a significantly higher rate than a control group with lower GFR and normal albumin excretion rates. This study cannot single out the independent contribution of glomerular hyperfiltration to the progression of renal damage and loss of glomerular function but it is compatible with the view that an elevation of the GFR may play a role in the sequence of events leading to diabetic renal failure. Whether the nephromegaly that invariably accompanies the high GFR has an independent predictive significance or simply represents an epiphenomenon is as unsolved as its temporal relationship with glomerular hyperfiltration.

Thus, markers of persistent proteinuria can be identified early in diabetes: they consist of microalbuminuria, probably glomerular hyperfiltration and, potentially the most important, subclinical elevations of arterial pressure.

## CORRECTION OF EARLY RENAL AND SYSTEMIC PRESSURE ANOMALIES

In sharp contrast to the relative insensitivity to treatment of established diabetic nephropathy, abnormalities in the early phase respond to a number of therapeutic manoeuvres. Intensified insulin treatment and strict metabolic control can correct hyperfiltration (28) and microalbuminuria (29) (Table 5) or at worst prevent the progressive rise of albumin excretion rates in individuals at risk (26). Correction of the marginal elevations in arterial pressure by diuretics or selective beta-blockers also reduces microalbuminuria (26), though results of controlled trials are awaited.

In the diabetic rat, lowering of blood pressure by an angiotensin-converting enzyme inhibitor seems to afford special benefits to the kidney by preventing, through a reduction of intraglomerular pressure, the development of albuminuria and renal histological damage (13).

Moreover, short-term studies in microalbuminuric diabetic patients show that a diet containing approximately 45 g of protein per day is capable of reducing both albumin excretion rate and the GFR independently of blood glucose or arterial pressure changes (30). This is consistent with findings in the diabetic rat; indeed, at similar levels of hyperglycaemia, a protein-restricted diet protects the rat kidney from hyperfiltration, albuminuria and the consequent histological lesions (26). Recent observations in humans with different protein intakes indicated interestingly that vegans, who eat less protein, all of which is vegetable origin, have significantly lower GFR, albumin excretion rates and arterial blood pressure values than those who eat more proteins largely of animal origin (31). A vegan diet, therefore, seems to be associated with renal and systemic changes that should confer protection against nephropathy in diabetes.

Table 5. Effect of strict glycaemic control on glomerular filtration rate (GFR) and albumin excretion rate (AER) in hyperfiltering and microalbuminuric insulin-dependent diabetic patients respectively

| | Ordinary BG control | Strict BG control | Level of significance ($p$ value) |
|---|---|---|---|
| GFR (ml/min/1.73m$^2$) ($n$ = 6) | 151 ± 6 | 129 ± 4 | <0.001 |
| AER ($\mu$g/min) ($n$ = 10) | 30 ± 9 | 10 ± 3 | <0.01 |

Data are mean ± SEM. For AER geometric means are used. BG = blood glucose.

Other kinds of pharmacological intervention may well be possible in the future, and preliminary reports in the diabetic animal model suggest that the administration of aldose reductase inhibitors, which block the sorbitol pathway, may have a beneficial effect in preventing the occurrence of—or reducing—proteinuria (32).

Thus, effective measures of correction of early renal abnormalities in diabetes mellitus are available, making diabetic nephropathy a potentially preventable condition. However, the correction of an early indicator of disease does not necessarily imply that disease itself will be abolished, and the results of long-term trials are now eagerly awaited. Moreover, from a careful analysis of the existing data on the treatment of microalbuminuria it would appear that approximately 30% of patients do not respond to treatment. This could be due to different subsets of patients or to different stages of the disease, and raises the question as to whether patients susceptible to diabetic nephropathy could be identified by some marker, probably genetic, present well before microalbuminuria or other risk indicators appear, at diagnosis of diabetes.

## PERSPECTIVES FOR PRIMARY PREVENTION: DETECTION OF SUSCEPTIBLE PATIENTS

It is now evident that only a subset of patients develops nephropathy. The curve distribution of the annual incidence of persistent proteinuria displays a peak at 16–20 years of diabetes and is followed by a considerable reduction in risk thereafter, with patients who survived 30 or more years with diabetes almost free of risk (15). This is consistent with the curve distribution of the cumulative incidence of persistent proteinuria, which levels off when duration of diabetes is longer than 25–30 years and only 30–40% of patients have developed nephropathy (3).

The finding that arterial pressure is elevated in microalbuminuric diabetic patients without renal hypofunction and that long-term diabetic survivors have unusually low arterial pressures has led us to formulate the hypothesis that an inherited predisposition to raised arterial pressure may confer the susceptibility to nephropathy if diabetes is present. In a recent family study we have shown that parents of proteinuric diabetic patients have significantly higher blood pressure levels than parents of non-proteinuric diabetic subjects matched for age and body mass index (33). A strong correlation was found between arterial pressures in the diabetic patients and those in their respective parents. These results have been complemented by the finding that the activity of red blood cell $Na^+/Li^+$ exchanger—a system the activity of which is thought to be genetically determined and is known to be associated with the risk of essential hypertension—is significantly higher in the proteinuric than in non-proteinuric insulin-dependent diabetic patients (34). We also found that the exchanger activity was not increased in matched, non-diabetic renal patients with renal function and blood pressure levels comparable to diabetic patients with clinical proteinuria, suggesting that high $Na^+/Li^+$ countertransport activity is not a feature of nephrogenic hypertension. These data would futher support the view that elevations of blood pressure may play a causal role in the development of diabetic kidney disease, rather than being a mere consequence of deteriorating renal function. If these preliminary findings are supported by further studies it may be possible in the future to identify diabetic patients at risk of nephropathy by a positive family history for arterial hypertension or by a cell marker associated with it well before microalbuminuria—indicative of early diabetic renal disease—develops. At this stage primary prevention would then be possible.

## REFERENCES


1. Andersen AR, Sandahl Christiansen J, Andersen JK, et al. (1983) Diabetic nephropathy in Type I (insulin-dependent) diabetes: an epidemiological study. Diabetologia 25: 496–501
2. Thomsen AC (1956) The kidney in diabetes mellitus. Thesis, Munksgaard, Copenhagen
3. Krolewski AS, Warram JH, Christlieb AR, et al. (1985) The changing natural history of nephropathy in Type I diabetes. Am J Med 78: 785–794
4. Rettig B, Teuch SM (1984) The incidence of end-stage renal failure in type I and type II diabetes mellitus. Diabetic Nephropathy 3: 26–27
5. Viberti GC, Bilous RW, Mackintosh D, et al. (1986) Monitoring glomerular function in diabetic nephropathy. Am J Med 74: 256–264
6. Parving HH, Anderson AR, Smidt UM, et al. (1983) Early aggressive antihypertensive treatment reduces rate of decline in kidney function in diabetic nephropathy. Lancet ii: 1175–1179

7. Viberti GC, Keen H (1984) The patterns of proteinuria in diabetes mellitus. Diabetes 33: 686–692
8. Viberti GC, Bilous RW, Mackintosh D, et al. (1983) Long term correction of hyperglycaemia and progression of renal failure in insulin-dependent diabetes. Br Med J 286: 598–602
9. Bending JJ, Viberti GC, Watkins PJ, Keen H (1986) Intermittent clinical proteinuria and renal function in diabetes: evolution and effect of glycaemic control. Br Med J 293: 83–86
10. Bjorck S, Nyberg G, Mulec H, et al. (1986) Beneficial effects of angiotensin converting enzyme inhibition on renal function in patients with diabetic nephropathy. Br Med J 293: 471–474
11. Hommel E, Parving HH, Mathiesen E, et al. (1986) Effect of captopril on kidney function in insulin-dependent diabetic patients with nephropathy. Br Med J 293: 467–470
12. Taguma AC, Kitamoto Y, Futaki G, et al. (1986) Effect of captopril on heavy proteinuria in azotaemic diabetics. N Engl J Med 313: 1617–1620
13. Zatz R, Dunn T, Meyer S, et al. (1986) Prevention of diabetic glomerulopathy by pharmacological amelioration of glomerular capillary hypertension. J Clin Invest 77: 1925–1930
14. Bending JJ, Dodds R, Keen H, Viberti GC (1986) Lowering protein intake and the progression of diabetic renal failure. Diabetologia 29: 516A
15. Borch-Johnsen K, Andersen PK, Deckert T (1987) The effect of proteinuria on the relative mortality in Type I (insulin-dependent) diabetes mellitus. Diabetologia 28: 590–596
16. Keen H, Chlouverakis C (1963) An immunoassay for urinary albumin at low concentrations. Lancet ii: 913–916
17. Keen H, Chlouverakis C, Fuller JH, Jarrett RJ (1969) The concomitants of raised blood sugar: studies in newly detected hyperglycaemics. II. Urinary albumin excretion, blood pressure and their relation to blood sugar levels. Guy's Hosp Rep 118: 247–252
18. Mogensen CE (1971) Urinary albumin excretion in early and long-term juvenile diabetics. Scand J Clin Lab Invest 28: 79–90
19. Parving HH, Noer I, Deckert T, et al. (1976) The effect of metabolic regulation on microvascular permeability to small and large molecules in short term diabetics. Diabetologia 12: 161–166
20. Viberti GC, Mackintosh D, Bilous RW, et al. (1982) Proteinuria in diabetes mellitus: role of spontaneous experimental variation of glycaemia. Kidney Int 21: 714–720
21. Mathiesen ER, Øxenboll B, Johansen K, et al. (1984) Incipient nephropathy in Type I (insulin-dependent) diabetes. Diabetologia 26: 406–410
22. Viberti GC, Hill RD, Jarrett RJ, et al. (1982) Microalbuminuria as predictor of clinical nephropathy in insulin-dependent diabetes mellitus. Lancet i: 1430–1432
23. Mogensen CE, Christiansen CK (1984) Predicting diabetic nephropathy in insulin-dependent patients. N Engl J Med 311: 89–93
24. Close CF, on behalf of the MCS (1986) The prevalence of at risk microalbuminuria in a population of non-proteinuric insulin-dependent diabetic subjects. Diabetic Med 328a (personal communication)
25. Wiseman MJ, Viberti GC, Mackintosh D, et al. (1984) Glycaemia, arterial pressure and microalbuminuria in Type I (insulin-dependent) diabetes mellitus. Diabetologia 26: 401–405
26. Viberti GC, Wiseman MJ (1986) The kidney in diabetes: significance of the early abnormalities. Clin Endocrinol Metab 15:753–782
27. Rasch R, Rytter Norgaard JO (1983) Renal enlargement: comparative autoradiographic studies of $^{3}$H-thymidine uptake in diabetic and uninephrectomised rats. Diabetologia 25: 280–287

28. Wiseman MJ, Saunders AJ, Keen H, et al. (1985) Effect of blood glucose control on increased glomerular filtration rate and kidney size in insulin-dependent diabetes. N Engl J Med 312: 617–621
29. Bending JJ, Viberti GC, Bilous RW, Keen H, for the Kroc Collaborative Study Group (1985) Eight month correction of hyperglycaemia in insulin-dependent diabetes mellitus is associated with a significant and sustained reduction of urinary albumin excretion rates in patients with microalbuminuria. Diabetes 34 (Suppl 3): 69–73
30. Cohen DL, Dodds R, Viberti GC (1986) Reduction of microalbuminuria and glomerular filtration rate by dietary protein restriction in Type I (insulin-dependent) diabetic patients: an effect independent of blood glucose control and arterial dietary protein restriction in Type I (insulin-dependent) diabetic patients: an effect independent of blood glucose control and arterial pressure changes. Diabetologia 29: 528A
31. Wiseman MJ, Hunt R, Goodwin A, et al. (1987) Dietary composition and renal function in healthy subjects. Nephron (in press)
32. Beyer-Mears A (1986) The polyol pathway, sorbinil and renal dysfunction. Metabolism 35 (Suppl 1): 46–54
33. Viberti GC, Keen H, Wiseman MJ (1987) Raised arterial pressure in parents of proteinuric insulin-dependent diabetics (submitted for publication)
34. Mangili R, Bending JJ, Scott GS, Li LK, Gupta A, Viberti GC (1987) A marker for diabetic nephropathy: increased RBC $Na^+/Li^+$ exchanger activity. Diabetes (in press)

Diabetic Complications: Early Diagnosis and Treatment
Edited by D. Andreani, G. Crepaldi, U. Di Mario and G. Pozza


# CHAPTER 27

# *Current Status of Kidney and Pancreas Transplantation in Uremic Diabetic Patients*

G. Pozza and V. Di Carlo
*Clinica Medica VI, Ospedale San Raffaele, Milan, Italy*

Insulin therapy has improved the life expectancy of patients affected by insulin-dependent diabetes mellitus (IDDM) and drastically reduced mortality from ketoacidosis or intercurrent infections, but has not prevented the development of severe microangiopathic complications leading to blindness, neuropathy and end-stage renal disease (ESRD). To date optimized insulin treatments and pump systems for delivering exogenous insulin have decreased the incidence of these dramatic complications, but life expectancy for the diabetic patient is still one-third less than that of the general population.

Disordered carbohydrate metabolism is considered the major cause of the late complications of IDDM (1). The main aim of diabetic therapy nowadays is the prevention or the delay of the progression of microangiopathic complications.

The purpose of pancreas transplantation is not only to make the diabetic patient insulin independent, but to give the patient a pancreas which responds to physiological insulinogenic stimuli in order to restore normal glycemic homeostasis (2).

The first pancreas transplant was carried out by Kelly and Lillehei in 1966 and for many years remained an experimental procedure without a real clinical interest (3).

Only recently have improved results, consequent to more effective immunosuppressive therapy and to technical progress, promoted renewed interest in this surgical procedure as is demonstrated by the ever-increasing number of transplants performed annually and reported by the Pancreas Transplant Registry (Figure 1) (4).

Pancreas transplantation is usually combined with kidney transplantation or performed in diabetic patients who already have an established renal graft (30% of the individuals with IDDM develop ESRD).

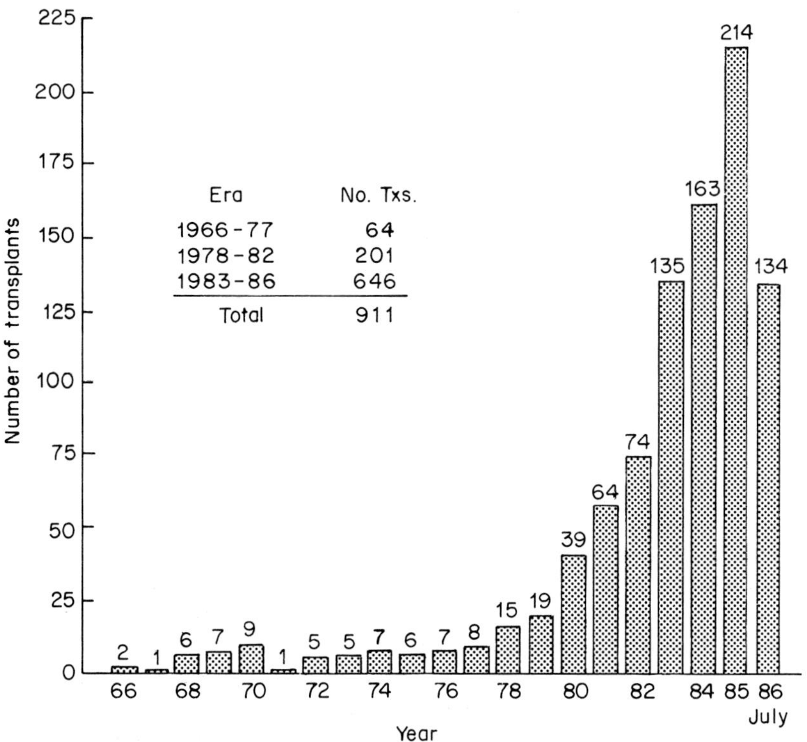


Figure 1. Number of pancreas transplantations by year reported to the Pancreas Transplant Registry.

Since microangiopathic complications cannot be predicted early and since almost every individual with IDDM may ultimately develop some manifestations of microangiopathy, it may be suggested that the surgical procedure should be performed at an earlier stage before renal, or other organ, damage has occurred. Some groups have already performed single pancreatic transplantations in patients in whom the threat of severe secondary complications is imminent, but in whom uremia has not yet developed (4). Kidney transplantation is also the elective therapy for ESRD in the diabetic patient as it allows an improvement in both the survival rate and the quality of life. At present, clinical experience shows a 1-year functional survival rate of more than 80% of kidney grafts.

## TECHNICAL PROBLEMS

Although results of clinical pancreas transplantation have significantly improved in the period 1983–1986 (42% 1-year functional survival rate for pancreas graft), they are still disappointing when compared with those obtained with other organs, such as kidney, heart and liver. One reason for this gap is the high incidence of surgical technical complications, the major ones being exocrine leakage and graft thrombosis.

These complications have led to the continuous search for a better and safer surgical technique which has still not been optimized because results are easily misinterpreted and controversial.

The first technical problem is which part of the pancreas to transplant. In segmental pancreas transplants, using the body and the tail of the gland, the vascular anastomosis is made between the donor splenic vessels and the recipient iliac vessels. This kind of transplantation is technically easier, since the graft can be taken from a living related donor and it can be removed faster from cadavers when multiorgan donation is required. Whole pancreas transplants, using the entire gland with a patch of aorta and portal vein anastomosed to the recipient iliac vessels, provide a much more functional islet mass and a larger vascular bed. Small segmental pancreatic transplants are in fact claimed to be more likely to undergo thrombosis. The reason for thrombosis is believed to be the abnormal hemodynamic situation created by the removal of the spleen. The large splenic artery is then left to drain via the small pancreatic branches and this low outflow may promote thrombosis (10–15% of the loss of function). Modifications of the standard surgical procedures have been also proposed (arteriovenous fistulas, splenic artery interposition or inclusion of the spleen in the graft), but despite all these measures thrombosis may still occur.

Results from the Pancreas Transplant Registry do not show a significant difference between the two techniques (40% of 1-year functional survival rate for the whole organ compared with 43% for segmental pancreas transplant).

The risk of the leakage of the highly digestive exocrine secretion, a well-known problem in pancreatic surgery, has resulted in the development of different surgical procedures. There are principally three effective methods to control the pancreatic secretion: diversion of the secretion to the gastrointestinal tract (pancreatico-jejunostomy), urinary tract diversion (ureter or bladder), and duct injections of polymers to occlude the ductal system and suppress the exocrine function. Each approach has its disadvantages and results still do not indicate which of the three methods is the most advantageous (44% of 1-year functional survival rate for duct injection, 41% for enteric drainage, and 50% for urinary drainage).

Our group preferred the technique of segmental pancreas transplantation with exocrine function suppression through Neoprene duct injection as it was developed in Lyon by Dubernard et al. (5). This method reduces postoperative complications (pancreatic fistulas, pancreatitis, digestive anastomosis leakages, and infections) but the ductal filling causes fibrosis and atrophy of the exocrine pancreas which may lead to an impairment of the endocrine function. In 40 patients, metabolic tests were used by our group to study the endocrine function of the pancreatic residual stump, injected with Neoprene after duodenocephalopancreatectomy, and no insular function derangement was observed at a 3-year follow-up (6).

Orthotopic transplantation has been completely abandoned and all authors now agree on performing a heterotopic transplantation with anastomosis on the recipient iliac vessels. Using the latter solution, insulin is released into the systemic and not the portal circulation, as happens physiologically, but this difference does not seem to be particularly relevant.

Finally, those problems connected to pancreas removal and preservation should be considered. The anatomical situs of the pancreas is the cause of considerable difficulties and its removal must be performed with the greatest accuracy. The pancreas is particularly sensitive to ischemia: clinical experience has shown that periods of cold ischemia lasting more than 6 hours are associated with primary graft failures (there is a 47% 1-year functional survival rate when the cold ischemia time is shorter than 6 hours, whereas a 35% functional survival rate is obtained when the cold ischemia time is longer than 6 hours) (4). It is likely that periods of warm ischemia could also have a similar importance.

## IMMUNOSUPPRESSION AND REJECTION

In those patients who receive grafts from the same donor, the monitoring of creatinine levels in order to follow kidney transplant provides a good marker for rejection. In fact rejections occur without a concomitant increase in the blood glucose level, meaning that either pancreas rejection follows kidney rejection or that blood glucose measurements are a less sensitive measure of graft damage. The opportunity of monitoring kidney function as a sign of impending rejection is also confirmed by the better results obtained from simultaneous kidney and pancreas transplants according to the Registry data (47% of 1-year functional survival rate of kidney + pancreas compared with 30% for pancreas alone).

In patients undergoing transplantation of pancreas alone or after a kidney transplantation from a different donor, rejection is monitored by blood glucose levels. Plasma insulin, peptide-C levels, biopsy of the graft, angiography or scanning have only a confirmatory role in the diagnosis of rejection. In this situation rejection is still a considerable obstacle to success; it is, however, difficult to distinguish on clinical grounds from a pancreatic fibrosis resulting in a total loss of pancreatic function.

This complication, which can be diagnosed only through a biopsy sample, may be related to the inflammatory reaction following polymer injection or to pancreatitis autodigestion.

According to the Pancreas Transplant Registry, cyclosporin improved the results and offered an advantage over the conventional immunosuppressive drugs (47% of 1-year functional survival rate for cyclosporin + azathioprine + prednisone compared with 41% for azathioprine + prednisone). As prednisone has an unfavourable effect on glucose homeostasis, the use of cyclosporin alone would seem to be particularly attractive but the results are still lower than those obtained using the triple therapy (39% of 1-year functional survival rate) (4).

## EFFECT ON GLUCOSE HOMEOSTASIS AND SECONDARY COMPLICATIONS

Nowadays, since the number of pancreas transplantations is rapidly increasing, the success rates in terms of presence or absence of function may be taken into consideration. In other words, one wonders whether normoglycemia achieved with pancreas grafting prevents, stops or reverses late diabetic complications (7–9). Accumulated data are still insufficient to answer the question of whether pancreas transplantation can cure IDDM, and whether diabetic complications are reversible; the results are nonetheless very encouraging.

### Short-Term Endocrine Function

The revascularization of the pancreatic graft leads to an immediate release of pancreatic hormones, mainly insulin and glucagon. C-peptide levels, which are virtually undetectable at the beginning of surgery, rise immediately after the graft revascularization (Figure 2).

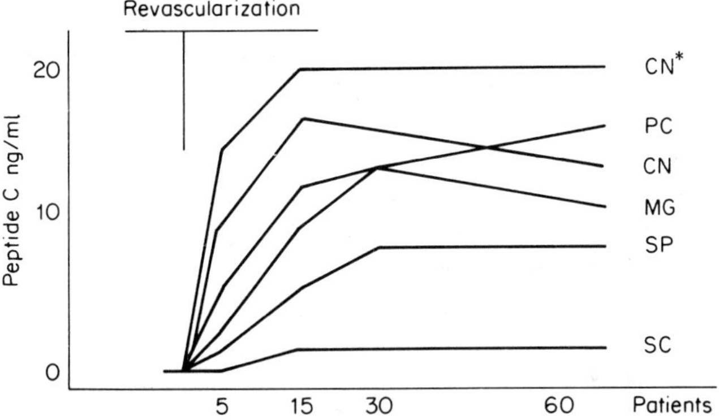


Figure 2. The intraoperative peptide-C levels after revascularization of the pancreas.

A contemporary reduction of exogenous insulin requirement is observed when patients are connected to an artificial beta cell.

### Medium-Term Endocrine Function

The transplanted pancreas restores satisfactory metabolic control within a few weeks.

During the first days after surgery, high blood glucose levels are often present along with high peptide-C levels. This condition can be explained by the high doses of steroids administered for immunosuppression, and by parenteral nutrition containing high levels of glucose and triglycerides which respectively increase blood glucose and insulin resistance.

Early postoperative hyperglycemia can also be an alarming sign of rejection; the assessment of endocrine function in these conditions by measurement of plasma and urinary C-peptide levels is warranted. High peptide C levels prove a preserved endocrine function, but the time-consuming radioimmunoassay is still an effective limitation to immediate assessment. Over the following weeks blood glucose levels, both fasting and postprandial, are restored and during this period beta cells show a satisfactory response to several insulinogenic stimuli.

The oral glucose tolerance test (OGTT) shows a good but delayed insulin release, while blood glucose levels show an impaired glucose tolerance. Insulinogenic stimulation of the pancreas (intravenous glucose tolerance test (IVGTT), arginine and tolbutamide tests) give a prompt insulin release which is similar to that in non-diabetic control subjects.

C-peptide levels, nearly undetectable at the beginning of surgery, rise and the response to arginine appears to be normal. Transplanted alpha cells respond correctly to the physiological inhibition although the mass of alpha cells is doubled, including those from both the original and the transplanted pancreas.

In conclusion, the transplanted pancreas retains the possibility of secreting insulin, but its release is delayed due to its paraphysiological condition. Several explanations may be put forward to account for this metabolic behaviour. First of all, the mass of transplanted beta cells is reduced by the segmental technique and may be further reduced as a consequence of undetected rejections and of warm ischemia, producing both necrosis and damage to endocrine tissues. Furthermore, pancreas exocrine suppression may reduce insulin secretion and impair glucose tolerance, as shown in animals. It should also be considered that the pancreas is denervated and that, because of the heterotopic position of the organ, insulin reaches the liver—the target organ of its action—only after a total body circulation.

Some weeks after surgery the patient is completely insulin-independent while endocrine and metabolic patterns remain within the normal range (Figure 3). Blood glucose levels show minimal variations in fasting and in the postprandial state. Insulin levels show a physiological increase, although delayed, in the postprandial period, while a mild hyperinsulinemia is present in the fasting period (probably due to steroid administration and to peripheral insulin delivery). A mild hyperketonemia is also present because of a low concentration of insulin at the hepatic levels unable to control the ketone body production.

## Long-Term Endocrine Function

As is frequently observed, several technical and immunological factors could be responsible for late failures.

The chronic rejection of the pancreatic tissue and the suppression of the exocrine function were considered to be the main causes of long-term insufficiency.

One- and 2-year metabolic studies show a normal glucose tolerance, insulin secretion closer to physiological levels, and the capacity of the transplanted pancreas to restore control over ketone body production.

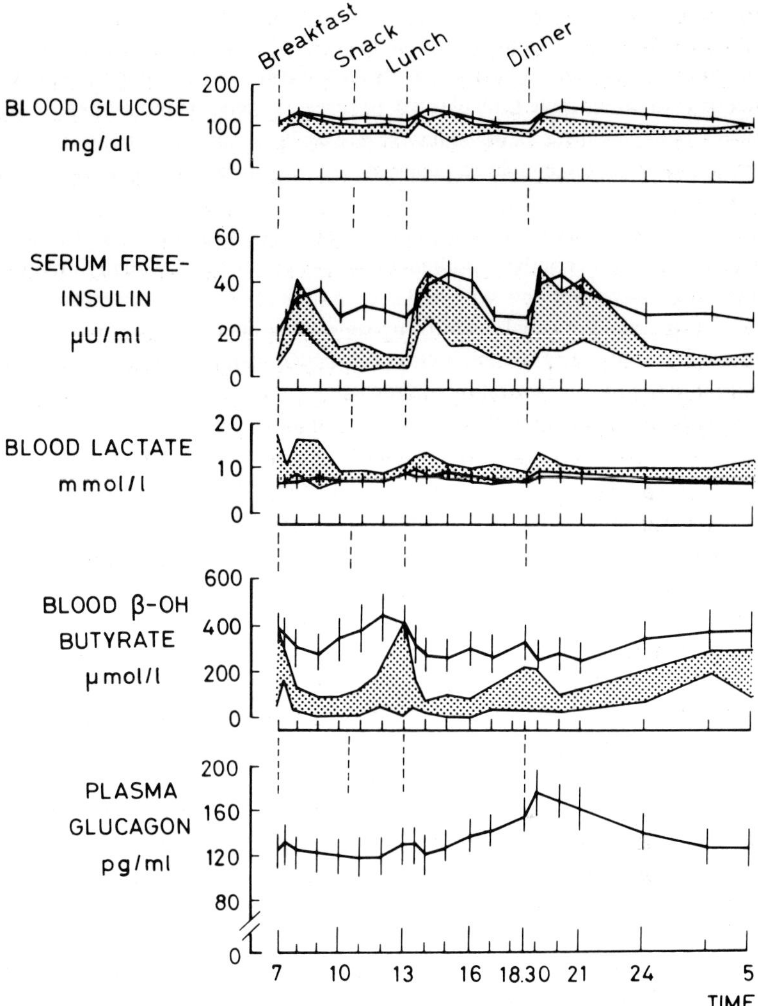


Figure 3. Metabolic profiles in 10 pancreas plus kidney transplantation patients

The availability of cyclosporin led to the reduction or suppression of steroid administration in the long-term period, thus reducing a potential diabetogenic stress on the transplanted pancreas. Metabolic studies showed improved glycemic control in patients treated with cyclosporin alone, in comparison to those treated with cyclosporin and steroids.

### Secondary Complications

Only preliminary conclusions can be drawn regarding the effects of pancreas transplantation on secondary complications (10). In fact, the number of patients who have retained pancreatic grafts for any length of time is still small (approximately 100 patients with functional transplanted pancreas surviving more than 1 year in all centres). Many of these patients had severe diabetic vascular changes at the time of transplantation, changes whose progress could probably be halted but could not be reversed.

Clinical assessment of the course of diabetic retinopathy as well as neuropathy suggests that the secondary diabetic lesions which are clinically manifested are slightly regressive. Patients who had severe subjective peripheral neuropathy report the relief of symptoms such as burning sensation, hyperesthesia, paresthesia.

Motor and sensory nerve conduction velocity and signs of autonomous neuropathy (postural hypotension, sexual disturbances, etc.) are reported to improve.

The ophthalmological follow-up showed that visual acuity did not decrease in patients with preproliferative or proliferative retinopathy. An improvement is also reported for signs of preproliferative retinopathy. A rarer recurrence of diabetic nephropathy has also been reported in patients receiving combined renal and pancreatic grafts.

## CONCLUSIONS

Although the surgical techniques currently used are still not completely satisfactory on account of the high incidence of technical complications, the long-term functional survival for pancreas transplantation is progressively improving.

Severe late complications may be markedly improved by glucose normalization, thus transplantation at a much earlier stage of IDDM might prevent the development of microangiopathic complications. This will be possible when a relatively high incidence of successful pancreas transplantations is attained.

## REFERENCES


1. Sutherland DER, Goetz FC, Ramsay RC, Fryd DS, Najarian JS (1983) Clinical and experimental kidney and pancreas transplantation for diabetics. In: Little HL, Jack RL, Patz A, Forsham PH (eds) Diabetic retinopathy. Thieme-Stratton, New York, p 199
2. Groth CG (1985) Clinical pancreatic transplantation. Transplant Proc XVII (1): 324–330
3. Kelly WD, Lillehei RC, Merkel FK, Idezuki Y, Goetz FC (1967) Allotransplantation of the pancreas and duodenum along with kidney in diabetic nephropathy. Surgery 61: 827–832
4. Sutherland DER, Moudry K (1986) Pancreas Transplant Registry report. Transplant Proc (in press)
5. Dubernard JM, Trager J, Bosi E, Gelet A, El Yafi S, Devonec M, Piatti PM, Chiesa R, Martin X, Mongin-Long D, Touraine JL, Pozza G Transplantation for the treatment of

insulin-dependent diabetes: clinical experience with polymer-obstructed pancreatic grafts using Neoprene. World J Surg 8: 262–266

6. Di Carlo V, Chiesa R, Pontiroli AE, Pozza G, Carlucci M, Staudacher C, Secchi A, Cristallo M (1984) Intraductal injection of Neoprene to suppress native pancreatic exocrine function in humans: clinical and metabolic evaluation. Transplant Proc XVI (3): 736–738
7. Dubernard JM, Traeger J, Bosi E, Secchi A, Piatti PM, Gelet A, El Yafi, Kamel G, Touraine JL (1985) Advances in human Neoprene-injected pancreas transplantation: experience with 47 cases. Transplant Proc XVI (5): 1267–1269
8. Di Carlo V, Chiesa R, Pontiroli AE, Pozza G, Carlucci M, Staudacher C, Secchi A, Cristallo M (1984) Intraductal injection of Neoprene to suppress native pancreatic exocrine secretion in humans: clinical and metabolic evaluation. Transplant Proc XVI (3): 736–738
9. Pozza G, Bosi E, Secchi A, Piatti PM, Touraine JL, Gelet A, Pontiroli AE, Dubernard JM, Traeger J (1985) Metabolic control of type 1 (insulin-dependent) diabetes after pancreas transplantation. Br Med J 291: 510–513
10. Land W, Landgraf R, Illner WD, et al. (1985) Improved results in combined segmental pancreatic and renal transplantation in diabetic patients under cyclosporin therapy. Transplant Proc XVII (1): 317–324

The editorial assistance of Dr Lucy Byatt is gratefully acknowledged.

# Index